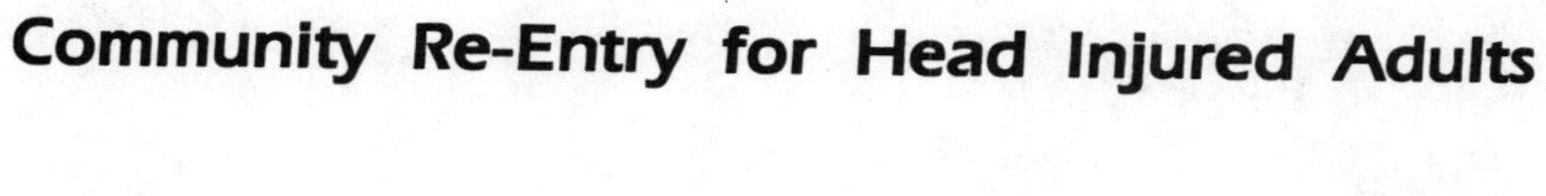

Community Re-Entry for Head Injured Adults

Community Re-Entry for Head Injured Adults

Edited by

Mark Ylvisaker, M.A., C.C.C./Sp.
Eva Marie R. Gobble, Ph.D., C.R.C.
The Rehabilitation Institute of Pittsburgh
Pittsburgh, Pennsylvania

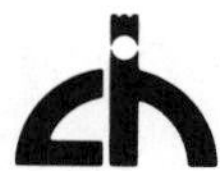

A College-Hill Publication
Little, Brown and Company
Boston/Toronto/San Diego

College-Hill Press
A Division of
Little Brown and Company (Inc.)
34 Beacon Street
Boston, Massachusetts 02108

Library of Congress Cataloging in Publication Data
Main entry under title.

Community re-entry for head injured adults.
"A College-Hill publication."
Includes index.
1. Brain damage — Patients — Rehabilitation.
I. Ylvisaker, Mark, 1944- . II. Gobble,
Eva Marie R., 1949- . [DNLM: 1. Brain Injuries
— in adulthood. 2. Brain Injuries — rehabilitation.
WL 365 C734]
RC87.5.C66 1987 362.2 87-4161

ISBN 0-316-96880-3

Printed in the United States of America

This book is dedicated to Mr. Charles H. Bisdee, whose career in rehabilitation set a standard of excellence and dedication to serving people in need.

Contents

Foreword, by Marilyn Price Spivack ix
Preface xi
Contributors xv

Chapter 1 Neuropsychological Deficits, Personality Variables, and Outcome **1**
George P. Prigatano

Chapter 2 Physical Rehabilitation **25**
Lillian J. Bray, Faith Carlson, Reed Humphrey, Joyce P. Mastrilli and Anne S. Valko

Chapter 3 A Framework for Cognitive Rehabilitation Therapy **87**
Shirley F. Szekeres, Mark Ylvisaker, and Sally B. Cohen

Chapter 4 Topics in Cognitive Rehabilitation Therapy **137**
Mark Ylvisaker, Shirley F. Szekeres, Kevin Henry, Deborah M. Sullivan, and Paula Wheeler

Chapter 5 Work Adjustment Services **221**
Eva Marie R. Gobble, Kevin Henry, James C. Pfahl, and Gloria J. Smith

Chapter 6 Treatment Aspects of Vocational Evaluation and Placement for Traumatically Brain Injured Adults **259**
James F. Wachter, Heidi L. Fawber, and Mason B. Scott

Chapter 7 Independent Living: Settings and Supports **301**
Al Condeluci, Sue Cooperman, and Barbara A. Seif

Chapter 8 Avocational Programming for the Severely Impaired Head Injured Individual **349**
Eva Marie R. Gobble, Lucille Dunson, Shirley F. Szekeres, and Jacquelin Cornwall

Chapter 9 Reactions of Family Members and Clinical Intervention after Traumatic Brain Injury **381**
Pamela Klonoff and George P. Prigatano

Chapter 10 Management and Advocacy **403**
William R. Bauer and Jan Titonis

Epilogue A Letter to Professionals Who Work with Head Injured People **421**
Beth B. O'Brien

Author Index **431**
Subject Index **439**

Foreword

As a parent and as the co-founder of the National Head Injury Foundation, I am very pleased to introduce this book and to recommend it to all those who are concerned with the struggle of head injured people to return to home and community at the highest possible level of functioning. As acute medical care and early rehabilitation programs improve and expand, professionals and family members alike are plagued by the question, "What's next?" The concerns and questions take many forms. At NHIF we encounter them daily in letters and calls from across the country: How do the patient and family cope? How do we maximize the remaining abilities of the patient in a practical and functional manner? What can we do that will be beneficial and practical outside of the hospital environment, when professional staff are no longer available? Is cognitive rehabilitation effective? What techniques should be used, for whom and by whom? When is the right time and what is the right place? What are meaningful vocational options? What are the long-term residential options? What can we do to make leisure time more meaningful and enjoyable? Is there hope for a positive outcome? Is the effort worth it?

This book addressed all of these issues. Its focus is the ultimate wish of every patient, family, and clinician — the return to the business of living in a way that is meaningful, satisfying, and productive. Returning to the community is the challenge of the next half decade for concerned professionals and for the National Head Injury Foundation as an advocacy organization. The editors of this book, Mark Ylvisaker and Eva Marie Gobble, and its contributors are to be thanked for making substantial progress toward meeting that challenge. The book includes useful reviews of background information and theories in many areas of interest to rehabilitation professionals. It is its *functional* and *practical* focus, however, that will make the book invaluable to clinicians in all disciplines, and to families working with adults who are in the rehabilitation phase following head trauma.

As a family member very involved with the rehabilitation of my daughter, I appreciate the timeliness of each topic and the clinical, "how to" approach of each contributor. The intervention techniques described in this book are meaningful and creative. They promote the *return* of the patient's functions and skills, and they rebuild energy, self-esteem, and self-understanding. I wish this book had been available to me five years ago. It is of practical value; it speaks to progress;

and it opens doors to encourage further innovative and creative rehabilitation because it gives valid direction and shares the rehabilitative successes and gains of patients.

Often, because of the complex array of physical, intellectual, and psychological disabilities caused by traumatic brain injury, the patient becomes a "package of disability." Professionals and even families can only view this person as an overwhelming challenge. The focus is on the losses and we lose sight of the person, of his or her personhood. It is high praise for this book that all of its authors have kept clearly in view the individual human beings with whom they work — their hopes and dreams; their unique personalities; their fundamental personhood; the people they are rather than the disabilities they have.

Successful return to the community will only be possible when society as a whole fully understands and is willing to deal with the complexity of the problems caused by traumatic brain injury. As of this writing, community-based services, opportunities, and long-term care programs are still unavailable to the vast majority of survivors. Funding, public awareness, public policy, and professional training are all factors contributing to this public health and societal problem. The NHIF and all concerned professionals *must* make a difference. Otherwise, the positive effects of early medical and state-of-the-art rehabilitative care will be diminished over time.

Community Re-entry for Head Injured Adults should be basic reading for those who believe that head injury rehabilitation is not defined by "length of time" but by ongoing challenge and opportunity in a creative and responsive community setting.

Marilyn Price Spivack
Founder and Executive Director
National Head Injury Foundation

Preface

The past decade has witnessed a long-overdue development of rehabilitation programs for survivors of traumatic brain injury. The level of interest in the professional community is not, however, out of proportion with the dimensions of the tragedy that each head injured person represents. The events that produce traumatic brain injuries occur most commonly during adolescence and early adult years — a time during which preparations for a career are completed, that career is begun, and new family commitments are made. For most people, this phase of life is characterized by high hopes and unlimited expectations. None are prepared for the personal struggle and familial disruptions that commonly follow severe head injury.

Head injuries are more common than spinal cord injuries and all neurologic diseases with the exception of stroke. Despite this, a relatively small commitment of resources has been made in this country to unravel the puzzles that many head injured individuals represent and to create meaningful long-term services and supports for those patients and their families, whose lives are permanently altered. Developments in the acute medical management of patients with traumatic brain injuries have increased the rate of survival. Evidence is beginning to accumulate that rehabilitative efforts can enhance recovery or help patients to compensate for skills that are irretrievably lost. It is only very recently, however, that professionals have recognized and accepted the staggering challenge of equipping patients with those skills that are required in the communities that they will re-enter, and creating in those communities vocational options, meaningful leisure-time alternatives, and independent living programs that are appropriate for survivors of severe closed head injury.

Our goal in selecting topics for this book was to bring together in one volume information and treatment perspectives that focus in a *practical* way on those needs of traumatically brain injured patients that relate directly to their successful reintegration into community life. Furthermore, we recognized that the community that head injured patients re-enter may range from home, family, and previous job to a long-term care facility and a dramatically altered domain of possible activities. Literature in the field of head injury rehabilitation has blossomed in recent years. For the most part, however, this literature deals with medical management, the natural history of recovery, outcome, and the rehabilitation of patients *up to* the point at which the very difficult problems of community re-entry become paramount.

It has long been recognized that cognitive and psychosocial sequelae, often unaccompanied by more readily observed physical deficits, pose the most stubborn obstacles to vocational and social success for head injured individuals as a group. Chapter 1 serves as a useful introduction to the book by describing those characteristic long-term cognitive and psychosocial problems. Chapters 5 and 6 explore the vocational implications of these deficits, present a model of work adjustment and vocational rehabilitation appropriate for traumatically brain injured patients, and present techniques of rehabilitation that show promise for this group. Chapters 7 and 8 fill a major gap in the existing literature by presenting frameworks and techniques of rehabilitation for head injured individuals in the often neglected areas of independent living and avocational rehabilitation. Again, cognitive and pyschosocial themes are stressed. The very difficult process of helping family members through the bewildering nightmare that often persists for years following traumatic brain injury is discussed in practical terms in Chapter 9.

In keeping with the theme of community re-entry, the discussion of physical rehabilitation in Chapter 2 focuses on two issues that frequently have the greatest impact at the point of re-entry: physical conditioning and compensatory devices that may enable an individual to function effectively in vocational, avocational or social activities despite persistent motoric impairments. This practical focus also dominates the discussions of cognitive rehabilitation in Chapters 3 and 4. Cognitive rehabilitation, which brings together under one label goals and intervention techniques that have traditionally been addressed separately by psychologists, speech–language pathologists, occupational therapists, and special educators, has come to be accepted as a cornerstone of rehabilitation for most severely head injured individuals. The authors of Chapters 3 and 4 present a framework and treatment techniques that highlight the functional and integrative aspects of cognitive functioning and the "real-life" needs of cognitively impaired patients.

Chapter 10 includes a summary discussion of the programmatic needs of this population, some proposals for systems that can deliver the needed services most efficiently, and an agenda for our advocacy efforts. The book concludes with a deeply moving letter written by a parent of a head injured young adult. The letter is addressed to the professional community and dramatically underscores a fundamental fact that should serve as the beginning and end of all discussions of rehabilitation: a head injury is a tragic event that occurs in the life of an individual human being and his or her family, that produces consequences that may change those lives forever, and that cries out for untiring efforts to help those individuals resume satisfying and dignified lives.

This book will be of interest to all rehabilitation professionals and family members concerned with head injury. Because of its focus on community re-entry, we expect the book to be of special interest to community advocates, staff of community facilities that serve neurologically impaired individuals (e.g., community recreation programs and adult day care or day treatment programs), staff of long-term care facilities, and administrators of programs for head injured patients. We are particularly hopeful that this book will be useful for those who work for community agencies or programs. Family members frequently report deep frustration in seeking appropriate community programs for their loved one following discharge from early medical rehabilitation. This frustration is poignantly described in the epilogue to the book.

The importance of an integrated, interdisciplinary approach to head injury rehabilitation emerges as a dominant theme throughout the chapters of this book. As with our previous book, *Head Injury Rehabilitation: Children and Adolescents,* we have attempted to promote and illustrate this interdisciplinary approach through the selection of authors. Most of the chapters are a product of the collaborative efforts of clinicians from several rehabilitation professions. For example, the discussion of physical rehabilitation represents the collaboration of a physiatrist, occupational therapist, physical therapist, speech–language pathologist, and exercise physiologist; cognitive rehabilitation is discussed jointly by members of an interdisciplinary cognitive rehabilitation therapy team with backgrounds in speech–language pathology, occupational therapy, and special education; a rehabilitation counselor, recreational therapist, and speech–language pathologist combine their expertise to produce a well integrated and innovative discussion of avocational rehabilitation.

The authors have attempted to incorporate into their discussions useful theoretical frameworks and the most recent research findings in their respective fields. However, the overall focus of the book is practical. With few exceptions, the contributors are active clinicians whose working days are spent working with and learning from head injured patients. Their goal is largely to share with colleagues and family members clinical tools and strategies that have evolved over many years of intervention with head injured patients. Research activity in the years ahead should help to identify those intervention strategies that have greatest value and enable clinicans to fine tune their intervention by matching specific treatment objectives and techniques to an individual patient's unique constellation of strengths, weaknesses, goals, and social and vocational settings.

There are many good people who deserve rich acknowledgment and thanks for their help in creating this book. The contributors are committed and hard-working clinicians who somehow found hours very early in the morning or very late at night to put their clinical insights into words. We must also thank our patients who continue to be the best teachers in the field of rehabilitation. The administrators of The Rehabilitation Institute of Pittsburgh continue to provide leadership in rehabilitation and have made this book possible through their active support and commitment of resources. John Rosenbek and Sean Monagle once again gave excellent editorial advice. We thank Ken Seibert for his expert graphics work, Tina Celender for her design consultation, Nancy Spears for her assistance in obtaining resource materials, Roberta Houston, Melanie Grace, Carol Litzinger, and Edie Scales for their help in typing the manuscript, and Bernadette Deramus for reproducing more copies of manuscripts than she cares to remember. Finally, we thank our wonderful families — Kathy, Jessie, Ben, John, John III, Elena — who have been far more supportive and patient than we have a right to expect.

Mark Ylvisaker
Eva Marie R. Gobble

Contributors

William R. Bauer, M.Ed., C.R.C.
Director of Education,
The Rehabilitation Institute of Pittsburgh,
Pittsburgh, Pennsylvania

Lillian J. Bray, L.P.T.
Physical Therapist,
The Rehabilitation Institute of Pittsburgh,
Pittsburgh, Pennsylvania

Faith Carlson, M.A., C.C.C./Sp.
Speech-Language Pathologist,
Augmentative Communication Project Leader,
The Rehabilitation Institute of Pittsburgh,
Pittsburgh, Pennsylvania

Sally B. Cohen, M.Ed.
Cognitive Rehabilitation Clinical Services Facilitator,
The Rehabilitation Institute of Pittsburgh,
Pittsburgh, Pennsylvania

Al Condeluci, Ph.D.
Program Director,
United Cerebral Palsy,
Pittsburgh, Pennsylvania

Sue Cooperman, M.S., O.T.R./L.
Director, Occupational Therapy Department,
The Rehabilitation Institute of Pittsburgh,
Pittsburgh, Pennsylvania

Jacquelin Cornwall, B.S., C.T.R.S.
Recreational Therapist,
The Rehabilitation Institute of Pittsburgh,
Pittsburgh, Pennsylvania

Lucille Dunson, B.A., C.R.C.
Clinical Team Leader,
Vocational and Career Services Department,
The Rehabilitation Institute of Pittsburgh,
Pittsburgh, Pennsylvania

Heidi L. Fawber, M.Ed., C.R.C.
Former Director, Head Trauma Program,
The Vocational Rehabilitation 15Center of Allegheny County, Inc.,
Pittsburgh, Pennsylvania

Eva Marie R. Gobble, Ph.D., C.R.C.
Director, Vocational and Career Services Department,
The Rehabilitation Institute of Pittsburgh,
Pittsburgh, Pennsylvania

Kevin Henry, M.Ed.
Cognitive Rehabilitation Therapist,
The Rehabilitation Institute of Pittsburgh,
Pittsburgh, Pennsylvania

Reed Humphrey, Ph.D.
Certified Exercise Program Director through the American College of Sports Medicine,
Pittsburgh, Pennsylvania

Pamela Klonoff, Ph.D.
Neuropsychologist,
Barrow Neurological Institute,
St. Joseph's Hospital and Medical Center,
Phoenix, Arizona

Joyce P. Mastrilli, O.T.R./L.
Assistant Director,
Occupational Therapy Department,
The Rehabilitation Institute of Pittsburgh,
Pittsburgh, Pennsylvania

Beth B. O'Brien, B.S.
Executive Director,
Pittsburgh Regional Chapter
National Head Injury Foundation
Pittsburgh, Pennsylvania

George P. Prigatano, Ph.D.
Chairman, Neuropsychology,
Clinical Director, Neurological Rehabilitation,
Barrow Neurological Institute,
St. Joseph's Hospital and Medical Center,
Phoenix, Arizona

James C. Pfahl, B.S., C.R.C.
Clinical Team Leader,
Vocational and Career Services Department,
The Rehabilitation Institute of Pittsburgh,
Pittsburgh, Pennsylvania

Mason B. Scott, Ph.D.
Supervisor of Clinical Services,
Consulting Psychologist, Head Trauma Program,
The Vocational Rehabilitation Center of Allegheny County, Inc.,
Pittsburgh, Pennsylvania

Barbara A. Seif, M.S. Ed., C.R.C.
Rehabilitation Specialist,
Vocational and Career Services Department,
The Rehabilitation Institute of Pittsburgh,
Pittsburgh, Pennsylvania

Gloria J. Smith, O.T.R./L.
Tutor, Lincoln Institute,
School of Health Sciences,
Melbourne, Australia

Deborah M. Sullivan, M.Ed.
Cognitive Rehabilitation Therapist,
Training Specialist,
The Rehabilitation Institute of Pittsburgh,
Pittsburgh, Pennsylvania

Shirley F. Szekeres, M.A., CCC/Sp.
Cognitive Rehabilitation Therapist,
Assistant Director, Speech-Language Therapy Department,
The Rehabilitation Institute of Pittsburgh,
Pittsburgh, Pennsylvania

Jan Titonis, M.P.H.
Senior Program Coordinator for Head Injury Programs,
The Rehabilitation Institute of Pittsburgh,
Pittsburgh, Pennsylvania

Anne S. Valko, M.D.
Physiatrist
Pittsburgh, Pennsylvania

James F. Wachter, Jr., M.Ed., C.R.C.
Vocational Rehabilitation Counselor,
Director, Head Trauma Program,
The Vocational Rehabilitation Center of Allegheny County, Inc.,
Pittsburgh, Pennsylvania

Paula Wheeler, O.T.R./L.
Cognitive Rehabilitation Therapist,
Staff Occupational Therapist,
The Rehabilitation Institute of Pittsburgh,
Pittsburgh, Pennsylvania

Mark Ylvisaker, M.A., CCC/Sp.
Director, Speech-Language Therapy Department,
The Rehabilitation Institute of Pittsburgh,
Pittsburgh, Pennsylvania

CHAPTER 1

Neuropsychological Deficits, Personality Variables, and Outcome

George P. Prigatano

Scientific investigation of higher cerebral deficits following traumatic brain injury has typically revolved around neurological criteria. That is, classification of patients with traumatic brain injuries is done according to neurological standards and then patients are studied by a variety of neuropsychological methods. For example, Sir Richie Russell (1971) classified patients according to the duration of post-traumatic amnesia (PTA) and then related this to presence or absence of later memory or calculation difficulties. Brooks (1976) related duration of PTA to performance on the Wechsler Memory Scale. Bond (1975) did the same thing for the Wechsler Adult Intelligence Scale. Levin and his associates (Levin, Benton & Grossman, 1983) produced a number of informative papers relating initial Glasgow Coma Scale scores to a variety of neurobehavioral problems secondary to traumatic brain injury.

Although this approach is certainly necessary, it is by itself not sufficient. Patients who suffer brain injury with neuropsychological sequelae have a personal reaction to their deficits (Prigatano, Pepping & Klonoff, 1986). Moreover, their premorbid intellectual, personality, and sociocultural characteristics interact with acquired brain injury to produce a complex symptom picture which often involves disorders of personality as well as cognitive functioning (Prigatano and others, 1986). As Ewing-Cobbs, Fletcher, and Levin (1985) have pointed out: "Statements attributing post-injury behavioral disturbance solely to the cerebral insult are probably simplistic explanations" (p. 79).

When one is confronted with the long-term outcome of traumatic brain injury, the premorbid characteristics often seem to be very important. For example, Shaffer, Chadwick, and Rutter (1975) reported that the psychiatric difficulties in children with localized brain injuries correlated better with the degree of psychosocial adversity in the home than with the actual length of coma. The recent work by Rimel, Giordani, Barth, and Jane (1982) gives clues that a history of maladaptive behavior may contribute notably to the extent of disability after traumatic brain injury.

Clinicians involved in the rehabilitation of traumatic brain injured patients are often impressed that personality variables, both pre- and post-injury, contribute greatly to the long-term rehabilitative outcome (Gans, 1983). In a recent clinical research project, patients who benefited most from an intensive form of neuropsychologically mediated rehabilitation had fewer psychiatric or personality disturbances *prior* to the onset of treatment (Prigatano and others, 1986).

EPIDEMIOLOGY OF TRAUMATIC BRAIN INJURY

While reports have appeared reviewing the epidemiology of head injuries (Thompson & Klonoff, 1975), there still is very limited data concerning the long-term psychosocial outcome of such injuries. In fact, in 1980 the National Institute for Neurological and Communicative Disorders and Stroke (NINCDS) began the National Traumatic Coma Data Bank Project in an effort to obtain systematic information on the outcome of severe head injuries and their neurological and non-neurological predictors. At this point we can only surmise, based on a few studies in the literature, the typical outcome of such injuries. The work of Gilchrist and Wilkinson (1979) seems fairly representative. Seventy-two patients were followed after having an injury which produced a period of post-traumatic amnesia of 24 hours or longer. Of these patients, 23.6 percent returned to their previous level of employment (not necessarily level of competency). Approximately 15 percent returned to a lower job. Close to 40 percent of the sample seemed to have adequate self-care skills but were unable to return to gainful employment. They "walked and talked" — but stayed home. The remaining individuals were either hospitalized or deceased at time of follow-up.

Interpreting these data, it appears the best estimate is that only about one-third of severe craniocerebral trauma patients return to gainful employment using traditional rehabilitative methods.[1] Of the remaining two-thirds, perhaps 40 to 50 percent literally walk and talk but do not return to gainful employment. The question is: to what degree could this subgroup of the population be helped to return to work? Recent research by Prigatano and others (1986) estimates that approximately half of these people might be able to return to gainful employment given intensive neuropsychologically oriented rehabilitation. Ben-Yishay and his colleagues in New York City (1985) have also reported that approximately 50 percent of their patients return to gainful employment given an intensive form of cognitively oriented rehabilitation.

Given these findings, one must ask the question: to what degree do personality variables contribute to long-term outcome? Studies in the literature suggest that personality variables play a major role in long-term outcome, particularly psychosocial adjustment. Personality variables seem to have a substantial impact on the degree to which there is distress in the family situation and problems in maintaining pre-trauma friendships. Understanding certain "key" neuroanatomical and neuropathological facts associated with both the cognitive and personality deficits seen after brain injury helps clarify the nature of these deficits. In this chapter, emphasis will be placed on the importance of the interconnection between cognitive and personality disorders and a model for conceptualizing personality difficulties after traumatic brain injury will be offered. The effects of personality deficits on overall psychosocial adjustment and capacity to return to work will be considered. Finally, the implications for treatment outcome studies will be briefly reviewed and two case examples of how pre-injury behavior may influence outcome will be presented.

NEUROANATOMICAL AND NEUROPATHOLOGICAL CONSIDERATIONS

Traditional ideas concerning the areas of the brain which are at "high risk" following craniocerebral trauma emphasize the tip (or prefrontal region) of the frontal lobes, the anterior portion of the tem-

[1]Recently at the Review Course in Physical Medicine and Rehabilitation at the University of Washington, Seattle, Washington, Dr. Nathan Cope stated that in his opinion only 10 percent of severely head injured patients actually got back to work. The figures reported by Gilchrist and Wilkinson, therefore, may be even more optimistic than we think.

poral lobes, as well as brain stem structures (see Levin et al., 1983; Prigatano and others, 1986). While these areas are prone to contusion injuries, other types of brain injury can also occur. These include ischemic injury in which brain tissue is deprived of blood and thereby oxygen and glucose. Graham, Adams, and Doyle (1978) studied 138 patients who died from severe craniocerebral injury and noted that 91 percent of the brains studied had evidence of ischemic brain injury. Hippocampal and basal ganglia structures had a very high incidence of involvement (88 percent and 86 percent, respectively). These findings are important because they emphasize that deep brain structures that are either a part of the limbic system (e.g., the hippocampus) or are closely connected to limbic and frontal lobe systems tend to be impaired following such injuries. The amygdala, for example, sits anterior to the hippocampus and is considered by some anatomists to be part of both the limbic system and the basal ganglia. The amygdala is well recognized for its role in the "interrupt" function of behavior. Emotion can be defined as the complex feeling state which has an arousal component and serves to interrupt an ongoing behavior for survival value (Prigatano and others, 1986). The amygdala may well be at high risk in cases of craniocerebral trauma and this may explain in part why these patients are often considered more "emotional" following their injuries and are generally described as having less frustration tolerance and being more irritable (Prigatano, in press).

Mesulam (1985) recently put forth some rather interesting ideas concerning the architechtonics, connectivity, and neurotransmitter neurochemistry of the brain which are relevant to this discussion. He suggested that the "entire cortical mantle can be subdivided into only five subtypes which display a gradual increase in structural complexity and differentiation" (p. 2). In Mesulam's analysis, the prefrontal regions of the brain and the anterior portions of the temporal lobe represent part of what he calls "heteromodal" association cortex and paralimbic cortex. These particular regions, according to his analysis, provide for a unique combination of intellectual and affective components of information processing. Mesulam (1985) stated:

> At least two essential transformations are likely to occur in heteromodal cortex. First, these areas provide a neural template for intermodal association necessary for many cognitive processes, especially language. Second, they provide the initial interaction between extensively perceived sensory information and limbic-paralimbic input. Thus, another distinction that is lost in heteromodal cortex is that between limbic and nonlimbic. This may initially come as a surprise since there is a tendency to think of heteromodal cortex as a higher order association area devoted to intellectual processes and hence impervious to limbic impulses. However, the evidence obtained in the

macaque brain unequivocally shows that heteromodal areas receive substantial paralimbic input. This anatomic arrangement explains how mood and drive can influence the manner in which the self and the world are experienced and also how thought and experience eventually influence mood.

Damage to heteromodal areas yields a set of complex deficits with cognitive as well as affective components. In lesions of the temporoparietal heteromodal fields, it is the disruption of transmodal integration that gains prominence. On the other hand, the additional affective and motivational components become conspicuous in lesions of the frontal heteromodal field. (p. 25)

The importance of these observations is that they help explain why the typical lesions encountered in severe closed head injury *by their very nature* tend to produce a combination of cognitive and personality problems. To date, neuropsychological research has primarily explored the cognitive components, but has not adequately addressed the affective or personality disorders which are also a part of these neuropathological insults. Moreover, the patients' and families' personal reactions to this class of deficits have not been adequately understood or treated. Consequently, many patients are discharged from rehabilitative programs because of their behavioral problems — yet these problems deserve as much attention as do hemiparesis or aphasia.

INTERCONNECTION OF COGNITIVE AND PERSONALITY DISORDERS AFTER TRAUMATIC BRAIN INJURY

As early as 1942, Goldstein emphasized the importance of personality disorders after brain injury and their interconnection with cognitive deficits. In his famous paper, "The Effect of Brain Damage on the Personality," Goldstein (1952) emphasized how problems of abstract reasoning or impairment of the abstract attitude predisposed patients to behave impulsively and socially inappropriately. He also outlined how patients can become overwhelmed with their cognitive (and motor and language) deficits and thereby produce what he called a catastrophic reaction. For various reasons, the importance of the catastrophic reaction has not been adequately recognized in scientific research or in the clinical management of patients with traumatic brain injuries. Yet it is an extremely important phenomenon and one that needs further evaluation (Prigatano and others, 1986).

In 1959, Chapman and Wolff investigated how the magnitude and location of discrete lesions influence both cognitive and person-

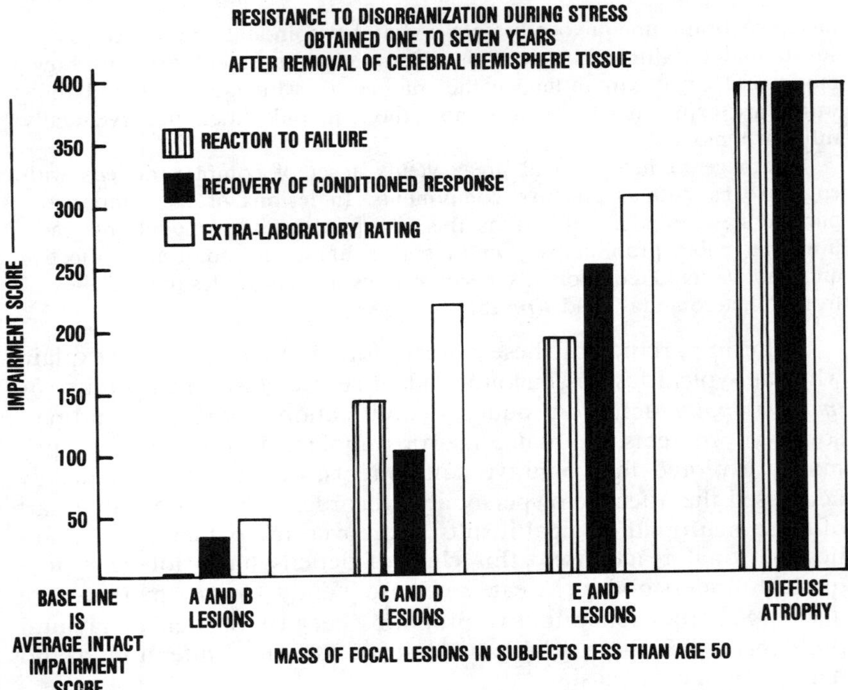

Figure 1–1. Demonstration in subjects less than age 50 that impairment of resistance to disorganization during stress increased with increased mass of cerebral hemisphere tissue loss. These impairment scores were obtained 1 to 7 years after removal of cerebral hemisphere tissue. The "reaction to failure" procedure is described in the text. The "recovery of conditional response" score is based on the number of trials required to re-establish a previously stable conditioned response after a period of induced failure. The "extra-laboratory rating" was based on two of the extra-laboratory criteria listed in Table 1, i.e., (1) reduction of the thresholds for deprivation and frustration and (2) longer-lasting and severer disorganization after frustration, deprivation, failure, or conflict. (Table 1–1 refers to the original manuscript.) (From "The Cerebral Hemispheres and the Highest Integrative Functions of Man" by L. R. Chapman and H. G. Wolff, 1959, *Archives of Neurology, 1,* p. 65.)

ality functions. Figure 1–1 (taken from a series of important tables and figures in that manuscript) shows how increasing amounts of brain tissue loss lead to increased difficulties in coping with failures and dealing with a disorganized environment.

Focusing on patients with slight diffuse loss of brain tissue from the cerebral hemispheres, Chapman and Wolff (1959) stated:

> These patients continued to work, but showed lessened ambition, initiative, or imagination. They attempted to deal with daily problems

> by constricting the fields of interest and habitually performing old routinized patterns, at work, at home, and in the community. Defense reactions were integrated less well and were modulated poorly, although the subjects often maintained relatively effective states for long periods by repeating old, previously learned patterns. Disinterested, detached behavior and the capacity to participate fell off concurrently. Several remained at home a good part of the day, staring into space, rarely seeking the company of others or the advantages of the community's entertainment facilities. Social responsibility was avoided, and athletic endeavors were diminished or absent. Recall was delayed; calculation was labored, and persistent effort was increasingly difficult. Frustration threshold and tolerance were lowered, and the subjects were irritable or showed outbursts of hostility. Situations which were new, which might lead to failures, or which required decision making or incisive action were avoided. Anxiety was sometimes conspicuous. The expression of affect often appeared inappropriate, and there was a paucity of expression of feeling. Examination of the patient revealed impairment in memory in regard to recent events, slowed calculation, and poorly performed serial 7's tests, but no significant loss in vocabulary or general information. (p. 65–67)

These observations are all too familiar to today's practicing clinicians who are involved in the evaluation and rehabilitation of patients with traumatic brain injuries. Unless the problems described by Chapman and Wolff are dealt with in a systematic rehabilitative program, many of these patients unfortunately remain inactive and nonproductive.

In assessing psychosocial outcome after severe head injury, Bond (1975) drew attention to the importance of memory and personality disorders for impaired social functioning. Later, Weddell, Oddy, and Jenkins (1980) reported a high correlation between personality change and memory disturbance. These patients tended not to work and were likely to lose pretrauma friendships.

Beyond this type of research, it has been difficult to systematically relate personality variables to various cognitive or intellectual deficits. Moreover, while cognitive deficits are often related to the severity of injury, Levin and Grossman (1978) failed to find a strong relationship between grade of injury and ratings of depression, hostility, or suspiciousness. Yet other variables such as conceptual disorganization and motor retardation were highly related to this variable. Similarly, Lishman (1968) reported poor association of many personality variables with length of PTA or estimates of amount of brain tissue destroyed. This is not to say that personality variables are unrelated to neurological or cognitive variables, but only that the relationship is a complex one. Part of the problem has been that we have lacked an adequate definition of personality to guide research in this area.

One approach is to consider personality as patterns of emotional and motivational responses that develop over the lifetime of the organism and are highly sensitive to biological and environmental contingencies. Prigatano and others (1986) and Prigatano (in press) elaborate on this definition. For purposes of this discussion, however, three types of personality disorders after traumatic brain injury can be conceptualized:

1. those that flow directly from the neuropathological lesions and therefore can be described as neuropsychologically mediated personality disorders;
2. personality disturbances which are in reaction to the brain injury and associated failures in coping. These could generally be labeled as reactionary personality problems; and
3. those personality disorders that existed prior to the onset of the brain injury and are therefore long-term or characterological in nature.

Reactionary problems may well increase in traumatic brain injured patients, even as cognitive, motor, and/or linguistic problems stabilize. For example, a few studies have reported that patients show more emotional distress 12 months following brain injury than during the first 6 months (Fordyce, Roueche & Prigatano, 1983). In contrast, other problems such as paranoia are likely to be more stable and less ready to change. This kind of deficit is more clearly related to temporal lobe pathology and often is considered a neuropsychologically mediated personality disorder (Leftoff, 1983; Lishman, 1968). Suggested strategies for assessing reactionary, neuropsychologically mediated, and characterological personality problems are discussed by Prigatano (in press).

PERSONALITY DISORDERS AND PSYCHOSOCIAL ADJUSTMENT AFTER SEVERE CLOSED HEAD INJURY

Brooks and McKinlay (1983) asked relatives to describe a group of patients with severe injuries using a series of bipolar adjectives. They asked for an assessment of the patient from the relatives' point of view both before and after brain injury. Nearly two-thirds of the relatives reported personality change one year after the trauma. Figure 1–2 illustrates the retrospective and post-injury descriptions by

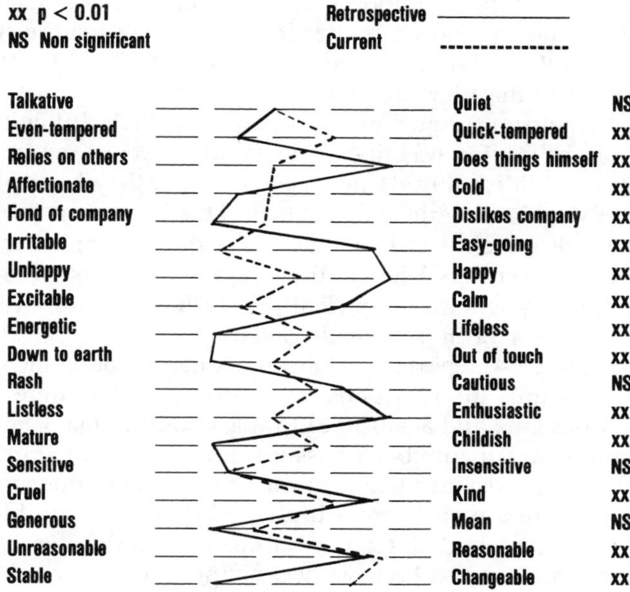

Figure 1–2. Retrospective (solid line) and current (dotted line) assessment at 12 months in cases with personality changes (33 cases). (From "Personality and Behavioural Change After Severe Blunt Head Injury — A Relative's View" by D. N. Brooks and W. McKinlay, 1983, *Journal of Neurology, Neurosurgery, and Psychiatry, 46,* p. 337).

relatives. Statistically reliable differences pre- and post-trauma are indicated by "xx." Not unexpectedly, patients are seen as more quick tempered, irritable, and childish post-injury. These clinical observations have now been documented for nearly 100 years.

Over time, these problems may increase or diminish depending on their biological basis and environmental factors. It is often the clinician's task to try to distinguish personality variables that are truly reactionary from these that are neuropsychologically mediated and long-term or characterological in nature. Such a separation may help establish more reasonable rehabilitation goals.

Oddy, Coughlan, Tyerman, and Jenkins (1985) described traumatic brain injured patients' psychosocial functioning some 7 years post-injury. Their data are interesting in that this is one of the longest follow-up reports to have appeared in the literature. One of the findings (which has considerable importance for rehabilitation outcome) is that families tend to report a higher incidence of difficulties than do patients themselves. For example, in Table 1-1, 79 percent of the families reported that the patients had problems in memory; in contrast, only 53 percent of the patients admitted to such difficulties. The other important finding was that patients often do not recognize that they are more childish and do not recognize that they have problems in objectively evaluating their difficulties. This important problem — unawareness of deficit — (which has both cognitive and personality components) is perhaps one of the major predictors of outcome. However, little systematic empirical research data supporting this point of view has been obtained to date.

Thomsen (1984) reported perhaps the longest group outcome data on severely brain injured patients. Forty patients were studied 2.5 years post-trauma and again 10 to 15 years post-trauma. Her findings are informative on a number of issues. First, physical impairment, dysarthria, and persistent memory problems were *not* the substantial deterrent to re-entering a normal lifestyle. While these problems are certainly important and deserve continued rehabilitative attention, the problems that seem to be most devastating to the patients' ultimate psychosocial adjustment centered around personality disturbances. Again, not unexpectedly, Thomsen reported that from the patients' point of view the single biggest problem 10 to 15 years following

Table 1-1. Symptoms Reported by Patients and Relatives 7 Years Post-Injury

Patients	%	Relatives	%
Trouble remembering things	53	Trouble remembering things	79
Difficulty concentrating	46	Difficulty concentrating	50
Easily affected by alcohol	38	Difficulty speaking	50
Often knocks things over	31	Easily affected by alcohol	43
Often loses temper	31	Difficulty in becoming interested	43
Difficulty in becoming interested	28	Becomes tired easily	43
Likes to keep things tidy	28	Often impatient	43
Sometimes loses way	28	Sometimes behaves childishly	40
Eyesight problems	28	Likes to keep things tidy	40
Difficulty following conversation	28	Refuses to admit difficulties	40

From "Social Adjustment After Closed Head Injury: A Further Follow-Up Seven Years after Injury" by M. Oddy, T. Coughlan, A. Tyerman, and D. Jenkins, 1985, *Journal of Neurology, Neurosurgery, and Psychiatry, 48,* p. 565.

traumatic brain injury is that of social isolation. These patients frequently lack the cognitive and personality resources for establishing and maintaining friendships. Sadly, many patients did not recognize that their personality difficulties systematically produce a turning away by family members and friends. Second, their data indicate that it is precisely the personality disorders that are most upsetting to the family members. Family members can live with motor deficits, language deficits, and cognitive deficits. They cannot, however, easily tolerate the belligerent, irritable, childlike, and emotionally labile relative who has suffered a brain injury (see Chapter 9 for further discussion of Thomsen's study).

Thomsen's data suggest that while some affective problems may actually improve with the passage of time (patients appear to be less childish according to their relatives some 10 to 15 years post-injury than they are 2.5 years post-injury), other problems seemed to remain at the same level or increase. For example, patients were judged to be more irritable 10 to 15 years post-trauma than they were 2.5 years post-trauma. This is an extremely important finding because it suggests two ideas. First, irritability (not emotional lability) may well be a reaction to limited cognitive, motor, and language abilities. Second, if patients are not taught to compensate for long-term or persistent problems, their ability to tolerate repeated failures decreases. This is understandable with and without brain injury. It is also interesting to note in Thomsen's data that with the passage of time patients report being more tired and having less tolerance for distress. This finding could be interpreted as patients becoming more depressed and unable to find methods of coping with their deficits with the passage of time.

Personality Variables and Treatment Outcome

In the course of our neuropsychological evaluation of patients with traumatic brain injuries, families are frequently asked to describe these patients on the Katz-R Adjustment Scale. This scale, which is described in greater detail elsewhere (Katz & Lyerly, 1963; Prigatano, Wright & Levin, 1984), consists in part of 127 items which basically describe behavioral characteristics, feeling states, interest patterns, cognitive capacities, and preoccupations. From the files of patients seen in the Department of Clinical Neuropsychology at Presbyterian Hospital in Oklahoma City, 137 patients with documented craniocerebral trauma and a complete Katz-R Adjustment Scale were identified and their Katz-R Adjustment Scale scores analyzed. To provide for a "rough" medical control group, older patients with chronic obstructive pulmonary disease (COPD) seen in another research project were also studied (Prigatano, Wright & Levin, 1984). Details are available in an unpublished manuscript concerning how the data were analyzed and how the two groups were compared (Prigatano, Klonoff, Zeiner & Pepping, 1985).

Of the 127 items sampled, 19 items were described more frequently as being true of traumatic brain injured patients versus COPD controls. The items that separated the two groups are listed in Table 1–2. As can be seen from this table, many of the items which separate the groups have to do with personality difficulties. Interestingly, when

Table 1–2. Katz Adjustment Scale-Relatives Form Items that Discriminate Head Injury from COPD Patients by at Least a 20 Percent Rate of Endorsement

		Percentage of Endorsement as Almost Always or Often True according to Relatives	
Item No.	**Item Content**	**COPD**	**HI**
4	Feels lonely	5.2	34.6
6	Is restless	24.7	52.3
15	Gets very sad, blue	5.2	34.6
32	Has mood changes without reason	5.2	27.3
42	Bossy	14.3	28.5
44	Argues	16.9	38.0
46	Is cooperative	88.0	58.1
48	Stubborn	18.2	40.9
55	Gets annoyed easily	18.5	48.2
62	Is dependable	92.3	68.4
63	Is responsible	92.3	65.7
66	Shows good judgment	83.2	43.8
75	Is independent	76.7	55.5
89	Remembers important things	80.6	50.4
91	Acts as if he can't get certain things out of his mind	6.5	31.4
92	Acts as if he can't concentrate on one thing	5.2	28.5
93	Acts as if he can't make decisions	5.2	30.0
104	Keeps repeating the same idea	5.2	25.8
121	Talks about big plans	1.3	21.3

examining traumatic brain injured patients who underwent a neuropsychological rehabilitation program on these 19 items, three items separated out treatment "successes" versus "failures." By and large, treatment successes were those individuals who were able to obtain and maintain gainful employment or at least a productive lifestyle (see Prigatano and others, 1986, for a more detailed description of the two groups). The items which reliably separated these two groups were: "bossy" ($p<.01$); "is cooperative" ($p<.05$); and "is responsible" ($p<.01$). Thus, patients who are bossy and argumentative clearly have a lesser chance of maintaining gainful employment than cooperative and responsible patients. Cooperativeness and responsibility are not characteristics which are totally a result of brain injury or the lack of it. These two characteristics seem to reflect both premorbid personality characteristics and residual abilities following injury. This type of data suggests, along with research that has been done on other populations (see Chapter 9), that personality variables have a profound impact on the capacity to return to work and to adjust within the family environment after significant brain injury.

PSYCHOTHERAPEUTIC AND LONG-TERM REHABILITATIVE EFFORTS WITH TRAUMATIC BRAIN INJURED PATIENTS

In light of the findings presented combined with our clinical experience with these patients, it becomes important to help educate and convince patients that the major problem they have to face over time is that of social isolation. Therapy may help them find ways to modify personality disorders to avoid this outcome. The fact that some problems, such as irritability, get worse with time implies that these may in fact be reactionary problems and consequently much more amenable to treatment than might have been previously thought. If patients can be taught to compensate for their deficits, can acquire a realistic view of what they can and cannot handle, and can obtain a level of employment which is compatible with their abilities, then they have a chance of re-establishing some meaning in their life, thereby creating the basis on which to conduct mutually satisfying interpersonal relationships (Prigatano and others, 1986). Therapists involved in the long-term care of these patients have to find the best medium or approach for helping patients deal with these personality deficits. While individual and group psychotherapy may be one avenue for approaching this class of problems, there are multiple ways of achieving this goal. Many brain injured patients have a difficult time conceptualizing important issues that are normally discussed in any form of psychotherapy. They may, therefore, appear resistant to psychotherapy, and attempts to deal with personality deficits may be prematurely abandoned.

If patients could be progressively educated as to the importance of personality deficits, then they may become more amenable to traditional forms of psychotherapy as practiced in a neuropsychologically oriented rehabilitation program. Another approach is to try to establish a therapeutic milieu or community in which the personality issues are dealt with on a day-to-day basis much like a family or small group. This can take the place, for some patients, of insight oriented psychotherapy or strict behavioral management techniques. A third option is to work with these patients on a variety of tasks in which the affective problems emerge and help them deal with those problems in a counseling or teaching manner during those times. Various rehabilitative clinicians, not just including psychotherapists, have to give more thought to how these personality deficits are going to be dealt with. New methods for dealing with these problems must be developed if patients are to be substantially helped, especially the more cognitively impaired patients.

As a guideline for helping further conceptualize the nature of personality deficits after these injuries, it may be useful to list those personality disorders which are currently believed to be neuropsychologically mediated rather than reactionary. These issues are discussed in some detail by Prigatano and others (1986).

Hypothesized Neuropsychologically Mediated Personality Disorders Versus Reactionary Problems

In the clinical setting in which the goal was to rehabilitate young adult brain injured patients, a number of personality problems emerged which appeared to have a clear organic basis (Prigatano and others, 1986). These neuropsychologically mediated problems included impulsiveness, socially inappropriate comments or actions, emotional lability (which includes poor tolerance for frustration), agitation, paranoia, a variety of childlike behaviors, and unawareness of the degree of neuropsychological deficits. In some patients there is also a clear lack of "motivation" and hypoarousal.

The neuropathological correlates for these diverse emotional and motivational disturbances are at best tentative. However, a review of the literature suggests the following correlations. Lesions which interrupt the corticobulbar motor pathways bilaterally may release reflex mechanisms for facial expression from cortical control. These lesions can result in "pathological" laughing and/or crying behavior (Poeck, 1969).

Lesions which interrupt the cortical-limbic reticular loop often produce hypokinesis and indifference. This is frequently associated with low arousal level and poor attention (Pribram & McGuinness, 1975).

Orbital-basal frontal cortex has rich connections with the septal area and the amygdala. Lesions of the orbital-frontal cortex can thus produce problems of disinhibition (i.e., inappropriateness, irritability, angry outbursts, at times inappropriate sexual activity) (Valenstein & Heilman, 1979) (see Chapter 9).

Conversely, dorsal lateral frontal cortex appears to have rich connections with the cingulate gyrus and the reticular activating system (Valenstein & Heilman, 1979). Thus, lesions of the dorsal lateral frontal cortex often seem to lead to deficits in arousal. This can produce a patient who has reasonably good cognitive responses to external stimuli but who may fail to adequately sustain arousal level in the absence of external stimulation. In previous work (Prigatano, Stahl, Orr & Zeiner, 1982), for example, it was noted that traumatic brain injured patients had sleep disturbances which suggested some disruption of the sleep/wake cycle. Often patients would wake several times during the course of the night but easily fall asleep. It was hypothesized that some of these disturbances may have resulted from dorsal lateral and/or reticular activating system disturbances.

Lesions of the anterior temporal lobe frequently produce a variety of affective disturbances which often appear psychiatric in nature. This may have to do with the low seizure threshold of the amygdala. It may also have to do with what is frequently described as paranoid, egocentric, and oftentimes aggressive characteristics of patients with temporal lobe epilepsy (Ferguson, Schwartz & Rayport, 1969) (see Chapter 9). Lesions of the anterior cortical area (involving particularly frontal-limbic systems) may interfere with the ability of the patient to use feeling states as aids in learning and memory. This frequently results in patients who are unable to learn by using arousal cues (Prigatano & Pribram, 1981).

Lesions of the left hemisphere, perisylvian area, notoriously produce language disturbances. Dysphasic disturbances may interfere with the ability to use propositional speech and therefore with the comprehension of affective meaning of the words that are used (Gardner, Ling, Flamm & Silverman, 1975). However, the comprehension of the affective meaning of intonation patterns may be adequately preserved. Thus the patient may not know what is said, but may get an idea of how something is said. In contrast, lesions of the right hemisphere, in comparable areas, may produce substantial difficulties in ability to perceive the emotional tone of language. Ross (1981) recently provided a stimulating description of what he calls the aprosodias.

Lesions of the right temporo-parietal area notoriously produce visuo-spatial and visual constructive difficulties. These deficits seem to relate to problems in facial recognition and the recognition of emotional expression on faces (e.g.,DeKosky, Heilman, Bowers & Valenstein, 1980). Both left and right temporo-parietal lesions seem to influence the ability to recognize facial emotion (Prigatano & Pribram, 1982). When the task requires matching visual stimuli, the right hemisphere patients do worse. When the task involves verbally describing the emotional expression, the right and left hemisphere patients have similar difficulties (Prigatano & Pribram, 1982).

In summary, it appears that lesions of the frontal-limbic system, the limbic system per se, and the limbic-reticular loop are especially important in producing disturbances of emotion and motivation. These disturbances seem to be reflective of problems in spontaneous control and expression of feeling states after the brain injury. Lesions involving the cortex, particularly posterior to the Rolandic fissure, appear to influence the perception of affective stimuli coming from others. Lesions anterior to the Rolandic strip seem to reduce the ability of the patient to properly utilize information; this frequently results in behavior which is considered "inappropriate" and childish. These are hypothesized neuropsychologically mediated disturbances with potential neuroanatomical correlates. Additional research is needed to confirm these notions.

In contrast to these neuropsychologically mediated problems, in the clinical setting the patient often shows a wide variety of affective reactions which do not seem to be related to neuroanatomical knowledge of memory and emotion. There are behavioral problems which simply seem to lack any correlation with amount of brain dysfunction or location of brain dysfunction. These affective problems are often considered reactionary in nature and may reflect the individual's premorbid personality characteristics as well residual cognitive capacity. While there is no definitive list of reactionary problems (or of neuropsychologically mediated problems for that matter), the following behavioral disturbances seem to be reactionary in nature (see Chapter 9): anxiety, depression, feelings of hopelessness and helplessness, anger, and possibly irritability. Irritability is frequently seen in patients who have no neurological difficulties per se, but who are overwhelmed by the environment. It is tentatively suggested that irritability may be reactionary in nature for many traumatic brain injured patients and not necessarily the result of brain dysfunction. This, of course, also awaits further evaluation and documentation.

THE ROLE OF PREMORBID FACTORS IN DETERMINING OUTCOME FROM TRAUMATIC BRAIN INJURY

It has long been recognized by clinicians that premorbid factors, particularly personality characteristics, are important determinants of long-term behavioral outcome of brain injury. There are, however, serious methodological problems evaluating these premorbid variables. Kozol (1945, 1946) attempted to do systematic interviewing of brain injured patients and their family members in order to correlate pre-trauma personality with post-trauma behavior. In general, his findings were disappointing. They suggested very little evidence for a close correlation between pre-trauma personality characteristics and post-trauma behavior. Nevertheless, in the clinical setting one is often convinced that such a correlation exists. When there is a change or deviation from premorbid personality or behavioral patterns, it is often thought to be a result of frontal lobe injury. The classic examples are those patients who act in a somewhat impulsive, socially inappropriate manner *prior* to brain injury and 2 years following the injury are considered by family and friends to be more congenial, satisfied with traditional roles, and generally calmer in their behavior. There are considerable methodological problems in assessing how these premorbid variables in fact influence outcome, and research in this area is badly needed. Another interesting question is whether or not premorbid variables may actually contribute to the likelihood of suffering a brain injury in the first place. Some psychological theories suggest that the pre-existing psychosocial state of the individual (as well as unconscious personality conflicts or characteristics) can put him or her at risk for brain injury. The methodological problems in measuring this are immense.

However, with children one may be able to more accurately approach these problems. In the case of children, there are school records to be evaluated which document the child's academic and psychosocial functioning for years preceding the accident. The child's academic performance may give a clue as to whether or not there were major academic or behavioral problems prior to the injury. For example, a 13 year old adolescent boy who suffered a traumatic brain injury in 1983 reported post-injury academic difficulties. When evaluating his school records as far back as 1981 (3 years prior to the injury), it was quite clear that this child, had difficulties in schoolwork which substantially predated his accident. Figure 1-3 summarizes this child's California Achievement Test scores between the years 1981 and 1985. There was a progressive decline in academic performance in the 3 years *predating* the injury. There is, of course, continued decline in academic performance after the injury. These findings, however, raise the question of whether or not some of the problems of adaptation following the brain injury in fact reflect a combination of pre-injury difficulties as well as post-injury cognitive and/or personality impairments. Certainly, in this case it is difficult to know what is causing what, but the findings are informative in so

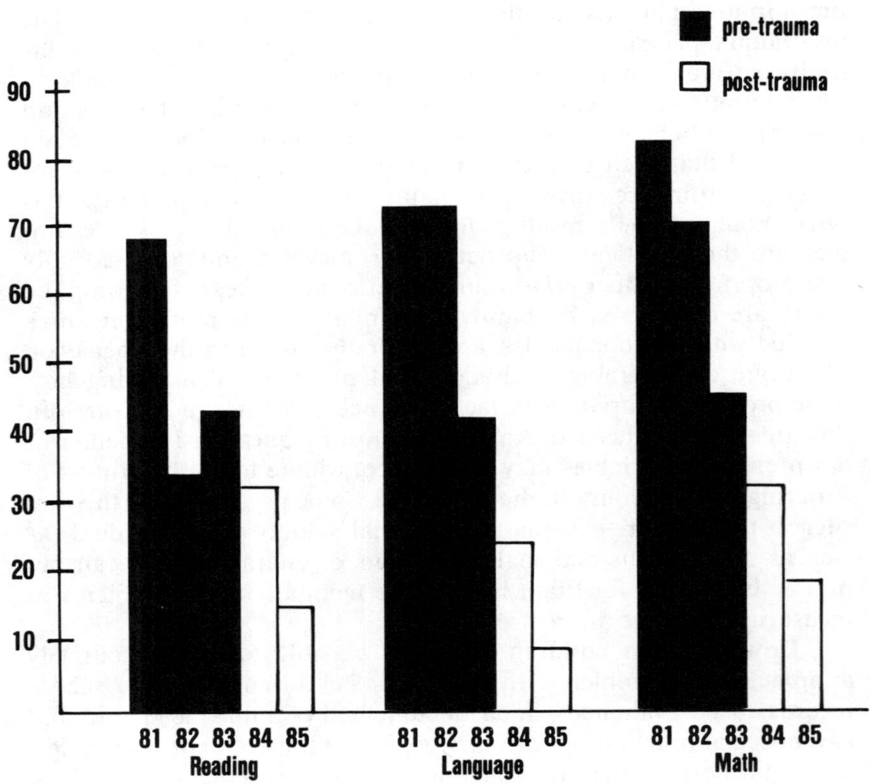

Figure 1–3. California Achievement Test scores of a 13 year old boy 3 years prior to and 2 years post brain injury. (Note decline in performance *prior* as well as post brain injury.)

far as they suggest that a more careful assessment of children's pre-injury behavior may give a clue to what variables are contributing to the overall symptom picture after brain injury.

A second child, who was 15 at the time of injury, had school records dating back approximately 9 years pre-trauma. This child had a history of learning disability and was given a Wechsler Intelligence Scale for Children-Revised Form (WISC-R) in 1977, 1981, and 1984. His accident occured in 1985. He suffered a significant brain injury with both right and left subdural hematomas being surgically removed. Table 1–3 lists this child's pre- and post-injury WISC-R scores. Again, there is evidence of below average performance *prior* to the onset of the injury and then precipitous decline in performance after the injury, particularly in the ability to recall long-term verbal information (Information scale score), verbal reasoning (Similarities scale score), and Vocabulary. It is interesting to note though that if this child's post-injury performance were compared to his performance 7 or 3 years prior to injury, there would not be substantial change in many of the areas. In 1981 this child had moved to Phoenix and there was a general decline in certain aspects of intellectual functioning at that time. Also, just prior to his injury (1981 and 1984), there was a decline in the speed of acquiring new information (note the Coding subtest scores of 6 and 7). Following his injury there

Table 1–3. WISC-R Scores for an Adolescent Boy Several Years Prior to Traumatic Brain Injury and 2 Months Following the Injury

WISC Subtest	1977*	1981**	1984†	1986‡
Information	6	8	11	4
Similarities	8	4	8	5
Arithmetic	8	7	10	7
Vocabulary	8	5	10	5
Comprehension	5	8	8	--
Digit Span	9	4	8	6
Picture Completion	12	7	8	6
Picture Arrangement	10	9	12	10
Block Design	8	7	9	9
Object Assembly	12	12	10	--
Digit Symbol (coding)	12	6	7	5

* 7 yr, 8 mo pre-trauma
** 3 yr, 1 mo pre-trauma
† 1 yr, 4 mo pre-trauma
‡ 0 yr, 2 mo post-trauma

was an even further deterioration in this dimension. This case study raises the question of how much decline in intellectual test findings after brain injury can be attributed solely to neurological factors. It appears that there are other important non-neurological determinants. Personality characteristics and psychosocial adversity prior to the injury may be important variables in the total outcome picture. Obviously this type of clinical observation needs to be thoroughly evaluated in both group and individual studies.

SUMMARY

Outcome from traumatic brain injury is often related to neurological variables and residual cognitive, linguistic, and motor deficits. The importance of personality variables for outcome seems relatively neglected, but in light of recent research, this neglect must be considered unjustified. While there are theoretical pitfalls in trying to separate so-called "organic" from "functional" personality disorders (as Goldstein pointed out years ago), such a distinction may in fact prove helpful in refining research and clinical care of the patients. While some gross clinical correlations can presently be made between region of brain injury and personality disorder, the role of premorbid and postmorbid personality characteristics seems inadequately explored. Personality variables have a profound influence on psychosocial adjustment of the patient and family and may not only influence outcome from severe brain injury, but in some cases may actually herald its occurence or at least increase its likelihood.

REFERENCES

Ben-Yishay, Y., Rattok, J., Lakin, P., Piasetsky, E. B., Ross, B., Silver, S., Zide, E. & Ezrachi, O. (1985). Neuropsychologic rehabilitation: Quest for a holistic approach. *Seminars in Neurology, 5*(3), 252–259.

Bond, M. R. (1975). Assessment of the psychosocial outcome after severe head injury. In CIBA Foundation, *Outcome of severe damage to the central nervous system* (pp. 141–157). New York: Elsevier-North Holland Publishing Co.

Brooks, D. N. (1976). Wechsler Memory Scale performance and its relationship to brain damage after severe closed head injury. *Journal of Neurology, Neurosurgery, and Psychiatry, 39,* 593–601.

Brooks, D. N. & McKinlay, W. (1983). Personality and behavioural change after severe blunt head injury — A relative's view. *Journal of Neurology, Neurosurgery, and Psychiatry, 46,* 336–344.

Chapman, L. R. & Wolff, H. G. (1959). The cerebral hemispheres and the highest integrative functions of man. *Archives of Neurology, 1,* 19–86.

DeKosky, S. T., Heilman, K. M., Bowers, D. & Valenstein, E. (1980). Recognition and discrimination of emotional faces and pictures. *Brain and Language, 9,* 206–214.

Ewing-Cobbs, L., Fletcher, J. M. & Levin, H. S. (1985). Neuropsychological sequelae following pediatric head injury. In M. Ylvisaker (Ed.), *Head injury rehabilitation: Children and adolescents.* San Diego: College-Hill Press.

Ferguson, S. M., Schwartz, M. L. & Rayport, M. (1969). Perception of humor in patients with temporal lobe epilepsy. *Archives of General Psychiatry, 21,* 363–367.

Fordyce, D. J., Roueche, J. R. & Prigatano, G. P. (1983). Enhanced emotional reactions in chronic head trauma patients. *Journal of Neurology, Neurosurgery, and Psychiatry, 46,* 620–624.

Gans, J. S. (1983). Psychosocial adaptation. *Seminars in Neurology, 3,* 201–211.

Gardner, H., Ling, P. K., Flamm, L. & Silverman, J. (1975). Comprehension and appreciation of humorous material following brain injury. *Brain, 98,* 399–412.

Gilchrist, E. & Wilkinson, M. (1979). Some factors determining prognosis in young people with severe head injuries. *Archives of Neurology, 36,* 355–358.

Goldstein, K. (1942). *Aftereffects of brain injury in war.* New York: Grune & Stratton.

Goldstein, K. (1952). The effect of brain damage on the personality. *Psychiatry, 15,* 245–260.

Graham, D. I., Adams, J. H. & Doyle, D. (1978). Ischemic brain damage in fatal nonmissile head injuries. *Journal of Neurological Sciences, 39,* 213–234.

Katz, M. M. & Lyerly, S. B. (1963). Methods of measuring adjustment and social behavior in the community: I. Rationale, description, discriminative validity and scale development. *Psychological Reports, 13,* 503–535.

Kozol, H. L. (1945). Pretraumatic personality and psychiatric sequelae of head injury. *Archives of Neurology and Psychiatry, 53,* 358–364.

Kozol, H. L. (1946). Pretraumatic personality and psychiatric sequelae of head injury. *Archives of Neurology and Psychiatry, 56,* 245–275.

Leftoff, S. (1983). Psychopathology in the light of brain injury: A case study. *Journal of Clinical Neuropsychology, 5*(1), 51–63.

Levin, H. S., Benton, A. L. & Grossman, R. G. (1983). *Neurobehavioral consequences of closed head injury.* New York: Oxford University Press.

Levin, H. S. & Grossman, R. G. (1978). Behavioral sequelae of closed head injury: A quantitative study. *Archives of Neurology, 35,* 720–727.

Lishman, W. A. (1968). Brain damage in relation to psychiatric disability after head injury. *British Journal of Psychiatry, 114,* 373–410.

Mesulam, M. M. (1985). *Principles of behavioral neurology.* Philadelphia: F. A.

Davis Co.
Oddy, M., Coughlan, T., Tyerman, A. & Jenkins, D. (1985). Social adjustment after closed head injury: A further follow-up seven years after injury. *Journal of Neurology, Neurosurgery, and Psychiatry, 48,* 564–568.
Poeck, K. (1969). Pathophysiology of emotional disorders associated with brain damage. In P. J. Vinken & A. W. Bruyn (Eds.), *Handbook of Clinical Neurology* (Vol. 3). New York: Elsevier-North Holland Publishing Co.
Pribram, K. H. & McGuinness, D. (1975). Arousal, activation, and effect in the control of attention. *Psychological Review, 82,* 116–149.
Prigatano, G. P. (in press). Psychiatric aspects of head injury: Problem areas and suggested guidelines for research. In H. S. Levin (Ed.), *Neurobehavioral recovery from head injury.* New York: Oxford University Press.
Prigatano, G. P. and others. (1986). *Neuropsychological rehabilitation after brain injury.* Baltimore: The Johns Hopkins University Press.
Prigatano, G. P., Klonoff, P., Zeiner, H. & Pepping, M. (1985). Katz-R adjustment ratings on traumatic brain injured patients and COPD controls. Unpublished manuscript.
Prigatano, G. P., Pepping, M. & Klonoff, P. (1986). Cognitive, personality, and psychosocial factors in the neuropsychological assessment of brain-injured patients. In B. Uzzell & Y. Gross (Eds.), *Clinical neuropsychology of intervention* (pp. 135–166). Boston: Martinus Nihoff.
Prigatano, G. P. & Pribram, K. H. (1981). Humor and episodic memory following frontal versus posterior brain lesion. *Perceptual and Motor Skills, 53,* 999–1006.
Prigatano, G. P. & Pribram, K. H. (1982). Perception and memory of facial affect following brain injury. *Perceptual and Motor Skills, 54,* 859–869.
Prigatano, G. P., Stahl, M. L., Orr, W. C. & Zeiner, H. K. (1982). Sleep and dreaming disturbances in closed head injury patients. *Journal of Neurology, Neurosurgery, and Psychiatry, 45,* 78–80.
Prigatano, G. P., Wright, E. C. & Levin, D. (1984). Quality of life and its predictors with mild hypoxemia and chronic obstructive pulmonary disease. *Archives of Internal Medicine, 144,* 1613–1619.
Rimel, R. W., Giordani, B., Barth, J. T. & Jane, J. A. (1982). Moderate head injury: Completing the clinical spectrum of brain trauma. *Neurosurgery, 11*(3), 344–350.
Ross, E. D. (1981). The aprosodias. Functional-anatomic organization of the affective components of language in the right hemisphere. *Archives of Neurology, 38,* 561–569.
Russell, W. R. (1971). *The traumatic amnesias.* London: Oxford University Press.
Shaffer, D., Chadwick, O. & Rutter, M. (1975). Psychiatric outcome of localized head injury in children. In CIBA Foundation, *Outcome of severe damage to the nervous system.* New York: Elsevier-North Holland Publishing Co.

Thompson, G. B. & Klonoff, H. (1975). Epidemiology of head injuries. In P. J. Vinken & G. W. Bruyn (Eds.), *Handbook of clinical neurology — Injuries of the brain,* Part I, #23, (pp. 23–24). New York: Elsevier Science Publishers.

Thomsen, I. V. (1984). Late outcome of very severe blunt head trauma: A 10–15 year second follow-up. *Journal of Neurology, Neurosurgery, and Psychiatry, 47,* 260–268.

Traumatic Coma Data Bank Project, NINCDS-OBFS, 1980, Bethesda, Maryland.

Valenstein, E. & Heilman, K. M. (1979). Emotional disorders resulting from lesions of the central nervous system. In K. M. Heilman & E. Valenstein (Eds.), *Clinical neuropsychology.* New York: Oxford University Press.

Weddell, R., Oddy, M. & Jenkins, D. (1980). Social adjustment after rehabilitation: A two-year follow-up of patients with severe head injury. *Psychological Medicine, 10,* 257–263.

CHAPTER 2

Physical Rehabilitation

Lillian J. Bray
Faith Carlson
Reed Humphrey
Joyce P. Mastrilli
*Anne S. Valko**

Since the subject of this book is community re-entry, we have chosen to give this chapter on physical rehabilitation a somewhat nonstandard focus. Intervention for motor disorders, including motor speech disorders, following head injury is essential during both acute and chronic phases of recovery. However, in this chapter we say very little about attempts to improve motor functioning. We chose rather to focus on two themes that, we believe are together a good answer to the question, "During the period of time that a head injured patient with motor impairments is preparing to leave a rehabilitation facility to return to work or to a vocational training or independent living program, how can the physical rehabilitation team best help that patient achieve his or her goals?" With this question in mind, our major theme is evaluation and treatment for compensatory devices that allow patients to function adaptively and independently despite residual motor impairments. Because physical conditioning enables patients to put their motor skills and compensations to work for themselves in vocational or avocational settings, we conclude the chapter with a discussion of this important and often neglected topic. We begin by briefly reviewing studies of physical outcome following head injury. Throughout the subsequent assessment and treatment sections, we emphasize the extent to which ultimate

*Authorship listed alphabetically at the authors' request.

functional outcome is affected by the patient's level of cognitive recovery, psychosocial abilities, communicative skills, family supports, and conditions in the environment.

PHYSICAL OUTCOME

Traumatic brain injury may result in a wide variety of physical deficits. In this section we summarize motor outcome as described in the literature. Frequently, studies of physical outcome do not address postconcussion syndrome, chronic pain syndrome, and decreased physical conditioning. Each of these affect physical abilities and ultimately have a major impact on community re-entry. Therefore, a brief discussion of these dimensions of physical outcome is also included.

Motor Outcome

Outcome following head injury in adults has been studied by several investigators using the Glasgow Outcome Scale (Jennett & Bond, 1975), which categorizes overall recovery on the basis of physical functioning, economic dependence, and social reintegration. The five outcome categories are: death, vegetative state, severe disability, moderate disability, and good recovery. Patients are said to be in a persistent vegetative state if they remain unresponsive to external stimuli. Severe disability includes patients who are awake but totally dependent because of physical and/or cognitive problems. Moderate disability refers to patients who are independent in daily activities but impaired to some degree vocationally and in the community due to residual cognitive, communicative, or physical problems. Good recovery includes reintegration into society with ability to pursue normal occupational and social activities. Patients whose recovery is rated good may continue to have subtle neurological or cognitive deficits (Blyth, 1981). Table 2–1 summarizes several outcome studies.

Physical deficits often have less impact on the patient's ultimate functional outcome than cognitive deficits. Physical disabilities following head injury rarely occur without some degree of accompanying cognitive impairment (Griffith, 1983). The interaction of physical and cognitive problems markedly reduces the patient's ability to be independent. Heiden, Small, Caton, Weisst, and Kurze (1983) found that cognitive problems were the primary contributors to disability in 67 percent of a group of moderately disabled patients and in 53 percent of severely disabled patients. Cognitive and physical

TABLE 2–1. OUTCOME FOLLOWING HEAD INJURY

					GLASGOW OUTCOME SCALE				
STUDY	Number of Subjects	Median Age (yrs.)	Duration of Coma (hrs.)	Post-Injury Time (mo.)	Death (%)	Vegetative State (%)	Severe Disability (%)	Moderate Disability (%)	Good Recovery (%)
Heiden, Small, Caton, Weisst, & Kurze, 1983	213	35 (mean)	>6	12	52	2	11	16	19
Young et al., 1981	170	26.2	>6	12	26	3	7	10	54
Bowers & Marshall, 1980	200	25–29	>6		36	4	8	10	42
Jennett et al., 1977 (Glasgow Group)	593	35	>6	6	48	2	10	18	23
Jennett et al., 1977 (Netherlands Group)	239	32	>6	6	50	2	7	15	26
Jennett et al., 1977 (Los Angeles Group)	168	35	>6	6	50	2	14	19	12

factors contributed equally to the patient's disability in 47 percent of those with severe disabilities. None of the severely disabled patients had physical problems which were more debilitating than their cognitive deficits. These results seem to be quite representative of groups of head injured patients. We cite these data not to deemphasize physical sequelae, which can be profoundly impairing and are often the primary concern of patients, but rather to remind clincians who are responsible for the physical restoration of head injured individuals that it is essential to integrate a sensitivity to cognitive and psychosocial themes into the process of physical rehabilitation.

Motor dysfunction following head injury may range from mild to severe and include any of the following neuromuscular disorders: spasticity, ataxia, rigidity, dyskinesia, tremors, and flaccidity. Involvement may be unilateral or bilateral. Sensory impairments, including visual and auditory deficits, may also compound the disability. Mills (1985) studied 24 patients with traumatic head injuries who received rehabilitation between 1981 and 1983. She found that, on discharge from the rehabilitation unit, 16.7 percent were quadriparetic, 41.7 percent were hemiparetic, and 41.7 percent had intact voluntary movement. Furthermore, 12.6 percent of these patients had peripheral nerve injury and 41 percent had impaired coordination. Lewin, Marshall, and Roberts (1979) evaluated 291 patients who were at least 10 years post-trauma. They found that 5 percent of the patients had athetoid pseudobulbar movement patterns, 20 percent exhibited brain stem cerebellar patterns, 40 percent were hemiparetic, 21 percent had no detectable motor impairment, and 14 percent did not fall into any of these categories. Functional implications of these disorders are described in Jaffe, Mastrilli, Molitor, and Valko (1985).

Recovery following head injury may continue, but at a decelerated rate, for several years. Thomsen (1984) followed 40 head injured patients first at 4 to 5 months after the injury, then approximately 2.5 years, and finally at 10 to 15 years post-trauma. All had post-traumatic amnesia of at least one month in duration, the majority at least 3 months. Despite a lack of significant improvement in motor functioning between 2.5 and 10 to 15 years post-injury, improvements were noted in independence in activities in daily living (40 percent independent at 2.5 years and 65 percent at 10 to 15 years following their injury). This study shows that some improvment in functional physical abilities can occur long after the injury and initial rehabilitation even in patients whose underlying neuromotor functioning remains unchanged.

Postconcussion Syndrome

The postconcussion syndrome, resulting from apparently minor brain injuries, includes some combination of the following symptoms: dizziness, impaired concentration, fatigue, depression, alcohol intolerance, irritability, headaches, insomnia, and memory deficits. Each of these can cause problems, separately or in combination with other aspects of the syndrome, for the patient's vocational, psychosocial, or educational adjustment (Griffith, 1983).

It is often assumed that recovery from simple concussive injuries will be complete and without residual neurological deficits. However, some of these patients do experience one or more of the postconcussion symptoms. Because these deficits are generally too mild to qualify the patient for therapy services, these patients are forced to cope on their own with the transition to home, work, or community, possibly with the advice of their doctor to "take it easy for awhile." These patients may have a reduced ability to adapt to changed circumstances, which adds to their anxiety and to the postconcussion symptoms. A feeling of being unable to cope further exaggerates the personal disability (Long, Gouvier & Cole, 1984).

Chronic Pain Syndrome

Chronic pain syndrome can occur as a secondary result of head injury and can be as incapacitating to the patient as primary motor deficits. Pain can compound the negative effects of motor deficits on activity and mobility which, in turn, generally increases the pain, thus setting in motion a vicious cycle which interferes with rehabilitative efforts, vocational pursuits, and resumption of previous lifestyle. Since motor deficits are more readily observed and recognized by physicians, insurance representatives, patients, and families, treatment may be concentrated on these symptoms to the exclusion of functionally significant symptoms like chronic pain which are less observable.

Headache or head pain is a common complaint of patients following head injury. Van Zomeren and van den Burg (1985) found that 23 percent of the 57 patients they followed 2 years post-injury suffered from headaches. These headaches are unlike other headaches in duration, frequency, origin, intensity, and distribution. Their effects range from mild occasional inconvenience to a near total incapacitation several days per week. They can be diffuse in orgin and are described with a range of descriptors including "dull ache," "throbbing pain," "knifelike pain," or "burning sensation." Generally, they are aggravated by tension, but often respond to treatments such as relaxation exercises, biofeedback, acupuncture, or medication. Medications that have shown some success with these patients are Elavil, Inderal, Midrin, or Fiorinal.

Chronic neck and back pain, also reported by some patients following head injury, may be secondary to a soft tissue injury which occurred at the time of the initial accident. Patients with neck and back pain can experience feelings such as anxiety, frustration, or guilt which increase muscle tension in these areas. Alternatively, muscle overactivity in the neck and back can result from abnormal patterns of muscle tone, bad posture, or poor body mechanics. Methods of treatment, which may vary with the cause of the pain, include therapeutic modalities, such as heat and cold, traction, postural relaxation exercises, biofeedback, electrical stimulation (Calliet, 1977), and medication.

Decreased Physical Conditioning

Prolonged inactivity during the initial hospitalization and rehabilitation process may lead to excessive muscle weakness and cardiopulmonary deconditioning both of which impede subsequent efforts to restore functioning (Perry, 1983). The incorporation of structured physical activity into the total rehabilitation plan confers several important benefits. Aside from improved general health and the reduced risk of illness that is associated with regular exercise, a properly designed program can provide desired physical outcomes to enhance the patient's ability in vocational or avocational tasks. Because physical strength and cardiopulmonary conditioning have a major influence on the success of community re-entry after severe head injury, extended discussion of exercise programs for these patients has been included at the end of this chapter.

INTERRELATIONS AMONG PHYSICAL, COGNITIVE, AND COMMUNICATIVE FACTORS IN RECOVERY

Motorically impaired head injured patients may have cognitive and communicative problems which interfere with their physical rehabilitation and exaggerate their functional deficits. Many of these patients are unable to monitor their behavior and therefore continue to use habitual nontherapeutic motor patterns. Furthermore, they often do not remember strategies that could faciliate more effective functioning. For example, patients with impaired memory easily forget to lean forward when transferring from a wheelchair. This results in loss of balance and therefore makes the patient unsafe for independent transfers, despite being physically able to manage the task. Attentional and perceptual problems, memory problems, impulsivity, weak problem-solving skills, weak self-awareness and self-appraisal of deficits, and catastrophic reactions to stressful situations, separately or in combination, exaggerate physical deficits.

Conversely, motor impairments can exaggerate cognitive weakness. For example, patients with limited attentional "space" (restricted working memory) are additionally impaired if they are forced to dedicate part of those limited attentional resources to maintaining their balance, producing fine motor acts, or remembering strategies for normalizing muscle tone. This is illustrated by the head injured patient who was able to understand and use fairly complex language structures when the demands on his motor system were minimal, but who produced at best telegraphic language when using a motorically demanding communication device.

Communicative functioning is dependent on both cognitive and motor recovery. Neuromuscular involvement of the speech mechanism (dysarthria) or inability to sequence oral movements for intelligible speech (apraxia) can result in the need to acquire another means of communication. Gross and fine motor problems as well as depressed cognitive functioning may severely restrict the domain of communicative options that are open. Perceptual and learning impairments may prevent the patient from acquiring a communicative system that is motorically feasible. Patients with limited self-awareness and impaired self-monitoring may not recognize the need to communicate more effectively. J.P., a head injured patient who was unable to talk, illustrates several of these problems. She attempted to write as an alternative to speaking; however her writing was illegible. Despite repeated demonstrations that her writing could not be read, even by herself, she refused to try a keyboard.

Communication impairments may, in turn, exaggerate the effects of motor or cognitive deficits. For example, individuals with weak communication skills are deprived of many of the most effective strategies for compensating for physical or cognitive deficits. They may be unable to ask for help or give instructions to others who may assist them, both effective strategies to compensate for their difficulties. In addition, communication breakdowns may cause severe stress which can increase abnormal muscle tone and precipitate further deterioration of already weak cognitive skills.

Although these examples do not exhaust the many interrelationships among motor, cognitive, and communicative deficits, the clinical implication should be apparent. These problems do not exist in isolation. Programs of physical rehabilitation, whether focused on neuromuscular re-education or on compensation, must be carefully integrated with a coherent package of rehabilitation services that addresses the needs of the total person.

INTERRELATIONSHIPS BETWEEN PSYCHOSOCIAL FACTORS AND PHYSICAL RECOVERY

In Chapter 1, Prigatano emphasizes his belief, based on empirical research as well as clinical experience, that personality and psychosocial variables are often the strongest predictors of successful community re-entry. These variables include the patient's motivation, attitude, level of initiation or inhibition, self-concept and self-awareness, as well as personal characteristics like cooperativeness and responsibility. These factors not only influence the ability to obtain and maintain employment, but also affect the therapy process. It has been our experience in physical rehabilitation that those patients with a reasonably accurate self-appraisal of their deficits, achievable goals, and a positive and realistic attitude toward therapy and compensatory devices have the best chance of achieving their potential. A positive attitude toward rehabilitation among family and community members also contributes to this achievement.

Initiation problems, typically associated with damage to the frontal lobes which are especially vulnerable in closed head injury (see Chapter 1), confound intervention for physical deficits and functional independence. The patient may simply fail to initiate movement or activity without physical prompting or verbal cuing. For example, we have worked with patients who were able to feed themselves, but remained inactive until a staff member physically prompted the movement of the spoon toward the mouth. Other patients, who have the linguistic and motor ability to use a communication device and who do use it functionally in a highly structured therapy context, do not attempt to use the device in natural settings, even to express basic needs, without consistent cues.

Head injured patients often demonstrate decreased *inhibition* and *impaired judgment* which result in inappropriate behaviors (see Chapter 1). The patient may therefore be unsafe in using available motor skills unless closely supervised. For example, patients who use an electric wheelchair may endanger themselves or others by maneuvering into traffic on a busy street or by running into other people when angry with them. Patients who are otherwise good candidates for a sophisticated computerized communication device may not be given the device because of legitimate fears that they will use it inappropriately, lose it, or damage it. The complicating effects of impaired judgment on the use of communication devices are illustrated by the head injured young man who repeatedly hit keys on the device that aborted the program, rendering the device unusable until the program was reloaded by a staff person. This pattern of behavior dramatically reduced the functionality of the communication system.

Following a head injury, a patient's *self-concept* is often based on pre-traumatic ideas and abilities. Patients may have decreased awareness of their current condition, rooted in specific damage to the brain (see Chapter 1). Alternatively, they may be emotionally unable to accept the loss that the injury has caused. In either case, the predictable result is resistance to essential therapy activities and to use of assistive or compensatory devices. In physical rehabilitation, it is often necessary to work toward personally meaningful goals (e.g., walking) by beginning with developmentally early activities (e.g., rolling) in order to develop the musculature needed for later ambulation. The patient's combination of weak self-awareness of deficits and concrete thinking, which does not support an understanding of complex relations between current activities and ultimate goals, presents therapists with a fundamental challenge. Furthermore, family members often reinforce the patient's resistance and focus only on what they wish their loved one could do rather than on the events that are necessary to accomplish this goal. Creativity, patience, and skillful communication are required to ensure the patient's acceptance of short-term therapy objectives. Clear and simple explanations of the rationale for treatment activities may need to be offered repeatedly. Written instructions, written and illustrated training materials, and frequent contact with family members are extremely valuable. (Issues in family training are further discussed in Chapter 4.)

Acceptance of equipment and compensatory devices is strongly influenced by patients' and family members' attitudes toward "gadgets." Many people have had little or no experience with such things and are suspicious of and intimidated by such everyday products as remote controls for the television and home computers. Others are comfortable with such devices and may even be intrigued by rehabilitation technology. Preconceived notions about a specific apparatus that is used by handicapped people may also color decisions. Furthermore, initial failure and frustration with a device, or an awareness of other patients' lack of success, can easily make a patient unwilling to try equipment like electronic wheelchairs, communication devices, or environmental controls. Strong aesthetic feelings about devices may have the same effect. Some have stated that they will use an electric wheelchair only if it is small and looks like a go cart, braces only if their pants cover them, and a communication device only if it looks like a calculator and does not sound like a robot. Some patients and families feel that devices accentuate rather than reduce the handicapping condition. For example, the inhibitory casts used to hold feet in a position to make standing possible may be seen by family as too heavy and as the cause of an awkward gait rather than a factor in the resolution of the motor problem. Families may resist a communication device because of the natural assumption that having a way to communicate that is easier than talking will interfere with the recovery of speech. In the studies that Silverman (1980) reviewed, augmentative communication strategies appeared to enhance the potential for speech or leave speech unaffected. Augmentative intervention did not interfere with speech development or reacquisition.

These powerful attitudinal factors are illustrated by a head injured adolescent who was unable to walk or talk, but refused to use either an electric wheelchair or a communication device with speech output since, in her view, they were unacceptable substitutes for abilities which she felt she would soon reacquire. The only compensatory equipment that she agreed to use was an electric typewriter, since she had typed prior to her injury and therefore did not see the typewriter as a substitute for speech.

Attitudes toward independence play a particularly strong role in facilitating or inhibiting the rehabilitation process. The goal of therapy at this stage is to promote community re-entry at the highest level possible by helping the patient to become increasingly independent. However, independence carries with it the risk of failure or at least temporary setbacks and frustrations. Often it is very difficult for family members to wait patiently while the patient struggles to grasp a spoon and orient it properly for eating. Because of their strong temptation to help, they fail to recognize that they are doing the work, not the patient. Grasping the spoon may be the patient's first step toward independence and the family member's assistance may only increase the period of dependence. Similarly, family members, friends, and fellow workers often guess at messages rather than let the patient struggle with a device or communication board to communicate independently his or her thoughts and intentions.

REHABILITATION OF PHYSICAL DEFICITS

Techniques of physical rehabilitation for head injured individuals generally focus on either remediation of motor deficits deficits or compensation for motor skills not yet recovered or permanently lost. Therapeutic techniques that aim at regaining abilities in all areas of motor functioning are an important part of rehabilitation following head injury. However, these techniques are probably familiar to most speech-language pathologists, physical therapists, and occupational therapists working in the field of rehabilitation and have been described in excellent textbooks on the subject. Therefore, therapeutic approaches to restoration of motor function will be discussed only briefly in this chapter, with references to other sources.

The two prominent themes of this chapter — compensatory techniques and devices that can substitute for delayed or absent motor skills, and cardiovascular conditioning and training to increase endurance, strength, and flexibility — were selected because of their capacity to increase the individual's potential for vocational and avocational activities and for independent living. It should be stressed that therapy to regain motor skills generally continues during the time that compensatory techniques and devices are explored and trained, and during the conditioning program. It is the combination of these three dimensions of physical rehabilitation that most effectively promotes community re-entry. In each of these areas of physical rehabilitation, we will discuss evaluation and treatment methods as well as the need for follow-up when the individual returns to home, work, and the community.

Therapeutic Approaches to the Restoration of Motor Skills

There is a substantial literature on treatment approaches to neuromuscular disorders associated with stroke, cerebral palsy, and other causes of motor dysfunction. Since the gross motor, fine motor, and motor speech deficits associated with closed head injury, considered in isolation from cognitive and psychosocial concommitants, resemble motor deficits seen in other central nervous system disorders, this literature is relevant to head injury rehabilitation. Pharmacologic intervention, bracing, neurodevelopmental treatment, and other intervention strategies have all been used successfully with selected individuals recovering from head injury.

Evaluation

Evaluation includes both discovering which motor and cognitive skills remain after head injury and which are impaired and also selecting intervention techniques and an appropriate sequence of treatment objectives by means of exploratory diagnostic therapy. Finally, ongoing monitoring of the patient's response to treatment is used to refine the program and ensure that intervention keeps pace with the patient's progress.

Evaluation of motor skills includes assessment of gross motor, fine motor, and oral motor skills. In the area of gross and fine motor skills, clinicians should assess range of motion, sensation, muscle strength, flexibility, postural tone, active movement, coordination, and balance. The ability to control the muscles of the oral, respiratory, and phonatory mechanisms in a coordinated fashion (as is needed for speaking) should also be evaluated. Functional use of available motor skills should also be determined, including assessment of activities of daily living or self-help skills such as dressing, bathing, or feeding. Functional assessment is ideally performed in a natural setting.

Treatment

Therapeutic approaches such as neurodevelopmental treatment (Bobath, 1978), proprioceptive neuromuscular facilitation (Knott & Voss, 1968), neurorehabilitation techniques (Farber, 1982; Rood, 1962; Umphred, 1983), and sensory integration (Ayres, 1972) all are based on the notion that the technique will facilitate the recovery of normal or more normal gross motor, fine motor, and motor speech function. It has been our experience that all of these techniques have value in treating patients with head injuries, assuming wise matching of patient, deficit, therapist, and technique. Adjuncts to therapy such as serial and bivalve casting (Booth, Doyle & Montgomery, 1983), splinting and bracing, biofeedback (Basmajian, 1981), and functional electrical stimulation (Baker, Parker & Sanderson, 1983) have also been effective with this population. Pharmacological regimes (e.g., adminstration of Baclofen, Dantrolene, or Valium to reduce spasticity) may be established in the early stages of rehabilitation. Anti-spasticity medication needs to be carefully monitored in terms of its effects on the patient and also the results of new research (Young & Delwaide, 1981a,b).

Follow-up and Maintenance

It is an unjustified, but all-too-common practice to terminate physical rehabilitation after a short period of plateau or after discharge from inpatient rehabilitation. As mentioned earlier in this chapter, the period of spontaneous recovery from head injury is often very long and recovery is frequently characterized by periods of plateau followed by periods of improvement. Furthermore, changes in the patient's cognitive or psychosocial functioning may open intervention possibilities which, prior to those changes, were not available, and changes in environmental demands may require a focus on new skills or compensations. Finally, in the absence of maintenance therapy, motor skills and corresponding functional abilities may be lost, thereby decreasing vocational or community independence. For these reasons, a plan for maintaining skills and monitoring the patient's status needs to be established at the time of discharge from the medical rehabilitation facility. This plan may include treatment in the home or self-programming as well as follow-up visits to appropriate professionals. New research or newly developed techniques may make improvements possible for patients who had previously reached their highest level of motor functioning.

Patients who are long-term post head injury and who have not received intervention for a period of years may benefit from renewed intervention to retrieve lost or neglected skills and to address previously untreated problems. For example, a patient whose head injury had occurred 6 years earlier and whose residual deficits included severe left hemiplegia gained improved ankle stability and an active gross grasp and release with the reinitiation of therapy. This enabled her to stand and carry out homemaking tasks (e.g., washing dishes) with both hands. Sometimes motor skills that are initially perceived to be insignificant, such as rolling over in bed, achieve a more elevated status after the patient has experienced the frustrations of disability and has consequently come to set more realistic goals. Other patients neglect their home exercise program and lose important functional abilities such as independent transfers. Furthermore, new equipment or techniques which could benefit the patient may have been developed since active treatment was terminated. There are, therefore, many considerations that support long-term follow-up for motorically impaired individuals after head injury.

Compensatory Devices and Techniques

For many severely head injured individuals, the recovery of functional skills occurs over a prolonged period. During that period it may be possible to perform the functions subserved by that skill through the use of adapted equipment or compensatory devices. Other patients may never recover lost skills and therefore may require permanent use of compensatory devices. For example, an individual unable to walk can achieve independent mobility with a power wheelchair; those unable to speak may be able to sign, point to messages on a communication board, or "talk" by means of an electronic communication device.

Available Aids

MOBILITY AIDS. For individuals who are unable to walk or self-propel efficiently in a standard wheelchair, power wheelchairs provide independent mobility. The many types of power wheelchairs that have been designed to meet individual needs can be divided into three major categories. The more familiar power chair has a built-in power drive system. Also available are adaptable add-on power units which can convert a manual wheelchair into a power chair. Finally, there are battery-powered 3-wheel carts that are easier to maneuver and lighter weight when dismantled (for easier transport of the chair) than standard power wheelchairs.

All three power mobility systems are adjustable and have a wide variety of options that allow them to be individualized for a particular user. To achieve the best "fit" for an individual, therapists must be aware of the options that are available. Rather than describe specific systems, we have prepared a table (Table 2–2) that lists characteristics of chairs and the needs they were intended to accommodate. None of the systems has available all of the options listed in the table. The characteristics of power chairs are divided into five categories: performance, switches, positioning, durability, and miscellaneous considerations.

COMMUNICATION AIDS. Individuals who are unable to speak intelligibly, may, nevertheless, be able to communicate by means of some form of augmentative communication. "Augmentative communication" refers to methods of communicating that supplement or substitute for absent or unintelligible speech. This includes expressive options that are as familiar as writing, typing, and gesturing and as sophisicated as computer-based speech output devices activated by eye movements.

Table 2–2. Power Mobility

Chair Characteristics	Patient Needs/Problems
Performance	
1. Variable Speeds: Low/medium/high with adustability within each range.	Patients need to practice at slower speeds initially; speed needs vary according to terrain and environment.
2. Acceleration/Deceleration Control: This allows the chair to gradually reach its selected speed and gradually come to a stop.	Patients who startle easily need a slower rate of acceleration/deceleration. This makes the chair start and stop more smoothly.
3. Turning: a. Speed b. Radius c. Acceleration/deceleration	Patients with abnormal movement patterns and poor control of the joy-stick benefit from slower speeds in turns and in acceleration/deceleration into and out of the turn.
4. Tremor Dampening: The adjustability delay between the activation of a switch and the movement of the wheelchair allows for accidental switch activation.	This is for patients with abnormal movement patterns or extraneous movements. The chair can be finely adjusted to the user.
5. Trim Forward/Reverse: This allows for balancing of the motors for straight line travel.	This is advantageous for all users so that if the motors are not equal in charge, the chair does not pull to the stronger side.
6. Automatic Course Correction: This allows for the traversing of rough terrain without continuously adjusting the controls.	For the patient with good control only on level terrain, this makes possible control on rough terrain.
7. Self-Aligning Casters: The front casters align them-selves facing straight ahead when stopped.	Without this feature, when patients driving chairs at lower speeds stop the casters turn in different directions making starting again difficult because the tires are facing the wrong direction.

(continued)

Table 2–2 (*continued*)

8. Freewheeling: This makes the chair easy to push when the motors are disengaged.	This is for patients who will be in situations in which caretakers, attendants, or family will need to push the electric chair some of the time.
9. Braking System: A dual or two-stage system stops the chair completely, even on an incline.	This is a safety feature for all users, especially those operating chairs on an uneven surface.
Switches	
1. Latching Mode: This gives continuous operation with only a momentary activation of a switch. The timing can be adjusted.	This is for patients who are unable to maintain pressure on the switch or who make frequent starts and stops to turn.
2. Momentary Mode: The chair is operated only when the switch is held in an activating position.	This is for patients with good motor control who need to operate the switch smoothly and quickly.
3. Proportional Drive: The speed of the chair is directly related to the amount of excursion of the joystick.	This is for patients with good motor control who can provide pressure changes on the switch needed for slower or faster driving.
4. Nonproportional Drive: Regardless of the force on the joystick, the speed remains the same.	This is for patients who are unable to grade changes of pressure on the joy-stick for speed control.
5. Ability to Accept Other Interfaces: Some power chairs accept a variety of interfaces without changes in existing circuitry.	This is for patients with degenerative, regressive, or changing symptomatology who might later need access to interfaces other than a joystick control.
6. Inductive Joysticks: This joystick uses a magnetic field rather than a mechanical (contact) as in earlier joysticks.	This is for patients who, because of hand positioning, place greatest force in one direction in a mechanical ballbearing joystick creating stress and the need for frequent replacement of the joystick.

Chair Characteristics	Patients Needs/Problems
7. Placement of Control Switch, Speed Control, On/Off Switch: Some chairs offer options in placement of the control switches, the speed control, and the on/off switch on either the right or left side of the chair.	This is for patients who need to reach the control switch, speed control, and on/off switch for complete independence. Because of judgment problems, some patients may be unsafe with access to the on/off switch or speed control.
Positioning	
1. Optional Seating Packages: These range from the traditional sling seat to modular systems.	Alternative seating is useful for patients who require modifications such as firmer cushions, slightly reclined backs, or cushioning for pressure relief.
2. Manual or Electric Recliner: The back of the chair can be moved from a vertical to a horizontal positon.	This is for patients who, because of size or muscle loss, need frequent changes of positon for pressure relief or who, for medical reasons, need to be reclined; this feature can be controlled by the patient if electric.
Durability	
1. Direct Drive Motors: This eliminates the need for drive belts.	For all users, this eliminates costly replacement of belts.
2. Friction Drive System: This uses drive belts on motors.	This is for patients who are able to replace drive belts as needed.
3. Warranty: Warranties on the main frame vary from six months to the chair's lifetime. (Altering the chair's switching mechanism may negate the warranty contract.)	An extended warranty is important for all users.

(continued)

Table 2-2 (*continued*)

Durability *(continued)*	
4. Repair Record: Some chairs have an established history of reliability and low maintenance costs.	The patient should ask the dealer about the chair's repair record.
Miscellaneous Considerations	
1. Quad Ease Engagement Lever: This requires 20% force to engage or release the drive belts.	This is for patients with limited strength who need independence in engaging and disengaging the drive belts to the motors.
2. Carpet Switch: This gives better traction on carpet.	This is for patients who get stuck in deep pile carpet.
3. Battery Level Indicator Light: This indicates when the battery is low.	It is helpful to the user to know when the battery needs to be recharged.
4. Horn: This is similar to an automobile's horn.	A horn is useful to sound an alarm or gain attention.
5. Tires: Tires can be pneumatic, semi-pneumatic, or solid.	Pneumatic tires are ideal for patients who need a smooth ride on a variety of terrain; however, they require regular maintenance.
6. Portability: Some chairs dismantle or fold to fit in the trunk of a car.	This is very useful if the cost of a lift van is prohibitive.

Sign language and other gestural systems, such as Amerind developed by Skelly (Skelly & Schinsky, 1979), have been successfully used by individuals unable to speak intelligibly. Gestural methods, often referred to as unaided techniques, are convenient because they do not require the assistance of a device; however, the family, friends, and others communicating with the individual must be trained in the system. A second significant disadvantage of sign language for head injured patients is that they are asked to learn an essentially new system of communication including new types of symbols at a time when their learning efficiency may be severely depressed.

Communication aids may take the form of a communication board or book with letters, words, symbols, or pictures to which the individual points to convey a message. Although simple communication boards have been used for years, it has only been recently that more complex boards, displaying the potential for more complete messages, have been developed (McDonald & Schultz, 1973; Vicker, 1974). Basic letter or word boards, while not novel or technologically sophisticated, hold a large number of advantages for head injured patients. They are easy to make and replace; they are inexpensive; they are flexible, allowing for a systematic progression from simple to complex as the patient recovers perceptual, cognitive, and linguistic skills; and they embody a system of communication which is generally easy for communication partners to understand and use.

For patients with severe upper extremity involvement, Eichler and Neale (1978) developed an eye "pointing" device, called an ETRAN, which many of these patients can use. It consists of a clear plastic display with letters or other communications on the perimeter. The receiver of the message sits opposite the sender, separated by the ETRAN board. The receiver then determines the message by watching the eye movements of the sender. Ten Kate, Duyvis, and Le Poole (1984) made it possible to more easily interpret eye movements by adding prisms/mirrors to the communication display.

In recent years, electronic devices have been developed which compensate for poor gross and fine motor skills. The devices require that the patient have a consistent movement of some part of the body to gain access to the system. Movements can vary from touch with a body part to eye movement to a controlled breathstream or voice. Electronic communication aids are available which produce a variety of different signals, including light-indicated, graphic, printed, or electronically spoken messages. Since new communication aids or devices are being developed with regularity, the characteristics of individual aids will not be covered in this chapter. Kraat and Sitver-Kogut (1985) created a chart that listed the commercial devices available at that time and the characteristics of each. The Trace Research and Development Center on Communication, Control and Computer Access for Handicapped Individuals, affiliated with the University of Wisconsin-Madison, regularly provides information about new devices.

The form of augmentative communication that is selected for a patient depends on the patient's remaining abilities (motor, perceptual, cognitive, linguistic, academic, and psychosocial) following head injury. The choice also depends on the patient's current and projected communication needs, communicative style and preferences, and the availability of resources. These resources must include both devices and the personnel to provide training in the use of the device as an interaction tool. Professionals providing this training must be aware of both the characteristics of individual communication devices and the demands they place on users and their communication partners. Table 2–3 presents an overview of the characteristics of augmentative communication aids or devices and the relationship of these characteristics to user skills and listener requirements.

ENVIRONMENTAL CONTROL. An environmental control system gives individuals with physical disabilities independent control over their immediate surroundings (Symington, Batelaan, O'Shea & White, 1980), thereby promoting independence at home, at school, and/or in the work place. Environmental aids range from low cost adaptive equipment like gooseneck phone holders to sophisticated control systems for a large number of devices. Patients who are motorically impaired following head injury are often able to use adaptive equipment that was developed for patients with other central nervous system disorders, or, in some cases, for the general public. The development of environmental controls for use by the general public has increased alternatives for disabled individuals and has significantly decreased the cost of environmental controls. Commercially available items like "touch on" lights, speaker phones, and remote control televisions are often sufficient to allow independence. Controller module systems developed for public use have been modified with switch interfaces giving access to those unable to activate the small buttons on the control box. Other devices, such as page turners, have been specifically developed for disabled individuals. Future advances in technology and robotics will greatly influence the type and sophistication of environmental controls available.

Almost any electronic or battery-operated device can be modified for switch activiation. Those individuals who have sufficient mobility to reach the device may be able to access it with simple adaptive equipment like door knob extenders or push-type light switches. Those who have limited mobility will need a remote device or a controller module system which transmits commands over house wiring. Some environmental controls are specific to a single device whereas others can be used to access many devices. Table 2–4 lists selected environmental aids which may be used by individuals with physical disabilities for increased independence. Detailed information on this topic is presented in Enders (1984) and Symington et al. (1980).

Table 2–3. Augmentative Communication Device Characteristics

Device Options	User Demands
Access Mechanism	
1. The switching system is built into the device itself and can be accessed through visual movements, sound, or body movements.	The user must be able to move his/her eyes, produce sounds, or move some other part of the body in a way that activates the switch which is standard equipment on the device.
2. The device is activated by an external switch which can be selected to match the user's skills.	The switch selected for use with the device must be compatible with the device and with the user's skills.
Input Message Storage/Display	
1. A fixed set of symbols, words, or letters (representing the exact messages) are stored on the switches or the surface of the device.	The user must be able to read or remember the locations of the symbols, words, or letters that are stored on the device, or it must be possible to change the locations or symbols to meet the user's demands.
2. A fixed set of symbols, words, or letters (representing a code rather than the exact message) are stored on the surface of the device.	The user must be able to remember what messages the codes represent or read a directory listing the codes and the corresponding messages.
3. Auditory signals or spoken messages are repeated by the device in a fixed sequence until one is selected by the user.	The user must be able to hear and understand the auditory signal or spoken message. (Many people have difficulty understanding electronically produced speech.)
4. A computer monitor displays a fixed or variable set of words, letters, or symbols.	The user must be able to see and read the display in the situations where communication will take place. (Bright lights often obscure the message and some display characters are hard to read.)
5. Lights are mounted on the device on or near the messages, or codes, or symbols.	The user must have the visual-perceptual and cognitive skills to associate a light going on with the appropriate message.

(continued)

Table 2-3 (*continued*)

Device Output	
1. A light turns on or is left on beside the designated message to be read by the "listener."	The user must realize that the "listener" needs to be close enough to read the message and must wait until the listener has completed receiving the message before continuing.
2. Electronically produced or reproduced speech "says" the message.	The user and listener must understand the device's speech.
3. The message is displayed on a screen.	The user must have adequate reading skills and judgment to tell if the "listener" can understand printed matter.
4. The message is printed on paper.	The user must have adequate reading skills and judgment to tell if the "listener" can understand printed matter.
Process of Selecting	
1. With *direct selection,* the user directly indicates the desired message for output (e.g., the user touches the switch marked hat and the device says "hat").	The user must be motorically, visually, and cognitively able to handle the number, size, and arrangement of the array on the device.
2. *Scanning* is a method that presents messages in a sequence and the user indicates when the desired message is indicated in the sequence.	The user must understand the scanning process, have the ability to wait until the desired item is indicated, and activate the switch before the scan continues.
3. *Encoding* is a method of selecting a large number of messages using a smaller set of symbols in sequence. Messages are stored in the device by code (e.g., Morse code, a sequence of letters, numbers, or symbols) that represent an entire message and are accessed using that code. Direct selection or scanning are used to input the code.	The user must be able to remember codes or look them up in a directory. Many devices permit the users to program their own codes and messages into the device. The user or someone in the environment must know how to enter new codes and messages.

INPUT OPTIONS. A switch or interface is the link through which the individual controls electronic equipment thereby gaining access to aids for mobility, communication, and control over the environment. One switch or several switches may be needed to control the chosen equipment. From a clinical perspective, the primary differences among switches are in the means of activation. For example, some are triggered

Table 2–4. Environmental Control Options

Task or Device	Environmental Control	Patient Characteristics
Feeding	*Electronic Feeders:* Generally have one switch which rotates the plate and one that moves the spoon to scoop food from the plate and raise the spoon to a predetermined level.	Patient unable to self-feed, but has adequate oral motor skills to eat food brought to the mouth; must have fair to good head control.
Telephone	*Goose Neck Phone Holder:* Holds telephone receiver in space; the patient uses a switch or lever to control access to phone lines; can also use commerically available speaker phones.	Patient unable to raise the telephone receiver or to hold it at an adequate height.
	Enlarged Pushbutton Phones: Commercially available.	Patient unable to use standard dial or pushbutton phones due to decreased fine motor control.
	Automatic Dialers: Commercially available; have a memory which stores frequently used numbers which can be accessed by pushing one or two buttons.	Patient has decreased endurance, or motor control which decreases with successive attempts.
	Telephone Command Controller Modules: Makes possible answering the phone and dialing the phone from a dual switch.	Patient able to access/control two switches.
Television	*Remote Control:* Commercially available.	Patient unable to maneuver to or reach TV switch/dials; able to use small pushbutton switches.
Lights	*"Touch-on" lamps:* Commercially available.	Patient unable to turn on a lamp but has gross movement to touch lamp.
	Remote Control or Electronic Control Module: Can be used with any electric appliances.	Patient unable to maneuver to the lamp or light switch.

(continued)

Table 2–4 (*continued*)

Tape Recorder	*Voice Activated:* Control of on/off.	Patient unable to access a tape recorder via switch, but able to speak.
	Remote Control: Control of on/off.	Patient able to access a single switch.
Turning Pages in Book or Magazine	*Electronic Page Turners:* Turn the page of a book which has been placed in a book holder. Some turn pages only in one direction while others in both directions. Accessed via multiple switch or a single switch scan system.	Patient unable to turn pages in a book or magazine.
Multiple Appliances	*BSR X-10 Standard:* Several models available to control up to 32 appliances; either a master control which must be plugged in or ultrasonic remote; requires appliance, lamp, or wall switch modules.	Patient needs access to multiple lamps or appliances; able to use small pushbutton.
	Modified BSR: Functions as above but modified for switch access.	Patient unable to access standard BSR unit.
	Computer Environmental Controls: Use computer to access BSR.	Patient using computer keyboard.
Misc. Items	Controls available for radio, electric bed, power drapery, electronic lifts, call buttons, intercoms, device monitors.	

by moving a lever through space, some by touching a surface, some by breaking a light beam, and some by vocalizing or making some other noise. Sensory feedback to the user is provided by switch activation. Feedback may be auditory (e.g., a light), or somatosensory including tactile kinesthetic and proprioceptive feedback (e.g., a feeling of one's hand touching the switch and moving it). Each of these characteristics may be essential to the success or failure of the individual's ability to use a device. For example, feedback in the form of a relatively quiet click may cause some patients to startle but for other patients be insufficient to indicate that the device has been activated.

Controls may be classified by the number of independent signals that are available for use (i.e., "flexibility" of the control). Controls range from single switches to small switch arrays (e.g., joystick or arm slot control) to keyboards of varying sizes (Williams, Csongradi & LeBlanc, 1982). Characteristics of switches and controls have been described in several sources, including *A Guide to Controls* (Williams et al., 1982) and the *Technology for Independent Living Sourcebook* (Enders, 1984). Flexibility, activation, and feedback are all important features for consideration in choosing a switch. Other variables include size, resolution, durability, cosmetic features, and comfort. Table 2-5 provides an overview of switch characteristics and the skills required of users.

Compatibility of Devices

When selecting electronic devices and other adaptive equipment for a patient, their compatibility must be considered. Some patients may require specialized seating equipment, power mobility, an augmentative communication device, computer access, and environmental controls. The need for interdisciplinary team interaction is necessary to avoid fragmentation and the purchase of expensive pieces of equipment that are not compatible with each other. Some systems are designed so that they are readily compatible with other devices. Using an integrated system, one switch or switch array may be used to access several devices. The Lainey System (University of Tennessee Rehabilitation Engineering Program, Memphis, TN) is an example of an integrated system in which power mobility, communication devices, and computer access are controlled by means of an optical sensor. The Fortress electric wheelchair (Fortress Scientific, Downsview, Ontario, Canada), also an integrated system, has built-in compatibility with environmental controls and tape recorder use. The Du-it control module (Du-it Control Systems Group, Inc., Shreve, Ohio) attaches to an electric wheelchair and enables alternative switch access and compatibility with augmentative communication devices and environmental controls. There are two ways in which devices can be compatible with one another. On the one hand, two or more devices may be integrated electronically. On the other hand, devices may be configured in such a way that they can be used together although they are each independent electronic systems. Figure 2-1 shows a young woman with severe neuromuscular impairment positioned in a power wheelchair which accommodates an environmental control unit and a communication device (each independent systems).

Table 2–5. Device Activation

Access Mechanisms	Switch Characteristics	User Skills Required
Visual/Oculomotor	1. A light beam is moved across the chosen message.	User must be able to move the light beam.
	2. The switch detects the located light on a device.	User must be able to move the switch into alignment with the device light.
	3. The device lens detects the reflected light on the eye itself.	User must be able to move at least one eye steadily.
	4. The "listener" reads eye gaze.	User must be able to fixate on one item long enough for the "listener" to read the selected item.
Auditory/Sounds	1. The switch detects the movements created by voicing.	The user must be able to produce voice on demand and control unwanted voicing.
	2. The switch detects movements made by pounding or the sounds the user creates.	The user must have sufficient motor control to pound or make other sounds only when wishing to activate the switch. (Random movements can be controlled.)
	3. The device recognizes spoken utterances the user has programmed into it.	The user must be able to repeat words (whether understandable or not) the same way each time so the computer recognizes them.
General Movement	1. The switch is moved through a space, its angle is changed, it is activated by the presence of moisture, or the beam is broken.	The user must be able to make one consistent movement with some part of the body, avoiding accidental activations.
	2. A series of switches are activated.	The user must be able to activate only one switch at a time, given the space between the two switches.

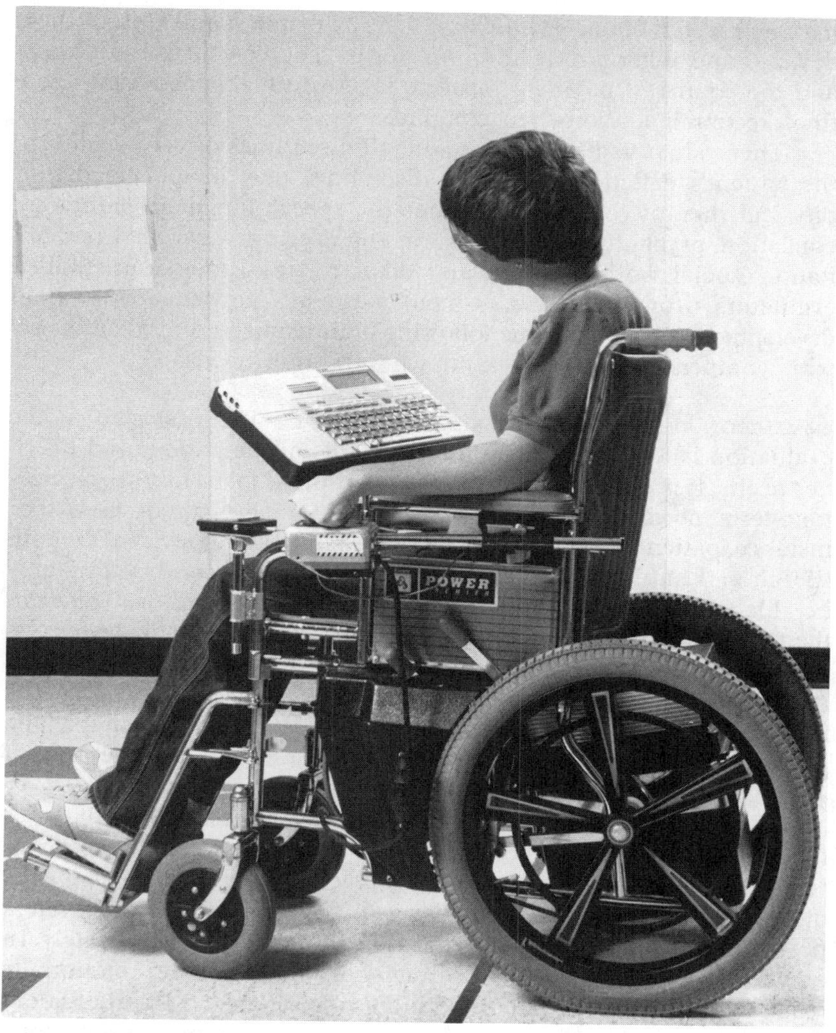

Figure 2–1. A woman following head injury using a power wheelchair, electronic communication device, and a remote control switch for a tape recorder.

Evaluation for Compensatory Devices

The evaluation includes determining the patient's existing skills and needs, matching these skills to the characteristics of potential devices, gaining at least provisional acceptance of the devices from the patient, assessing the environment in which they will be used, making recommendations for trial therapy or for acquisition of these devices, and determining training needs. The cost of these devices and the source of payment must be taken into consideration before final recommendations are complete.

The evaluators need to represent all disciplines directly related to the patient's deficit areas. These disciplines may include medicine, physical therapy, occupational therapy, speech-language pathology, education, psychology, rehabilitation engineering, vocational rehabilitation, social work, nursing, and other related professions. Skilled evaluators bring to the assessment a broad knowledge of normal development and of outcome following brain damage, and a familiarity with compensatory devices and with training needs.

EVALUATION OF THE PATIENT'S SKILLS AND NEEDS. The first step in the evaluation is to determine the *existing* skills of the patient and his or her needs. It is easy to yield to the temptation to focus on the patient's long-term needs rather than on what he or she can do now. For instance, patients who will require a communication device with both speech and hard copy output when they return to a work setting may be able to start with a simple call button to gain attention. They can then proceed in small steps toward more sophisticated devices as their motor, cognitive, and communication skills improve. Looking at immediate and long-term needs is a dynamic process that changes as the patient changes. A technological device can, for example, be introduced early into the rehabilitation process with the intention of adding or subtracting components as the patient changes.

Evaluating existing skills includes (a) assessing the patient's motor, cognitive, academic, emotional, communicative, and psychosocial skills and (b) determining how each skill area impacts on the others. For example, an individual with the motor skills to operate a power wheelchair may not have adequate judgment to use it safely. In other cases, patients or family members may not be emotionally ready at a given stage of rehabilitation to consider compensatory devices because they feel that such devices are only used when deficits are permanent. The true value of a team working together in an evaluation is that all team members have access to necessary information from the other disciplines in order to make their individual decisions functional. The physical therapist, for example, needs the psychologist's insight regarding the patient's potential for power mobility, while the psychologist or social worker can begin to help patient and family accept the role that adaptive equipment and devices can play in promoting independence.

Appendix 2–1 includes three screening forms (Communication; Seating and Mobility; and Visual Motor Functioning) used by the interdisciplinary Rehabilitation Technology Evaluation Team at The Rehabilitation Institute of Pittsburgh. These forms illustrate the parameters of assessment that we have found to be particularly important. The screening instruments are in the form of checklists that can be completed quickly with a patient, family member, or peer and provide information regarding the patient's functioning level in that area and the needs that must be addressed by the technology team. This information allows the team to create a plan of action for evalution, to assemble the devices needed for trial use, and to obtain further diagnostic information either through referral to another discipline or through contact with therapists previously involved with the patient.

THE NEED FOR PROPER SEATING AND POSITIONING. Prior to matching the patient's skills to potential devices, seating and positioning need to be addressed. Proper seating and positioning are the basis for the controlled movements needed to operate switches or devices. Because of changes in posture or because the patient's current equipment is inappropriate, the focus of this assessment is often *repositioning.* Pelvic stability is of primary importance, with a seat belt used to maintain this pelvic position. Second, we attend to the support and midline orientation of the trunk and head. Fixed deformities of the patient must be accommodated with positioning equipment with even weight distribution to limit pressure areas (Bergen & Colangelo, 1985). With proper positioning, the patient gains improved proximal stability and support, thereby promoting greater control over the extremities, which in turn makes possible more effective use of devices. Further adaptations to inhibit abnormal postural tone or to support weak extremities may be required. In addition, the therapist should ensure that neither the position of the patient nor his or her means of activating the switch will lead to further deformity.

The importance of seating and positioning is illustrated by a 43 year old head injured woman who was 13 years post-trauma. She had a regular adult wheelchair with a back insert and lateral supports. Unfortunately, in the past few years she had lost trunk and head control and had a fixed scoliosis and pelvic obliquity. In her chair, she fell forward and to the right and rested her head on her chest, tilted to the right. She required modification of her seating cushion to accommodate the pelvic obliquity and a three-point lateral support and back insert with cushioning to accommodate her scoliosis. She also needed a head support extending further on the right side than on the left. In addition, the seating in her chair was slightly reclined to align her head, trunk, and pelvis and to decrease her forward head and trunk position. This made her more available for communication and other activities vital to community re-entry.

MATCHING PATIENT CHARACTERISTICS TO DEVICE CHARACTERISTICS. Following evaluation of the patient's existing skills and determination of his or her needs (e.g., power mobility for indoor and outdoor use or a communication device with printed output for school), the team attempts to match the skills and needs to a device Unfortunately, the goal, which is to find the simplest device which includes all of the desired characteristics, is not always achievable. This is due in part to the fact that devices are not yet available to meet all possible needs and in part to conflicts that may exist within the interdisciplinary team's recommendations. Resolution of the latter problem requires frequent communication among staff and a willingness to negotiate priorities for and with the patient. In addition, the team needs to determine what switches the patient can use, what movement is used for activation, and under what conditions the communication, mobility, or environmental control devices are to be used. The goal, then, is to find the simplest system of devices that meets as many of the patient's needs as can be met and that helps him or her to be as functional and independent as possible in a chosen environment.

Equipped with knowledge of the patient's skills and needs, the evaluator makes a judgment regarding the device or devices that best fit those needs and skills. This judgment must be tested against the reality of the patient's performance in or with the actual equipment. However, since much of this equipment is expensive, to buy or to rent, it is frequently not available for actual trials. Under these circumstances, it is often more economical to construct a mock up of the device and evaluate the patient's performance in the mock up. For example, a power chair can be simulated by adding a switch to the manual chair and then pushing the patient only when the switch is activated, turning in the direction dictated by the patient's switch use. There are also computer programs that simulate interface control of various devices for mobility, communication, and environmental control (e.g., the Single Input Control Assessment developed by the Rehabilitation Engineering Department and Augmentative Communication Services, Ontario Crippled Children's Center, Toronto, Ontario).

The first use of a device may not be a good predictor of future success or failure. Patients often experience one of two opposing reactions. Some individuals are able to perform well beyond the skill levels anticipated by the isolated skill assessment because of the novelty of the device, the motivation that the patient has to succeed with the device, or the attention of evaluators. This may be the maximal performance that the patient achieves on that device. Others are unable to perform as well as predicted by the evaluation results because of their reaction to the stress associated with a new device or with the evaluation situation. For these reasons, repeated trials over multiple sessions or a prolonged period of time are needed to determine ultimate suitability of devices for individual patients.

CONSIDERATIONS FOR POWER MOBILITY. Considerations for power mobility begin with adequate motor skill for operating the controls of the power chair. However, other factors are equally crucial. These include additional physical factors (fatigue, reduced endurance, visual deficits, hearing deficits, startle reactions, tremors, impaired motor planning, and others) as well as cognitive/behavioral factors (selective attention, reasoning, judgment, behavioral self-control). It is necessary to begin by testing the patient's ability to perform simple maneuvers in the chair (e.g., "start," "stop," "drive a straight line down the middle of the hallway," and "right" or "left 90 degrees"). This assessment may be safely carried out during simulated power mobility exercises. Actual use of a power chair is necessary to complete the power mobility evaluation. Obstacle course driving, including weaving among objects and reversing into a small space, should be saved until the patient is more familiar with the operation of the chair or until training sessions are begun. Table 2–2 can be used as a reference in selecting characteristics of power chairs to promote success in operating the chair. If the patient's goal is to be completely independent with the chair, then it is additionally necessary to assess his or her ability to access the on/off switch and the controller as well as ease of transferring in and out of the chair. If the patient needs assistance operating the on/off switch, getting in and out of the chair, or operating the chair safely, then supervised mobility may be the goal. A separate control for attendants may be helpful if assistance is needed in the actual operation of the chair.

CONSIDERATIONS FOR COMMUNICATION AIDS. Evaluation of patients for the use of devices to augment communication is necessarily broad based. Current language levels must be thoroughly evaluated and the communicative demands of home, work, and recreation settings must be determined. For example, patients who are only able to communicate in single words, which are expanded into meaningful and appropriate sentences by family members and friends on the basis of contextual cues, will not benefit from sophisticated communication devices that produce sentence-level communication. For such patients, the device will only produce single words or consistently expand each word into a rote sentence without considering the contextual cues. Nonspeaking patients whose language is intact *will* benefit from such devices, but only if they have some consistent motor movement with which to activate a switch. The evaluator will need to determine each patient's output needs. Some need electronically produced spoken output whereas others need printed output or an indicator such as a light near or on the selected message.

Augmentative systems vary in the learning and processing demands that they place on the user. Systems that require efficient learning, storage, and quick retrieval of new codes may demand too much of the learning and processing skill of head injured patients. Although not invariant, it is common for head injured patients to experience fair recovery of pre-traumatically acquired knowledge and academic and linguistic skills despite severely reduced potential for new learning. In these cases, it is wise to explore communication systems that exploit those old overlearned skills (e.g., a communication device with a keyboard like that on a typewriter) rather than those that are essentially new (e.g., sign language or code-input communication devices). Patients with severe retrieval problems are predictably more successful with systems that present communicative options — either to be selected directly or selected through a scanning system — than with the systems that require the user to remember the options or codes. The ability to learn and to use codes and symbols (including letters and words) must be systemically explored.

Aesthetic judgments, in particular the patient's reaction to the sound of synthesized speech, should be elicited since the aesthetic features of a system are often the final determinants in its acceptance or rejection. Preferences of family members or other significant people in the patient's life are also important since their reaction to the patient's new communication device determines how often the system is used. The motor skills for optimal switch or keyboard activation should also be evaluated.

The patient's ability to interact communicatively with other people is vital to the functional use of any device or augmentative system. Many patients who have had a head injury are dependent communicators. They can carry on a conversation, but only if guided by questions or cued by family, friends, co-workers, or therapists. They are unable to control the interaction independently. An effective communication system must somehow give the patient the ability to start, continue, and terminate an interaction within any conversing situation. However, if patients do not possess the basic interactive skills, a device will not make them appropriately interactive. Devices do not communicate; people communicate. The INCH (*International Check-*

list for Augmentative Communication), developed by Bolton and Dashiell (1984), is a measure that attempts to look at the interaction of augmentative communicators.

The people who interact with the patient are also key to the evaluation outcome. Some devices or systems require trained listeners to assist in the communication process. Others require a considerable level of knowledge and commitment to maintain the system and trouble shoot when problems occur. In both cases, the evaluator must ensure that there are people to play these roles. Finally, the assessment should include consideration of the need for two or more devices or communication systems for different environments, for different communication partners, or for those times when the primary system breaks down.

CONSIDERATIONS FOR ENVIRONMENTAL CONTROLS. Special considerations in the evaluation of patients for the use of environmental controls include (a) the position that the patient will be in when using the device; (b) the place where the patient will be; (c) the devices that the patient needs or wants to control; and (d) the number and location of the devices. Evaluators should also routinely explore the patient's need for a signaling device in case of an emergency. Cognitively, the patient must understand the concept of using a switch to activate a device and be able to learn the use of the switch. In the case of a complex environmental control system, for example a scanning system, the patient needs to understand the process of using the device. Finally, behavioral parameters should be explored, since the inappropriate use of environmental control systems or signalling devices can be extremely disruptive in a home or residential facility.

ASSESSING THE ENVIRONMENT. In order to choose the most appropriate device or set of devices and to promote generalization in the use of the device to the community, the evaluators must consider the environments in which the devices will be used. The physical and psychosocial environment of the home, school, work place, and community should be assessed prior to making final recommendations. The physical parameters of space, size, and accessiblity of each environment will be factors in the practicality and ultimate use of any device. Acceptance and motivation factors in the family are often as significant as those in the patient. The cognitive abilities of family members and their philosophical orientation toward compensatory devices for disabled people are also fundamental in that it typically falls to the family members to maintain and repair the equipment and to encourage the patient to use the equipment functionally and appropriately.

The work place should be evaluated not only in terms of physical characteristics but also in the willingness of supervisors and co-workers to accept the use of assistive devices and to make recommended work site modifications if indicated. The community should be assessed for access and availability of vocational or avocational opportunities for physically disabled individuals. For example, an 18 year old male with moderate physical disability following head injury was limited in recreational activities. A visit was made with him and his brother to a local spa. With training in transfers to and from his electric wheelchair and simple adaptations, he gained access to the pool and the use of some of the exercise equipment.

FINANCIAL CONSIDERATIONS. The evaluation is not complete without giving the patient and family assistance in obtaining funding for the device. Potential funding resources include medical insurance, state departments of special education or vocational rehabilitation, government grants, charitable or service organizations, or private pay. A plan of action to make contact with funding agencies and fulfill the necessary requirements must be formulated as soon as a decision to recommend a device is made. Depending on a variety of factors, this plan could be implemented by family or staff members. In requesting payment for a device, careful attention must be paid to the terminology and statement of need. Selecting the proper terms to describe the product (e.g., "speech prosthesis" vs. "communication aid") and the need (e.g., "to communicate vital medical information to his physician" vs. "to enhance his social life") may mean the difference between acceptance and rejection of a request on the part of insurance carriers or agencies. For example, when requesting payment from a vocational agency the needs should be stated in the form of occupational opportunities the device would make available to the patient. For some equipment, a prescription signed by the appropriate professional is necessary. A description of the durability or lifespan of the equipment, a demonstration of cost effectiveness relative to comparable products, supportive medical or therapeutic information, and "before/after" photos may be necessary.

Perseverance is often the key to gaining approval by a funding agency. Research supported by the Office of Technology Assessment of the U.S. Congress found that funding is often denied even though it has been clearly demonstrated that a device is appropriate and beneficial (Office of Technology Assessment, 1982). The investigators also discovered that even when a device is approved, training in its use is often not funded. The denial appears frequently to be a result of the funding agency's unfamiliarity with new technology or the need for training in the use of the devices. Education of agencies and insurance companies can occur through the appeals process and will benefit not only the patient for whom the appeal was filed but other patients with similar needs as well.

Communities and states vary in their attitude toward and financial support of electronic devices for mobility, communication, and environmental control. If a community is truly committed to this important dimension of rehabilitation, resources can usually be created to obtain the devices. For example, Fort Collins, Colorado, dedicated some of its Public Service Community Development Block Grant Funds (awarded to cities by the federal government) to providing devices for individuals unable to speak (Montgomery, 1984). Pennsylvania, through its Department of Education, has set aside funds for providing electronic communication devices for personal and educational use by nonspeakers. Community awareness of the needs of individuals with handicapping conditions has gradually improved in recent years, but much progress remains to be seen.

THE DECISION PROCESS. The evaluation that we have described is complex. The interaction of a head injured patient's motoric, cognitive, and psychosocial deficits, combined with the complexity of community settings in which devices are used and the complexity of the devices themselves makes this inevitable. Figure 2–2 outlines the basic components of this process in the form of a decision-making tree. The figure outlines the progression from choosing an evaluation center and determining needs and options to making recommendations for purchase, training, and follow-up. This decision tree can be a useful tool for developing a systematic evaluation for compensatory devices. Although it is sometimes possible to make good decisions omitting one or more steps, it has been our experience that this often leads to inappropriate recommendations or to the acquistion of equipment that is underused or unused.

Treatment and Training for Compensatory Devices

Following acquisition of a device, the patient must be systematically and thoroughly trained in its use. Of equal importance, necessary instruction in the use of the device must be given to the family, teachers, other therapists, employers, attendants, or other involved community members. The effectiveness of these two processes contributes heavily to the eventual outcome. By pacing the introduction of each component of the device(s) and by gradually introducing

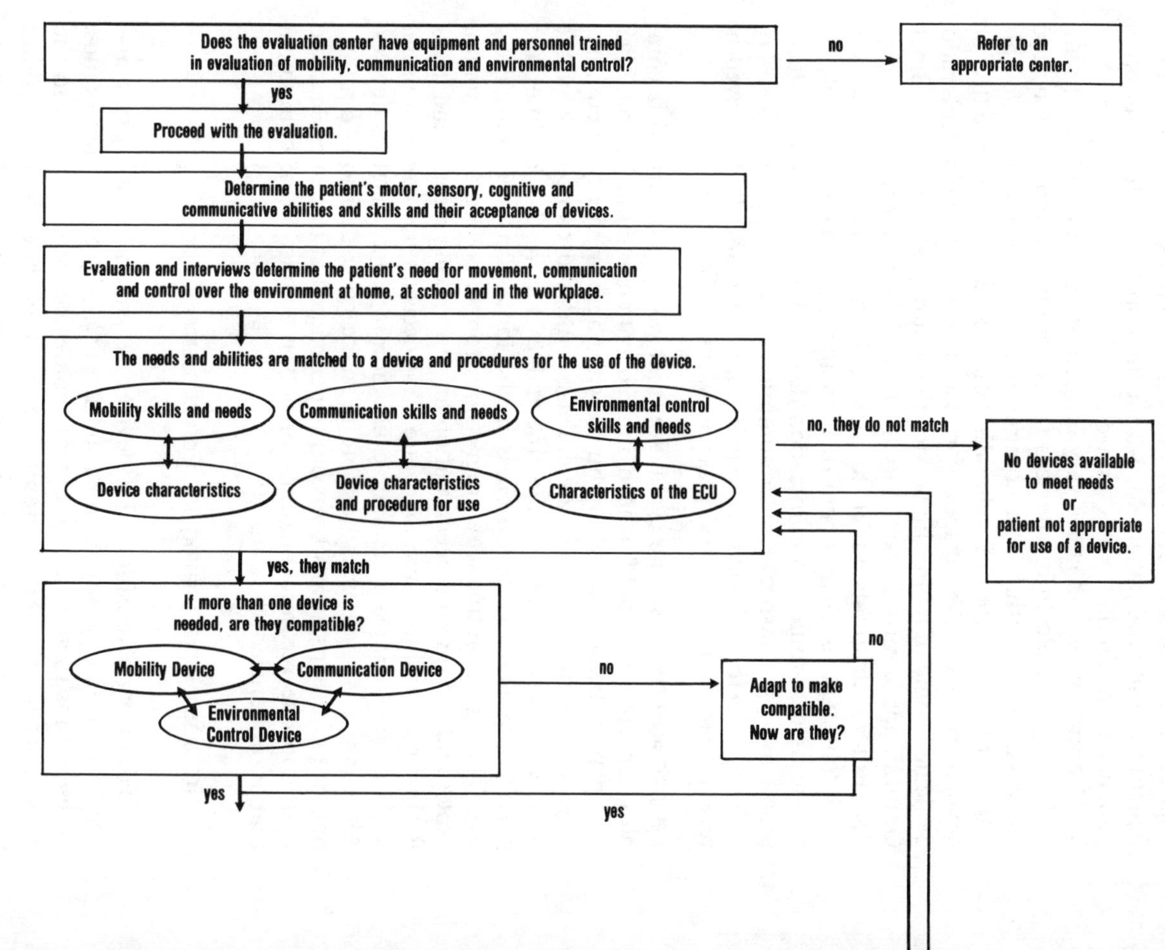
Does the evaluation center have equipment and personnel trained
in evaluation of mobility, communication and environmental control?
no
Refer to an
appropriate center.
yes
Proceed with the evaluation.
Determine the patient's motor, sensory, cognitive and
communicative abilities and skills and their acceptance of devices.
Evaluation and interviews determine the patient's need for movement, communication
and control over the environment at home, at school and in the workplace.
The needs and abilities are matched to a device and procedures for the use of the device.
Mobility skills and needs
Communication skills and needs
Environmental control
skills and needs
Device characteristics
Device characteristics
and procedure for use
Characteristics of the ECU
no, they do not match
No devices available
to meet needs
or
patient not appropriate
for use of a device.
yes, they match
If more than one device is
needed, are they compatible?
Mobility Device
Communication Device
Environmental
Control Device
no
Adapt to make
compatible.
Now are they?
no
yes
yes

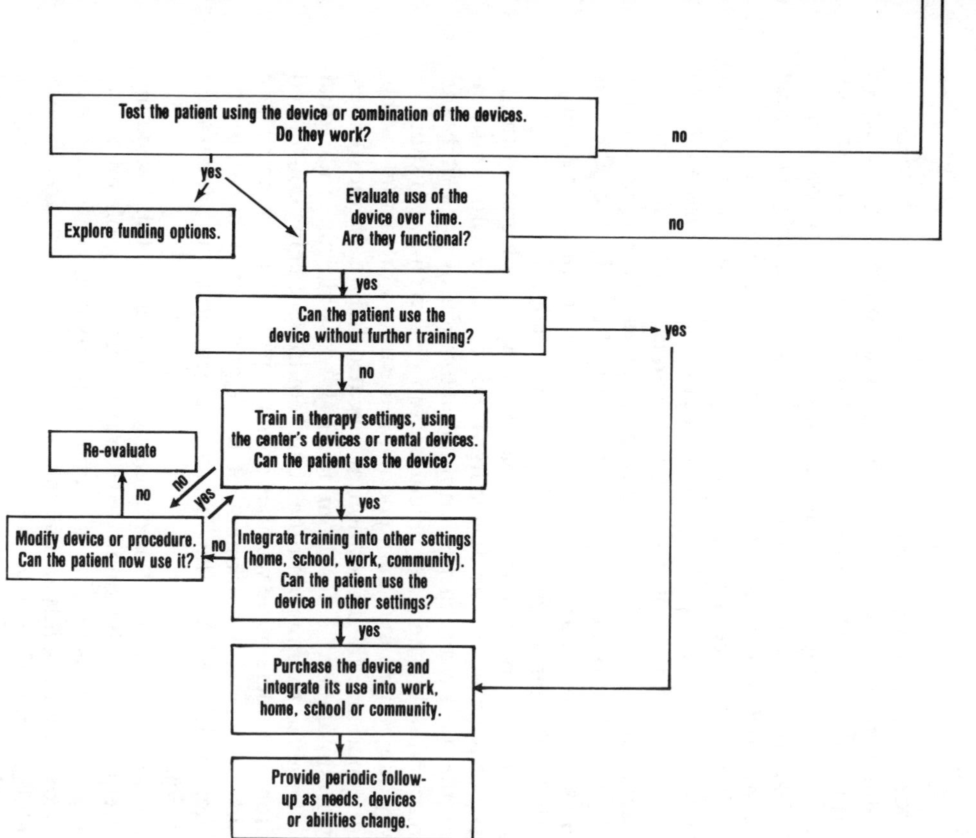

Figure 2–2. The evaluation process: a decision-making tree.

motoric and cognitive demands, therapists increase the efficiency of the training and also the likelihood that the patient will accept the device both socially and emotionally. The family should be involved during all phases of treatment and training. Work site personnel, if identified and available, should also be included. Efforts should be made to integrate training into the home, work site, and community to further ensure success. Often it is necessary to simulate home and work place conditions in the clinical setting. Simulation of the actual device is necessary if training must begin before the device is available.

SIMULATION. It is always best to use the actual devices, procedures, and settings in training. When this is not possible, an effective simulation of the device and of related procedures can be used for training. If, for example, a communication device with speech output is not available, an adapted tape recorder or one of the many new educational toys with electronic spoken output can be used in a controlled situation to see if the patient can communicate by means of electronically generated speech. Communication systems that use scanning as the method of selecting items can be simulated by having the patient activate a switch to indicate messages which the evaluator scans by pointing to a display. This prepares the patient for the process of using a device and decreases the chances of procuring equipment that will not be functional for the patient.

Simulation may also help the patient achieve a degree of initial success not possible on the device itself. For example, early in training, the therapist may react to minimal activation of the switch and later respond only when the patient uses more forceful activation. In this way, the patient may gain enough force to use the actual switch, but not experience the frustration of repeated failure. In most cases, however, simulation is far from ideal. If possible, the individual should be given training with the actual equipment being considered for purchase to determine whether or not it will be functional. There often is some small component of the equipment that cannot be simulated, which becomes the obstacle that prohibits the patient's use of the equipment.

The setting in which the patient will eventually use the equipment frequently can be simulated. An understanding of the setting can be gained by visiting the site and by interviewing relevant work site personnel and family or community members. Photographs may be useful. Devices that work well in the therapy setting may not be functional in the work place or at home because of environmental differences. In some cases, the patient must be trained in the specific environment in which the devices will be used. In other cases, only certain components of that environment need to be simulated. For example, practice driving an electric wheelchair through narrow doors, on carpet, or around sharp corners similar to those at home or work can occur in the clinical setting and may be vital to functional use of the power chair in the community setting. Use of a speech output device in a noisy work environment may need to be simulated with tape recorded background sounds so the patient can learn how to deal with auditory interference.

Despite the many advantages of simulations in assessing patients for use of a device, caution must be exercised when recommending a device solely on the basis of simulation.

PACING THE INTRODUCTION. The introduction of equipment to the patient and the family must be paced in order to optimize the patient's chance of success. The motoric, communicative, cognitive, emotional, and situational requirements of using a device should be analyzed and the demands graded to the patient's level of ability. Throughout the treatment phase, these demands are gradually increased by the therapist(s) toward the patient's maximal level of functioning. This promotes initial success and decreases the probability that the patient will be "turned off" to a particular device or to devices in general because the experience was too challenging or frustrating.

Devices often become "closet" items unless they are carefully and gradually introduced to the patient, family, work site personnel, and other community members. Without an adequate introduction to the use of devices, many families choose to leave the device in its case. If no one but the therapist can operate the device with a reasonable degree of efficiency, the family's choice may be perfectly reasonable. Since families of head injured patients often have many new rehabilitation and care tasks to learn in a very short period of time, it might be necessary to give the family extra time to adjust to the many changes in their lives. This may mean, for example, having the patient use an optimal communication device in therapy but continue for some time to use a less than optimal but functional system at home. This strategy is illustrated by a family that was unable to concentrate on a new computerized speech device for their daughter while attending to other aspects of the patient's rehabilitation. Therefore, it was decided that the family would continue to use gestural communication at home while practice with the new device continued at the rehabilitation facility. This arrangement continued until the family had mastered their other tasks and had gained greater acceptance of the consequences of their daughter's accident.

PACING THE MOTOR DEMANDS. Motoric requirements can be systematically increased by changing the actual control interface or by decreasing the amount of external stabilization or control provided to the patient. For example, a patient who has only gross arm movement may initially be able to trigger a large light pressure switch but, with practice and/or increased motor control, may be able to activate a smaller switch or several smaller switches. Initially, proximal stabilization (e.g., use of an elbow block) or distal splinting may be necessary for sufficient control. With time and practice, the patient may gain adequate stability and control so that external aids are no longer needed.

Frequently, the extraordinary effort that motivated patients produce in order to succeed in their initial trial use of a device causes increased abnormal muscle tone and patterns. This further reduces the patient's already impaired motor skills and results in failure with the device, frustration, and a vicious cycle of effort, reduced control, frustration, and further reduced control. Repositioning the patient or the device may help inhibit abnormal patterns and tone. More important, however, is the gradual introduction of components and demands so that the patient can exerience success from the outset. Fatigue is also a factor to consider in pacing the introduction of devices. For some individuals, any effort, even if successful, is fatiguing. By alternating the use of a device with rest periods or changes in position to a more relaxing one, there can be many short periods of successful use.

PACING FOR COGNITIVE DEFICITS. The cognitive demands of using a device should be matched to the cognitive abilities of the patient. Memory deficits, difficulty with new learning, and inefficient processing related to the amount and complexity of the information to be processed and the rate at which it is presented all affect the use of devices. For example, a patient who is unable to locate or remember messages related to every key of a communication device could use the device with all but a few keys covered. As facility with the device improves or memory and perceptual skills increase, more keys can be uncovered. The cognitive demands of power mobility are often not as obvious. For example, a decreased rate of processing visual or auditory information may be more of a factor in operating a power chair than motor skills for some patients. Reducing the chair's speed and introducing its use in a nondistracting environment may compensate for the cognitive processing problems and make the introduction of a power chair possible.

PACING FOR SOCIAL AND EMOTIONAL ACCEPTANCE. The introduction of technological devices or equipment should be paced to allow for social and emotional acceptance by the patient and the family. Individuals who have little experience with or tolerance for high technology products may need to be introduced slowly to one component at a time. By introducing more acceptance and potentially successful components first, the patient may be willing to try other more complex devices later. Because an individual's self-concept following head injury is often based on pre-traumatic abilities and attitudes, the patient may not be aware of residual physical deficits or may not be able to accept them. Environmental control devices may therefore be more acceptable than communication devices because they are similar to appliances used prior to the injury.

After a prolonged period of dependence, patients may exhibit signs of "learned helplessness." They may prefer the comfort or security of always having someone close to them. For this reason, patients who have been dependent for mobility have be resistive to power mobility even though it represents increased independence. They may fear being left to function independently and thus want the caretaker or family to be there to communicate with others and to care for their needs. Success for such patients may depend upon the introduction of a power chair in situations in which improved mobility clearly increases social contact with loved ones rather than decreasing this contact. Again, gradual introduction of the device with attention to successful, positive experiences is the key.

The introduction of an augmentative communication device may change in several ways established interaction patterns. For example, the rate at which messages are generated may be slower than the communication partners can tolerate. In this case pacing the introduction of the device may mean asking the communication partners to encourage the patient to use the device, but only for short periods of time. These periods can be lengthened as the communication partners become accustomed to the change in rate of communication.

GRADUAL INTRODUCTION TO COMMUNITY SETTINGS. The settings and situations in which devices are introduced and trained must be carefully selected to maximize success and demonstrate the full capacity of each device. Following success in the initial setting, the use of the device can be expanded to other settings. This process is important to ensure successful generalization to those settings in which the patient will ultimately need to function. For example, an electronic communication device may be introduced in therapy sessions with a knowledgeable communication partner and controlled communication activities that allow the patient to discover the full power of the device.

Success in the rehabilitation setting does not guarantee success when the patient returns to home, work, or other aspects of community life. The key to successful use of devices in the community is thorough training. For devices that have some dependency on those around the user or which require some degree of maintenance, training of family, teachers, friends, supervisors, or fellow workers will need to occur prior to expanding use of the device. Following training of the patient in therapy sessions and training of others involved with the patient, the use of the device should be gradually expanded to the home, school, work, or community setting, with as much supervision as is needed. Independent and unsupervised use of the device is appropriate only if its use has been thoroughly mastered. If introduced without sufficient training and practice, many problems may occur. For example, the user unable to maneuver a power chair out of a narrow doorway will not be independent even though given a potentially independent means of mobility. The individual who is able to communicate effectively with therapists and family members using an electronic device may have difficulty communicating with unfamiliar or untrained people in the work place.

The use of many devices requires judgment and effective processing of information. The safety of the patient and others is not only a factor when selecting a device and training the patient in its use, but also in identifying community settings in which the device can safely be used. Patients with severe deficits in processing or judgment may be able to use some devices safely only within a highly structured or supervised situation. Patients who are easily distracted or who become disoriented or overstimulated may endanger themselves and others. Busy sidewalks, emergency situations on the job, and other unstructured or out of the ordinary situations may place the individual in a dependent situation which he or she cannot handle. In treatment, the level of distraction can be gradually increased to challenge processing skills. Potentially dangerous situations can be simulated to assess and train safety judgment. Independent use of the device should then be recommended only in situations the patient easily handles. Later, if judgment and cognitive skills improve, more sophisticated devices or more challenging community situations should be considered.

REDEFINING THE TREATMENT APPROACH. In general, the goal of intervention is to provide patients with the most effective solutions possible to the problems that they face. A possible result of diagnostic intervention, however, is the decision to temporarily abandon the use of a device even though the device may serve an important functional purpose for the patient and even though the patient may demonstrate the ability to use it. It is at times necessary to "back down" to less sophisticated devices and procedures when the physical, emotional, and mental effort of using a device or procedure becomes too much for the patients or their families. The decision to back down is often a difficult one and requires a close working relationship between the family and other team members. In one case, for example, a young woman, fully capable of using an electronic device for communication and in need of special positioning within her chair for increased independence, refused both during the early months of her rehabilitation. The therapists judged that it would be therapeutically counterproductive to force the issue and therefore continued to use a limited gestural system of communication. Weeks later, when the communication system was reintroduced as a means of word processing (more comparable to activities in her previous work) rather than as a means of communication (which, in her mind, meant "substitute for speech"), it was received with much greater enthusiasm. To date she has not accepted additional chair adaptations.

THE NEED FOR MODIFICATIONS IN THE HOME, WORK PLACE, OR COMMUNITY. Physical modifications of the home, work place, or community may be necessary to care for the patient adequately and to maximize independence. Non-ambulatory individuals, for example, may be dependent in toileting only because of a lack of access. With a widened doorway and the addition of grab bars, these patients may achieve full independence in toileting. A visit to the home, community agency, or work place is usually necessary in order to determine needs and make recommendations. Chapter 7 details some common problems which need to be addressed for independent living. Housing and building modifications are described in other publications (American National Standards Institute, 1980; Wittmeyer & Barrett, 1980).

FOLLOW-UP AND MAINTENANCE. Following the acquisition of devices and training, the devices and their use need to be monitored over time to ensure that they continue to be appropriate in light of possible changes in skill levels or in life circumstances, including job needs. Monitoring is also needed to provide patients with information on newly developed devices that might satisfy their unmet needs or upgrade the quality of their present devices. Standard methods of follow-up include visits to professionals on a regular basis or consultation through a home health service. For some individuals, special arrangements for maintenance of devices may also need to be implemented in the work setting or at home. Finally, training staff members in nursing homes or health centers may be the most effective means of maintaining skills for patients discharged to those settings.

Some patients are unable to maintain levels of functioning, not because of a loss of underlying motoric skills, but rather because of changes in the home, work place, or community. For example, a communication system may be inadequate with a job change because of differences in computer systems. Job changes may also necessitate access changes. For example, the patient who receives a promotion to a job on the second floor may need a power mobility system and an elevator or ramp may need to be added to the work site. If a patient is no longer able to live independently, the family and work site personnel may need to be instructed in the how-to's of the device so that they can take responsibility for those aspects of care that the patient cannot handle. If family members or work site personnel are unfamiliar with the equipment, adaptations may need to be made before they can use or care for the system.

Endurance, Strength and Flexibility

In the introduction to this chapter, we distinguished among three areas within physical rehabilitation following head injury: (a) intervention to improve motor skills; (b) intervention to compensate for motor impairments; (c) intervention to improve overall physical endurance, strength, and flexibility. We chose to focus our attention on (b) and (c), not with the intention of questioning the value of intervention to improve underlying motor skills, but rather to highlight the importance of compensation and conditioning in relation to community re-entry. An important goal of physical rehabilitation is to have patients enter the work place or vocational training program or independent living program able to compensate in some way for their residual motor impairments. An equally important goal is to ensure that those patients have the strength and endurance to put their motor skills and compensations to work for themselves in demanding settings for adequate periods of time. This is the theme of the last section of the chapter. Its importance for head injured patients is underscored by the prolonged period of inactivity that typically follows severe head injury.

Evaluation

Assessment of cardiovascular health, endurance, muscular strength, flexibility, and body composition provides important information relative to a client's physical tolerance and specific health needs. An individual exercise treatment plan can then be tailored to maximize the desired physical outcomes for each patient.

The central component to the assessment is the estimation of cardiovascular endurance. It is essential to identify those patients who might be at risk for untoward cardiac events as a result of increased exercise. The American College of Sports Medicine (1980) has developed a simple classification system for this purpose. This test is generally performed on a cycle ergometer or motor-driven treadmill, but can be performed through a field test for groups of low-risk individuals. Criteria for test selection, procedures, and termination may be found in several sources, including Astrand and Rodahl (1977) and Pollock, Wilmore, and Fox (1984). The client's functional capacity, or maximal oxygen consumption, can be determined from this test. The oxygen requirements for nearly all vocational and avocational activities have been determined and are well documented (Astrand & Rodahl, 1977). Activities are rated in terms of net MET units which are an expression of the metabolic cost of activities. One MET unit is the energy required to sit comfortably, equivalent to approximately 3.5 ml O_2/kg/min. Two METS would be any activity requiring twice that amount. For example, the vocational activities of auto repair, janitorial work, or radio/television repair are at the 2-3 MET level. Welding and machine assembly are at the 3-4 MET level; painting, masonry, paper hanging, and light carpentry are at the 4-5 MET level. Most individuals work at about 50 percent of their functional capacity, so that the average physical demands of a job should not exceed 50 percent of the individual's physical capacity.

The relationship of physical conditioning to vocational function is illustrated by the patient whose functional capacity is measured at 6 METS and who wants a carpentry job which requires 4–5 METS. Unless this patient improves his physical condition, carpentry is not feasible since the energy required for that vocation would represent 65 to 85 percent of his capacity. However, a conditioning program will result in an increase in the functional capacity; an increase of just 2 METS would decrease the relative work load associated with light carpentry to 50 to 60 percent of capacity. As a result, this individual would function more effectively in his job with less fatigue. Indeed, in some occupations, the improvement in functional capacity resulting from physical conditioning may make the difference for a head injured patient between maintaining chosen employment and failing to do so. Although predictions based on this measure may be somewhat inaccurate as a result of individual differences in efficiency, functional capacity has been found to be a useful measure of an individual's ability to engage in various vocational and avocational activities.

Estimating functional capacity is useful in demonstrating the importance of improved fitness. Improvement in cardiovascular fitness results from very specific physiologic alterations that permit both increased oxygen delivery to muscle tissue and improved oxygen utilization. The improved efficiency translates to lower myocardial work (as measured by heart rate and blood pressure) at submaximal physical work loads, and an improved maximal physical tolerance.

Assessment of body composition allows for a determination of the percentage of total body weight that is fat and a realistic estimation of the patient's desirable weight. The feedback from this test is useful in helping patients understand their weight goals and in explaining fluctuations in weight, especially those due to exercise. For example, Table 2–6 represents normal changes in body composition as a result of regular exercise. There is a decrease in percentage body fat, but an adaptive increase in nonfat weight, principally in the form of muscle tissue. While total weight decreased only one pound, fat weight decreased 3.5 pounds, with an increase in nonfat weight of 2.5 pounds. The technique for assessing percentage of fat is inexpensive and relatively simple to learn and calculate (McArdle, Katch & Katch, 1981; Pollock et al., 1984). It is important that regression equations are used that are specific to the age and sex of those being tested, and that the same individual perform the tests, thereby enhancing reliability.

Additional tests of flexibility and muscular strength are helpful in identifying deficiences or targeting specific areas of physical improvement for vocational considerations. The reader is referred to Pollock and colleagues (1984) for a description of tests and techniques for these components of fitness.

Table 2–6. Results of Conditioning in One Patient

Evaluation Results	Pre-Conditioning	Post-Conditioning
Resting Heart Rate, beats/min.	94	84
Blood Pressure, mmHg	150/84	126/84
Weight, lbs	195	194
Percent Fat, percentage of total body weight	19.1	17.4
Recommended Body Weight	185	188
Cardiovascular Endurance, $ml0_2$/kg/min	34.0	39.5

Treatment

Because of their extended period of inactivity in addition to possible motoric impairments, head injured patients should be considered for a program of exercises designed to develop endurance, strength, and flexibility for vocational and daily living tasks. Physiological adaptation to exercise is dependent on the type of demands placed on the body during exercise. As such, the design of a patient's program must consider the desired outcomes. For example, if weight loss is a key consideration for a specific client, the activity plan should emphasize activities that result in maximum caloric output per unit of time. This concept of "specificity of training" underlies the development of an exercise treatment plan.

Although individual exercise plans may vary considerably to achieve specific outcomes, all plans include cardiovascular conditioning as a central component. Activities providing the greatest impact on cardiovascular endurance involve large muscle groups and have minimal interruption. The most commonly selected activities include walking or running, stationary or outdoor cycling, swimming, and aerobic dance, although rowing, rope-skipping, and bench stepping can be useful adjunctive cardiovascular activities when designing a total program. The arm ergometer is an example of a cardiovascular exercise for patients whose degree of motor involvement does not permit them to do more standard activities.

According to the American College of Sports Medicine (1978), the training "threshold" for cardiovascular adaptation appears to be participation in an aerobic activity for 20 to 30 minutes, 3 to 4 days each week, at an intensity close to 60 to 80 percent of the estimated functional capacity. Some patients have such limited exercise tolerance that 20 to 30 minutes of continuous activity is not feasible, even at a low intensity. A useful alternative is a circuit of activities that includes brief rest periods between exercise stations. As an example, the stations may be stationary cycling, walking or jogging, bench stepping, rowing, arm-cranking, rebounding, and calisthenics. Patients rotate through selected stations at determined intervals, resting between each station. The exercise-to-rest ratio should not exceed 2:1 and, as the patient's endurance improves, the ratio can likewise increase.

Improvement in strength requires specific activities that result in adaptation of the muscle fibers used in those activities. Hence, signicant improvement in muscular strength is brought about only through specific strength training exercises, such as weight lifting. While the focus of the treatment plan is a core of cardiovascular activities, muscle-strengthening activities may be added to enhance the plan or to improve specific muscle groups for vocational objectives. Isokinetic exercise, such as that which is done with Nautilus or Cybex equipment, can be used to provide strength training. This type of exercise provides variable resistance so that the patient's resistance is matched and the resistance is provided throughout the full range of motion. Weight training may be a useful adjunct to a cardiovascular exercise treatment plan, but should not supplant the aerobic exercise component; long-term health and weight management are much more likely to be achieved through cardiovascular activities.

Our experience in applying a cardiovascular fitness and weight training program to individuals with head injuries indicates that several specific areas should be closely monitored. *Posture* is of importance not only as observed in the patient at rest, but also in execution of each prescribed activity. For example, an individual with a hemiplegia tends to use the stronger side throughout all activities, thereby becoming asymmetrical and not receiving maximal benefit from the exercise. Unless the activity is designed to be bilateral, these patients tend to do more repetitions on the uninvolved side. In addition, faulty posture can lead to problems with chronic pain. Many patients have weak abdominal muscles and a lack of flexibility in their lumbar region; this combination can result in low back pain from any repetitive stressful activity such as weight lifting, rowing, or stationary bicycle riding. Improving or maintaining *flexibility* in head injured patients is, therefore, essential in the prevention of pain and the improvement of posture. Hamstring tightness or lack of trunk rotation may persist even with concentrated efforts to increase motion. *Fatigue* is another common characteristic following head injury and should be monitored on a regular basis. Finally, *increased muscle tone* (spasticity) raises questions about the appropriateness of certain types of exercises. Whether the patient with increased abnormal muscle tone should participate in a resistive weight training program has long been a subject of debate. Initial EMG studies done at the University of Maryland, which monitored muscle tone in spastic muscles during weight lifting exercises, show that muscle tone may increase only during the actual performance, and have no long-term effect (Fensterman, 1986). On the other hand, some patients clinically seem to become tighter with resistive exercises.

Table 2–6 shows physiologic changes that occurred in a specific patient over the course of an 8-week conditioning program. The resting heart rate decreased by 10 beats per minute, an expected result of cardiovascular conditioning. The individual had borderline systolic hypertension on entering the program. The systolic pressure decreased by 24 mmHg after the program, bringing blood pressure to well within normal limits. The diastolic blood pressure did not change, as might be expected since it was within normal limits. The body weight and percentage body fat measures indicate a typical adaptation to conditioning; body fat decreases and lean body mass increases due to the exercise. Cardiovascular endurance increased by 5.5 ml 0_2/kg/min or 1.6 METS.

Follow-up and Maintenance

Patients should be encouraged to engage in a regular exercise program following completion of their rehabilitation program. The well-structured and supervised experience that they receive during exercise treatment provides patients with the knowledge and skills necessary to effectively engage in their program without supervision. The program should include 3 to 4 days of vigorous cardiovascular activities per week (20 to 30 minutes per day). This level of activity should provide the stimulus necessary for maintenance of fitness and improved cardiovascular health over time. Follow-up assessment is not indicated unless a pre-existing medical problem warrants periodic re-evaluation.

The ultimate objective, of course, is for patients to maintain or to continue to improve their health and fitness following community reentry. Because adherence to a program of physical conditioning is highly dependent upon an individual's acceptance of the program as an integral part of his or her lifestyle, it is essential that the treatment plan be negotiated with the patient and be designed to fit that lifestyle. The end product should be an exercise program that the individual values while maximizing his or her health and vocational capabilities. There need to be parts of the program that patients can realistically do independently at home, at the local spa, or within the neighborhood.

SUMMARY

This chapter has focused on the physical deficits that often persist following head injury and their interrelationships with cognitive, psychosocial, and communicative skills. Treatment for such deficits, including traditional motor treatment, cardiovascular conditioning, and compensatory techniques and devices, has been reviewed. We have emphasized an interdisciplinary approach to treatment, a close working relationship with family members, and a focus on the ultimate goal of maximizing the patient's independence and effectiveness in home, work, and community settings.

REFERENCES

American College of Sports Medicine. (1978). Position statement on the recommended quantity and quality of exercise for developing and maintaining fitness in healthy adults. *Medicine and Science in Sports, 10,* 7–10.

American College of Sports Medicine. (1980). *Guidelines for graded exercise testing and exercise prescription.* Philadelphia: Lea & Febiger.

American National Standards Institute. (1980). *Specifications for making buildings and facilities accessible to and usable by physically handicapped people.* (ANSI 1–1980). New York: American National Standards Institute.

Astrand, P. O. & Rodahl, K. (1977). *Textbook of work physiology* (2nd ed.). New York: McGraw-Hill.

Ayres, A. J. (1972). *Sensory integration and learning disorders.* Los Angeles: Western Psychological Services.

Baker, L., Parker, K. & Sanderson, D. (1983). Neuromuscular electrical stimulation for the head-injured patient. *Physical Therapy, 63*(12), 1967–1974.

Basmajian, J. V. (1981). Biofeedback in rehabilitation: A review of principles and practices. *Archives of Physical Medicine and Rehabilitation, 62,* 469–475.

Bergen, A. & Colangelo, C. (1985). *Positioning the client with central nervous system deficits* (2nd ed.). Valhalla, NY: Valhalla Rehabilitation Publications.

Blyth, B. (1981). The outcome of severe head injuries. *New Zealand Medical Journal, 93,* 267–269.

Bobath, B. (1978). *Adult hemiplegia: Evaluation and treatment.* London: William Heinemann.

Bolton, S. D. & Dashiell, S. E. (1984). *The interaction checklist for augmentative communication.* Huntington Beach, CA: Inch Assoc.

Booth, B. J., Doyle, M. & Montgomery, J. (1983). Serial casting for the management of spasticity in the head-injured adult. *Physical Therapy, 63*(12), 1960–1966.

Bowers, S. & Marshall, L. (1980). Outcome in 200 consecutive cases of severe head injury treated in San Diego County. *Neurosurgery, 6*(3), 237–242.

Calliet, R. (1977). *Soft tissue pain and disability.* Philadelphia: F. A. Davis.

Eichler, J. J. & Neale, H. C. (1978). Etran eye signaling system. In G. C. Vanderheiden (Ed.), *Non-vocal communication resource book.* (pp. IIA). Baltimore: University Park Press.

Enders, A. (1984). *Technology for independent living sourcebook.* Bethesda, MD: Rehabilitation Engineering Society of North America.

Farber, S. D. (1982). *Neurorehabilitation: A multi-sensory approach.* Philadelphia: W. B. Saunders.

Fensterman, K. (1986, January). Aerobic exercise and dance for people with physical impairments. *National Handicapped Sports and Recreation Association Fitness Instructor Training Session.* College Park, MD.

Griffith, E. R. (1983). Types of disability. In M. Rosenthal, E. Griffith, M. Bond & J. D. Miller (Eds.), *Rehabilitation of the head injured adult* (pp. 23–32). Philadelphia: F. A. Davis.

Heiden, J., Small, R., Caton, W., Weisst, M. & Kurze, T. (1983). Severe head injury: Clinical assessment and outcome. *Physical Therapy, 63*(12), 1946–1951.

Jaffe, M., Mastrilli, J., Molitor, C. & Valko, A. (1985). Intervention for motor disorders. In M. Ylvisaker (Ed.), *Head injury rehabilitation: Children and adolescents* (pp. 167–194). San Diego: College-Hill Press.

Jennett, B. & Bond, M. R. (1975). Assessment of outcome after severe brain damage. *Lancet, 1,* 480–484.

Jennett, B., Teasdale, G., Galbraith, S., Pickard, J., Grant, H., Braakman, R., Avezaat, C., Maas, A., Minderhoud, J., Vecht, C. J., Heiden, J., Small, R., Caton, W. & Kurze, T. (1977). Severe head injuries in three countries. *Journal of Neurology, Neurosurgery, and Psychiatry, 40,* 291–298.

Knott, M. & Voss, D. (1968). *Proprioceptive neuromuscular facilitation.* New York: Harper & Row.

Kraat, A. & Sitver-Kogut, M. (1985). *Features of commercially available communication devices.* Flushing, NY: Queens College, Speech and Hearing Center.

Lewin, W., Marshall, T. & Roberts, A. (1979). Long term outcome after severe head injury. *British Medical Journal, 2,* 1533–1538.

Long, C., Gouvier, W. & Cole, J. (1984). A model of recovery for the total rehabilitation of individuals with head trauma. *Journal of Rehabilitation, 1,* 39–45.

McArdle, W. D., Katch, F. I. & Katch, V. L. (1981). *Exercise physiology, energy, nutrition, and human performance.* Philadelphia: Lea & Febiger.

McDonald, E. T. & Schultz, A. (1973). Communication boards for cerebral palsied children. *Journal of Speech and Hearing Disorders, 38,* 73–88.

Mills, V. (1985). Sensorimotor deficits in the traumatically head injured patient. *Neurology Report of the American Physical Therapy Association, 9*(1), 11–16.

Montgomery, J. (1984). Advocacy update. *Communication Outlook, 5*(3), 12.

Office of Technology Assessment. (1982). *Technology and handicapped people.* Washington, DC: U.S. Government Printing Office.

Perry, J. (1983). Rehabilitation of the neurologically disabled patient: Principles, practice and scientific basis. *Journal of Neurosurgery, 58,* 799–816.

Pollock, M. L., Wilmore, J. H. & Fox, S. M. (1984). *Exercise in health and disease.* Philadelphia: W. B. Saunders.

Rood, M. (1962). The use of sensory receptors to activate, facilitate and inhibit motor response, automatic and somatic in developmental sequence. In C. Sattely (Ed.), *Approaches to the treatment of patients with neuromuscular dysfunction.* Dubuque: Wm. C. Brown.

Silverman, F. (1980). *Communication for the speechless.* Englewood Cliffs, NJ: Prentice Hall.

Skelly, M. & Schinsky, L. (1979). *Amer-Ind gestural code based on universal American Indian hand talk.* New York: Elsevier North Holland.

Symington, D. C., Batellan, J., O'Shea, B. J. & White, D. A. (1980). *Independence through environmental control systems.* Toronto: Canadian Rehabilitation Council for the Disabled.

ten Kate, J. H., Duyvis, J. D. & Le Poole, J. B. (1984). Prism/mirror communicatior. *Communication Outlook, 5,*(3), 12.

Thomsen, I. (1984). Late outcome of very severe blunt head trauma: A 10–15 year second follow-up. *Journal of Neurology, Neurosurgery, and Psychiatry, 47,* 260–268.

Umphred, D. (1983). Conceptual model of an approach to the sensorimotor treatment of the head-injured client. *Physical Therapy, 63* (12), 1967–1974.

Van Zomeren, A. & van den Burg, W. (1985). Residual complaints of patients two years after severe head injury. *Journal of Neurology, Neurosurgery, and Psychiatry, 48,* 21–28.

Vicker, B. (1974). Nonoral communication system project, 1964–73. Iowa City, Iowa: Campus Stores, The University of Iowa.

Williams, J. R., Csongradi, J. J. & LeBlanc, M. A. (1982). *A guide to controls: Selection, mounting, applications.* Palo Alto, CA: Children's Hospital at Stanford.

Wittmeyer, M. & Barrett, J. E. (1980). *Housing accessiblity checklist.* Seattle: University of Washington Health Resource Center.

Young, B., Rapp, R., Pharm, D., Norton, J. A., Haack, D., Tibbs, P. & Bean, J. (1981). Early prediction of outcome in head injured patients. *Journal of Neurosurgery, 54,* 300–303.

Young, R. R., Delwaide, P. J. (1981a). Drug therapy: Spasticity (pt. 1). *New England Journal of Medicine, 304*(1), 29–33.

Young, R. R. & Delwaide, P. J. (1981b). Drug therapy: Spasticity (pt. 2). *New England Journal of Medicine. 304*(2), 96–99.

APPENDIX I. SCREENING FORM A.

The Rehabilitation Institute of Pittsburgh

Technology Team — Communication Screening

Name: ____________ Date: ____________ Examiner: ____________

Speech and Language

	No Problem Indicated	Documented Problem	Needs Assessment	Other
Hearing	☐	☐	☐	☐
Auditory Processing	☐	☐	☐	☐
Receptive Vocabulary	☐	☐	☐	☐
Memory	☐	☐	☐	☐
Speech	☐	☐	☐	☐
Speech Potential	☐	☐	☐	☐
Expressive Language	☐	☐	☐	☐

- ☐ Reflexive Communication
- ☐ Signal Communication
- ☐ Single Word
- ☐ Multiword
- ☐ Complete Sentences

NOTES:

RECOMMENDATIONS:

Significant Diagnostic Problem Areas

	No Problem Indicated	Documented Problem	Needs Assessment	Other
Word Finding Problems	☐	☐	☐	☐
Perservation	☐	☐	☐	☐
Distractability	☐	☐	☐	☐
Syntax Problems	☐	☐	☐	☐
Echolalia	☐	☐	☐	☐
Occasional Clear Speech	☐	☐	☐	☐
Variable Intelligibility	☐	☐	☐	☐
True Telegraphic Speech	☐	☐	☐	☐
Ritualistic Behaviors	☐	☐	☐	☐
Limited Subject Matter	☐	☐	☐	☐
Other	☐	☐	☐	☐

NOTES:

RECOMMENDATIONS:

Augmentative Communication Symbol Systems

Movement	In Use Now	Potential for Use	Questionable	Not A Consideration
General Body Movement	☐	☐	☐	☐
Gestures	☐	☐	☐	☐
Movement/Device	☐	☐	☐	☐
Hand/Arm	☐	☐	☐	☐
Head	☐	☐	☐	☐

Eyes	☐	☐	☐	☐
Legs/Feet	☐	☐	☐	☐
Sign				
Visual				
Objects in Context	☐	☐	☐	☐
Symbolic Objects	☐	☐	☐	☐
Pictures	☐	☐	☐	☐
Color photo	☐	☐	☐	☐
Color drawing	☐	☐	☐	☐
Black/White photo	☐	☐	☐	☐
Line drawing	☐	☐	☐	☐
Symbols:	☐	☐	☐	☐
Bliss, Mayer-Johnson PIC, PICSYMS, Rebus, Oakland, Other	☐	☐	☐	☐
Transitional reader	☐	☐	☐	☐
Reader/Speller	☐	☐	☐	☐
Auditory/Vocal				
Vegetative	☐	☐	☐	☐
Signal Call	☐	☐	☐	☐
Differentiated Signals	☐	☐	☐	☐
Word Approximations	☐	☐	☐	☐
Word + Jargon	☐	☐	☐	☐
Speech	☐	☐	☐	☐

NOTES:

RECOMMENDATIONS:

Interactive Process

	Visual	Vocal	Gestural	Manual Device	Electrical Device	Visual Device
Initiates Communication	☐	☐	☐	☐	☐	☐
Terminates Communication	☐	☐	☐	☐	☐	☐
Turn-Taking	☐	☐	☐	☐	☐	☐
Efficiency for System Type	☐	☐	☐	☐	☐	☐
Other	☐	☐	☐	☐	☐	☐

NOTES:

RECOMMENDATIONS:

APPENDIX II. SCREENING FORM B.

Seating and Mobility Summary

Patient: ____________ Date: ____________ Examiner: ____________

A. Present Position **Comments**

Pelvis:

neutral ☐ obliquity ☐

posterior tilt ☐ rotation ☐

Hips:

neutral ☐ windswept ☐

extension/adduction internal rotation ☐ abduction/external rotation ☐

Knees:

neutral ☐ excessive extension ☐

excessive flexion ☐ length discrepancy ☐

Feet:

neutral ☐ excessive plantar-flexion ☐

excessive dorsiflexion ☐

Spine:

straight ☐ kyphosis ☐

scoliosis ☐ lordosis ☐

Shoulder Girdle:

neutral ☐ scapular protraction ☐

scapular retraction ☐

Head:

midline ☐ rotation ☐

lateral flexion ☐ hyperextension ☐

Upper Extremities:

free ☐ required for support ☐

B. Influence on Position

Reflexes:

startle ☐ ATNR ☐ other ☐

Sensation:

intact ☐ impaired ☐ absent ☐

Areas of pressure concerns:______________________________
____

C. Gross Motor Skills	indep.	min. assist	mod. assist	max. assist	Comments
Sit	☐	☐	☐	☐	
Stand	☐	☐	☐	☐	
Walk	☐	☐	☐	☐	
Head/Trunk Control	☐	☐	☐	☐	
Transfers	☐	☐	☐	☐	
Bathroom Transfers	☐	☐	☐	☐	

D. Present Equipment Comments

Wheelchair, Manual: adequate yes ☐ no ☐

Wheelchair, Power: adequate yes ☐ no ☐

Seat: depth__________width__________back height__________

Footrest, type:______________________

Armrest, type:______________________

Joystick: right ☐ left ☐ other ☐

Other Control: right ☐ left ☐ other ☐

Inserts: seat ☐ back ☐

Headrest, type:______________________

Tray, type:______________________

Seatbelt, type:______________________

Custom:______________________

E. Equipment Recommended to Try

1. Wheelchair — Manual

a. Type — standard ☐ lightweight ☐

Power

Series H ☐ Du-It☐

other______________________________

b. Drive — one arm ☐ R ☐ L ☐

power drive ☐ R ☐ L ☐

c. Interface — joystick ☐ other______________________

2. Seating
   a. w/c cushion
      Jay ☐ Combi ☐ flat ☐ Otto Bock ☐ other ☐
   b. back inserts
      flat ☐ Combi ☐ Triwall ☐ other ☐
   c. lateral supports
      plywood ☐ Otto Bock ☐ other ☐
   d. vest
      bib ☐ upper chest belt ☐ other ☐
   e. seat belt
      type ____________________
   f. head support
      Otto Bock ☐ Foam Triwall ☐ other ☐
   g. MPI system
      size ____________________
   h. misc. straps
      type, location ____________________
   i. footrest
      extenders ☐ other ☐
   j. thigh support
      M-bar ☐ abduction wedge ☐ other ☐

APPENDIX III. SCREENING FORM C.

Visual Motor Screening

Patient: ____________ Date: ____________ Examiner: ____________

Visual Fields:

	Superior	Inferior	Left	Right
R	____	____	____	____
L	____	____	____	____

Tracking: Right Eye ______ Left Eye ______ Both ______

Tone Head/Neck ________ RUE ________ RLE________

Trunk ________ LUE ________ LLE________

Note those that influence active movement.

Reflexes ATNR________STNR________Moro________Other________

Voluntary Movement Code:

0 = unable
1 = attempts, gross movement
2 = moderate control
3 = controlled and isolated

Also Note:

Mid = midrange control
End = end range control
Stab = stabilization

Shoulder	Left	Right	Head	Left	Right
Flexion			Lateral Flexion		
Extension			Rotation		
Abduction			Head Nod		
Internal Rotation			Other Facial Mvmt.		
External Rotation			**Hip**		
Horizontal Adduction			Flexion		
Elbow and Forearm			Abduction		
Flexion			Internal Rotation		
Extension			External Rotation		

Voluntary Movement *(continued)*

Elbow *(cont.)*	**Left**	**Right**	**Knee**	**Left**	**Right**
Supination			Flexion		
Pronation			Extension		
Wrist			**Ankle**		
Flexion			Dorsiflexion		
Extension			Plantar Flexion		
Ulnar Deviation			Inversion		
Radial Deviation			Eversion		

Gross Arm Placement: ____________________

Localization/Resolution: ____________________

Dominance: Right ☐ Left ☐

Hands	**Left**			**Right**		
	grasp	sustain	release	grasp	sustain	release
Pincer						
Lat. Pincer						
Cylindrical						
Spherical						
Press Button						

Recommendations

________ Ophthalmology Eval. Needed

________ Other Motor Eval. Needed

3 Options for Motor Site for Switch

1. ________
2. ________
3. ________

CHAPTER 3

A Framework for Cognitive Rehabilitation Therapy

Shirley F. Szekeres
Mark Ylvisaker
Sally B. Cohen

Cognitive rehabilitation therapy (CRT) has, in recent years, become the keystone of many rehabilitation programs for young adults following traumatic brain injury. One explanation for this phenomenon is that researchers and clinicians alike have become increasingly aware that cognitive deficits and related psychosocial problems often pose the most stubborn obstacles to patients' return to satisfying vocational and social lives. Much of the research in this area is reviewed in Brooks (1984), Levin, Benton, and Grossman (1982), and Prigatano and others (1986).

Cognitive impairments that commonly persist among severely head injured young adults include, in varying combinations and degrees of severity: impaired attention and perception; inflexibility in attending, thinking, and acting; slow and inefficient processing of information; difficulty processing large amounts of information; difficulty processing abstract information; difficulty learning/remembering new information, rules, and procedures; inefficient retrieval of old information and of words; poorly organized behavior, verbal expression, and problem solving; impulsive and socially awkward behavior; and impaired "executive" functions, such as self-awareness of strengths and weaknesses, goal setting, planning, self-initiating or self-inhibiting, self-monitoring, and self-evaluating.

Even though head injured patients frequently display similar impairments, individual differences among the patients indicate the need for a flexible approach to cognitive intervention, one, that is, in which therapists customize treatment for each patient even as they work within very broad guidelines that are based on typical stages of recovery and on commonly occurring patterns of cognitive deficit. These individual differences result from differences in the types and severity of brain injury; from pre-traumatic differences in personality, intelligence, and educational level; and from differences in the support systems that are available to the patients, the coping styles they have, and rehabilitative intervention they receive after their injuries. Sensitivity on the part of clinicians to the variety of individual differences among patients should caution them not to assume too easily that head injured individuals *must* have certain cognitive characteristics simply because these characteristics are pervasive in the population. Even group studies occasionally fail to confirm received truths about head injury sequelae. For example, despite the frequent references to attentional deficits following head injury (Wood, 1984), Brouwer and van Wolffelaar (1984) failed to find a difference between mild-to-moderate head injured patients and control subjects on a measure of sustained attention.

The enthusiasm that professionals currently feel for the cognitive rehabilitation of head injured patients is based only in part on the recognition of the pervasiveness of cognitive problems in this population. There is, in addition, a small but interesting body of evidence that suggests that some consequences of brain damage that in the past were thought to be intractable are, in fact, remediable to some degree with intensive and appropriately targeted intervention (Ben-Yishay et al., 1982, Diller & Gordon, 1981; Gummow, Miller & Dustman, 1983; Prigatano and others, 1986). The enthusiastic proliferation of CRT programs is also based in part on the overall mistaken notion that techniques of cognitive rehabilitation are new weapons in the rehabilitative armamentarium. In fact, much that falls under this new label has for years been used in the fields of special education, speech-language pathology, occupational therapy, and psychology. In some cases, techniques that are now called "cognitive retraining" have been found to be relatively *ineffective* for other populations of cognitively impaired individuals (Kavale & Mattson, 1983). In addition to labels, novelty lies in some of the *packaging* of techniques (e.g., "CRT" computer programs that target specific cognitive deficits). Of greater moment than the new labels and packaging is the realization that cognitive and psychosocial issues must be addressed comprehensively and systematically in the context of tight interdisciplinary programming. A fragmented approach to cognitive rehabilitation simply contributes to the fragmentation that may already dominate the life of a head injured person.

In general terms, cognitive rehabilitation is simply the attempt to improve a person's cognitive processes and systems, or to improve the person's functional-integrative performance to the extent that this performance is impaired by a cognitive deficit. Disagreements about which functions lie within the province of cognitive rehabilitation are based on definitions of cognition that vary in scope. Verbal behavior may, for example, be considered an aspect of cognitive functioning (Anderson, 1976; Piaget, 1970) or a function that is relatively autonomous of cognition (Chomsky, 1968) or a function that is related dynamically to cognition (Sapir, 1921; Vygotsky, 1962). Other disagreements about the nature of cognitive rehabilitation derive from varying conceptions of the workings and interconnections of the cognitive mechanism and from varying degrees of emphasis on *restoring* functions with direct retraining and *compensating* for impaired functions (Prigatano and others, 1986; Szekeres, Ylvisaker & Holland, 1985).

In this chapter, we explore the field of cognitive rehabilitation by (a) describing in some detail those aspects of cognition which are central to CRT; (b) distinguishing forms of cognitive intervention; and (c) offering clinicians some guidance in their search for answers to the fundamental questions: How do I decide what it is that I am supposed to help this patient with? (selecting and sequencing objectives), and "How do I do it? (training procedures). The chapter concludes with a discussion of cognitive rehabilitation in a special education setting (since many head injured adolescents and young adults receive cognitive services in this setting) and key issues in the management of cognitive rehabiliation programs. Because parts of this chapter may be conceptually challenging to those clinicians new to the field of cognitive rehabilitation, we ask their perseverance so that they may explore the theoretical and conceptual bases of their clinical practice. Chapter 4 includes suggestions for treating many of the cognitive problems mentioned in this chapter.

COGNITION

Cognition is complex, and cognitive dysfunction that results from head injury is very difficult to map thoroughly. Without a conceptual framework of cognition, selection of goals may become somewhat random, and treatment may easily lapse into an inefficient "workbook" approach that lacks direction, structure, or rationale. A conceptual framework (a) enables professionals from diverse backgrounds to share a vocabulary and consistent perspectives which help them avoid conflicting approaches to treatment; (b) allows them to organize the assessment process so that diverse test data as well as data from informal observation and diagnostic therapy can be integrated within a consistent set of descriptive cognitive categories; (c) helps them to organize intervention, both at the programmatic level (e.g., deciding which aspects of cognitive functioning should be singled out as the focus of treatment groups) and at the level of selecting goals, objectives, and activities for individual patients (see Selecting and Sequencing Treatment Objectives); and (d) yields useful criteria for measuring progress that surpass those of standardized tests which may not represent all the dimensions of cognitive functioning that a comprehensive cognitive rehabilitation therapy program should address.

Aspects of Cognition

In developing a framework for CRT, we have relied heavily on information processing categories because they are comprehensive, clinically fruitful, and widely used in current theoretical discussions of cognition and cognitive dysfunction. Information processing theories of cognition are described in a number of excellent texts, including Crowder (1976), Dodd and White (1980), Hintzman (1978), Kausler (1974), Siegler (1983), Tarpy and Mayer (1978), and Weisberg (1980). Dodd and White (1980) noted that recent research in cognitive psychology has been dominated by three approaches: (a) studying the *structure* of cognition (i.e., components such as short-term memory, long-term memory, and the executive system, and their interrelationships); (b) studying the *processes* or *activities* or *operations* that are involved in taking in, interpreting, considering, and retrieving information and formulating output; and (c) studying *functional behavior,* including the purposes and goals of individuals dealing with available or potential information as they interact with an environment. We have chosen to follow Dodd and White in incorporating all three aspects into a working definition of cognition: "processing of information for particular purposes and within certain mental structures" (p. 8). Including component *processes* (attending, perceiving, learning/remembering, organizing, reasoning, and problem solving) and component *systems* (working memory, knowledge base [permanent or long-term memory], the executive system, and the response system) in the definition provides both the detail and comprehensiveness that are needed to delineate deficits in components and in their interactions. Including the dimension of functional-integrative behavior and purposes permits clinicians to focus on real-life performance as the measure of success of a treatment program. Ultimately, it is clinical usefulness of this sort that justifies the use of a particular set of categories to describe cognitive activity.

In the discussion that follows, we briefly define component processes and systems, and the variables that characterize functional-integrative performance. Table 3-1 summarizes these aspects of cognition. Mapping the bewildering array of dynamic interrelationships among these components is as important as listing and defining the components and variables, but this task is far beyond the scope of this book. In this chapter and the next, however, we illustrate some of the productive detective work that professionals should undertake to explore these relationships so that they may understand impaired cognitive functioning as well as the best ways to promote adaptive and successful cognitive behavior.

Component Processes

ATTENTION. Attention is the complex process of admitting and holding information in consciousness. Its components include: basic *arousal, directing* attention, *maintaining* attention, *selecting* particular objects of attention and *filtering* out irrelevant information, *shifting* attention from object to object, and *dividing* attention among two or more objects of attention. (The word "concentration" is often used to refer to the selecting and maintaining aspects of attention.) What one

Table 3-1. Aspects of Cognition

Component Processes	
Attending	Organizing
Perceiving	Reasoning
Memory/Learning	Problem Solving/Judgment
Component Systems	
Working Memory	Executive System
Long-Term Memory (Knowlege Base)	Response System
Functional-Integrative Performance	
Efficiency	Scope
Level	Manner

attends to is determined by the characteristics of the impinging stimuli (external or internal) and also by the level of arousal or alertness of the individual (Gummow et al., 1983) and by momentary intentions and long-term goals. On the one hand, attention may be captured by strong, novel, unexpected, and/or significant environmental stimuli (e.g., a loud noise or noxious odor) and is thus a phenomenon of considerable survival value. On the other hand, a person may *deliberately* direct attention to stimuli if this serves a particular purpose (e.g., studying a text or mentally reviewing information in preparation for an exam). Deliberate control over attention is necessary for effective and efficient processing.

Attentional problems resulting from traumatic brain injury have been emphasized as an important focus of cognitive remediation (Wood, 1984). Although our experience confirms that this concern with attentional deficits is often justified, we have also found that a given deficit must be carefully delineated before exercises are begun that specifically target basic-level attentional processes. Patients with similar symptoms may have quite different cognitive profiles and consequently quite different treatment needs. Two of our patients, B.N. and M.T., for example, both evidenced functional attention problems during conversation. Their conversation wandered from topic to topic, and they exhibited several signs of inattention, such as fidgeting, standing up, asking to leave, responding to other events in the environment, and failing to maintain eye contact. To isolate the underlying disturbance, we systematically varied the content and interest level of conversation, the conversation partner, and the modality of input (e.g., speech, speech with many gestures, written language, pictures). Despite these variations, B.N.'s conversational abilities and signs of inattention remained unchanged. By contrast, M.T.'s conversational skill and willingness to converse improved dramatically when the vocabulary level of the conversations was reduced, sentence structure simplified, and picture cues provided. The focus of treatment for B.N. became, therefore, basic attentional processes, whereas semantic knowledge and language comprehension became the focus of treatment for M.T., with the expectation that attending would improve as a result of improvements in these "higher" cognitive functions.

PERCEPTION. Perception is the process of detecting distinctive features, invariant relationships, and patterns in stimuli (Gibson, 1969). With experience, it is possible to differentiate more and more features and patterns of stimuli, and recognition may become automatic. If an array of stimuli is complex or unfamiliar, however, one must attend to it in detail until distinctive features and patterns emerge (e.g., learning to read aerial photographs) (Flavell, 1977). Pre-existing knowledge, attentional bias, and preferences make some features of stimuli more noticeable than others (Gibson, 1969). Developmental studies of perception in children 3 years old and older indicate that as attentional control and knowledge develop, it becomes increasingly inappropriate and misleading to isolate perception from other aspects of cognition, such as memory and organization (Flavell, 1977). Mature perceivers process specific kinds of information as circumstances require and, if necessary, search through stimuli for relevant information. Features also become perceptually salient when an environment is externally structured to highlight them.

The visual-perceptual deficits of head injured patients can be specific to perception (e.g., the neglect of a visual field or visual-spatial disorientation), or perceptual problems may result from more general cognitive deficits (e.g., inefficient perception relative to rate, amount, and complexity of the stimuli; difficulty shifting perceptual focus; and ineffective simultaneous processing of the object of perception and contextual cues). Perceptual symptoms may also be the consequences of impairments of "higher" level cognitive processes or systems. For example, perceptual inefficiency may result from generally weak organizing processes, from a shallow knowledge base, or from impaired executive control over attentional/perceptual processes. Furthermore, even in those cases in which perceptual problems are primary, effective treatment, if higher-level functions are relatively intact, may involve engaging the patient in meaningful higher-level tasks. For example, using interesting paragraphs as treatment materials rather than conceptually simpler, nonmeaningful materials may most effectively promote systematic scanning to the left for a person with left visual field neglect. Construing the meaning of sentences often facilitates the task of systematic visual scanning for patients whose language system is relatively intact.

LEARNING AND MEMORY. Learning/memory involves three stages: encoding, storage, and retrieval of information (Crowder, 1976; Hintzman, 1978; Tarpy & Mayer, 1978). The *encoding* or acquisition stage includes the constructon of an internal representation of a perceived event. The representation may include a nearly accurate replica (e.g., remembering a speaker's exact words) or an interpretation of the event, contextual information, concurrent internal experiences, and knowledge that is integrated with the event at the time of encoding. There are several interacting factors that determine which events are encoded and how much of a given event is encoded, such as the attentional focus and orientation of the individual (Postman & Kruesi, 1977), the social, emotional, and intellectual significance of the event (Smirnov, 1973), the depth of understanding or degree to which information is integrated into existing knowledge (Brown, 1975, 1979; Moely, 1977; Piaget & Inhelder, 1973), and the type and extent of deliberate elaboration the individual performs at the time of encoding (Craik & Tulving, 1975). People may thus encode the same event quite differently, some forming a shallow or incomplete representation of the event (possibly making the event less memorable) and others forming a deeper and more complete representation that is well integrated with other knowledge (possibly making the event more memorable). The *storage* stage of memory involves holding information over time in what is thought to be a highly organized long-term memory system (Smith, 1978).

At the *retrieval* stage of memory, information is transferred from long-term memory to consciousness. Retrieval may be deliberate and effortful, involving a strategic searching of memory and creative problem solving to reconstruct an event from the bits of information that have been retrieved (Norman, 1976). On other occasions, retrieval is automatic and effortless (e.g., retrieving words during relaxed conversation). Retrieval may even be out of control as, for example, when it is impossible to exclude stressful events and ideas from consciousness. Retrieval is referred to as *recognition* when the stimulus is present and one must only identify it (e.g., responding to yes/no or multiple choice questions, or identifying objects or pictures as having been seen before); *cued recall* when specific cues are given to prompt retrieval (e.g., wh-questions); and *free recall* when the stimulus is not present and must be recalled without cues (Hintzman, 1978).

Although "memory problems" may be inferred when retrieval failures occur, the specific source of failure could be inefficiency in any or all of the three stages of memory (encoding, storage, or retrieval) or in any of the other cognitive processes that influence learning efficiency. The literature suggests several possible explanations for memory failure. Some researchers attribute poor memory performance to ineffective retrieval processes (Ceci & Howe, 1978a; Kinsbourne & Wood, 1975; Tomkins, 1970). Tulving and Thompson (1973) emphasized the importance of being able to generate cues at retrieval that had been present at the time of encoding (e.g., constructing vivid images of the sequence of morning events in my attempt to later recall where I left my keys), with failure to reinstate these cues resulting in an inability to recall. Others emphasize inadequate semantic knowledge and problem-solving behavior in encoding and in reconstructing events at the time of retrieval (Bartlett, 1932; Ceci & Howe,

1978b; Cofer, 1977; Norman, 1976; Piaget & Inhelder, 1973); ineffective encoding (Huppert & Piercy, 1982) or inadequate active elaboration of information at the time on encoding (Cermak, Butters & Gerrein, 1973; Cermak, Butters & Moreines, 1974; Craik & Lockhart, 1972; Craik & Tulving, 1975); reduced durability of memory traces (Brooks, 1975); and interference from previously learned information (proactive interference) or subsequently learned information (retroactive interference) (Postman & Underwood, 1973). There is evidence that free recall and recognition involve different retrieval mechanisms (Anderson & Bower, 1972; Kintsch, 1968; Tulving, 1975). A differential performance of recognition and free recall in verbal functioning (word comprehension [recognition] versus word retrieval [free recall]) is commonly observed in head injured individuals (Levin, Benton & Grossman, 1982).

There is some support for all of these explanations and it is quite likely that they are all involved at one time or another in memory failures. Schacter and Tulving (1982) offer a critical review of these hypotheses in relation to amnesia research. The clinical value of these hypotheses lies in the direction that they give to the detective work that is necessary to isolate and define a specific memory problem and to target treatment correctly. In the vast conceptual territory covered by the term "memory," many additional distinctions are useful in analyzing memory deficits and designing individual treatment programs. These include:

1. *Episodic and Semantic Memory: Episodic memory* involves the encoding, storage, and retrieval of personally experienced events or episodes (e.g., remembering the meal one had at lunch or the ball game one attended with a friend after lunch). It has been described as a sort of autobiographical memory in that the memory traces include contextual information, such as the time, place, and conditions of an episode. In contrast, *semantic memory* is free of context. That is, information is stored independently of when, where, and how it was acquired (e.g., knowledge that baseball games have nine innings). A large quantity of general information as well as abstracted and organized knowledge about words, meanings, relations, concepts, rules, and strategies is thus stored in semantic memory (Brown, 1975, 1979; Kinsbourne & Wood, 1982; Tulving, 1972). Episodic and semantic memory interrelate in many ways. For example, some researchers presume that many items currently in semantic memory may first have been represented as specific episodes (Baddeley, 1982); furthermore, it is not uncommon that episodic elements are combined with abstracted knowledge. The distinction may not be entirely neat, but it is clinically useful nonetheless.

Wood, Ebert, and Kinsbourne (1982) and Parkin (1982) have described the episodic memory problems of amnesic patients as being characterized by grave difficulty remembering any personal experience despite their ability to learn new motor skills, procedures, and some general facts with repeated practice ("context free learning"). Normal learning and memory are thought to involve the interaction or collaboration of episodic and semantic memory processes (Parkin, 1982), but these episodic amnesic patients are apparently able to learn only through conditioning and the abstracting process that places information directly into semantic memory, in which there is no recollection of the context of learning. Although we have also observed these types of learning in head injured patients who have severe episodic memory problems, their learning is generally very slow and inefficient and requires much repetition or practice. Other patients reach a point in recovery at which their ability to automatically encode, store, and retrieve personally experienced events is well within normal limits, even though they learn new information or academic skills quite inefficiently.

2. *Input Modality:* Visual and auditory memory, or visual and auditory processing (and, less importantly, the other sensory input modalities) can be differentially impaired following closed head injury (Craine & Gudeman, 1981; Lezak, 1983).

3. *Verbal and Nonverbal Information:* There may be significant differences in the patient's ability to learn verbal and nonverbal information or in language processing versus visual-spatial-motor processing. In the latter category, memory for events, routes, faces, and newly taught procedures should be independently assessed (Brooks & Lincoln, 1984).

4. *Involuntary and Deliberate Memory: Involuntary memory* (or incidental learning, type I, Postman, 1964) refers to a condition in which an individual remembers information despite not having been oriented to learn it through the design of the task, or the task instructions, or external incentives. That is, the individual does not specifically intend to learn or remember the information (as is the case in studying for an exam or taking a memory test) but rather is simply engaged in an interesting or personally meaningful activity and learning is a by-product (Brown, 1979; Smirnov & Zinchenko, 1969). In a *deliberate memory* condition, the goal is specifically to remember some target information (e.g., studying for an exam). To be efficient, deliberate memory requires some degree of metacognitive awareness and planning. Strategies may be involved, ranging in sophistication from simply looking at information a little longer to rehearsing it mentally to creating an elaborate organizational framework that

ensures retrieval. Although motivation and initiation are prerequisites for efficient deliberate learning, these demands are reduced when the context of learning is a meaningful activity (Brown, 1975). Because of deficits in "executive functions," deliberate memory is often ineffective in head injured patients. In extreme cases, turning learning tasks into deliberate memory tasks by suggesting strategies and explicitly calling attention to the processes of learning can actually *reduce* a patient's learning ability. In these cases, treatment must focus on the design of the activity so that involuntary learning is enhanced. (This point is discussed in greater detail in Chapter 4.)

Measures of *post-traumatic amnesia* (PTA) are commonly used to chart recovery from closed head injury and to predict outcome (Brooks, 1984). As standardly defined, PTA includes elements of episodic memory and of orientation to person, place, and time (Levin, Benton & Grossman, 1982). In very severe cases, patients' confusion, disorientation, and severe memory problems can last months or continue indefinitely. Furthermore, the return of adequate orientation often does not coincide with that of continuous memory for ongoing events, and both faculties may recover so gradually that assigning a termination date to PTA is virtually impossible. Even in cases of mild head injury, there is evidence that continuous memory and orientation do not necessarily return to normal at the same time (Gronwall & Wrightson, 1980).

Memory impairments are among the most commonly reported deficits following closed head injury (Brooks, 1983), with inefficiency in new learning being the most typical and the most debilitating, at least for those individuals who return to academic or vocational settings that require new learning. In this brief discussion of various aspects of memory functioning, we have emphasized the complexity of memory, the variety of possible memory disorders, and, consequently, the need for very careful differential diagnoses that are much more discriminating than those that standard memory assessment instruments make possible.

ORGANIZING PROCESSES. Organizing processes relate and group stimuli with reference to information that is already stored in permanent memory. These processes include analyzing information; identifying relevant perceptual and conceptual features; comparing features and concepts; identifying similarities and differences; classifying and categorizing; sequencing; and integrating information into larger units (e.g., main ideas, themes, scripts). Organizing at the most basic level of processing involves "chunking" or grouping perceptual units (e.g., perceiving visual stimuli as a specific object or recognizing a sequence of sounds as a word). Most organizing at this basic level is automatic. At the highest level, organizing engages reasoning and problem-solving skills as well as the executive system in complex activities, such as organizing a table of contents for a book or organizing the process of constructing a house.

Functional organizational impairments following closed head injury are common and include difficulty analyzing a task into its components, sequencing ideas or steps in a complex task, arranging task materials and work space, seeing main ideas or central themes in a set of facts, and remaining on topic in conversation. (Organizational impairments and their treatment are discussed at length in Chapter 4.)

REASONING. Reasoning is the process of considering evidence and making inferences or drawing conclusions. In *deductive reasoning,* inferences are drawn on the basis of formal relations among propositions (i.e., if the premises are true, the conclusion *must* be true). The head injured patient who agreed that dentists require a college education, insisted that he had no intention of going to college, but declared nonetheless that he was going to be a dentist illustrates weakness in deductive reasoning. Since reasoning in daily life rarely takes the form of explicitly deductive arguments, training patients in deductive reasoning is of questionable practical value. However, patients' acceptance of the basis of deductive reasoning — namely, that a statement cannot at the same time be both true and false — is a necessary condition for rational thought and discussion.

Inductive reasoning involves *direct* inferences from experience, ranging from scientific generalizations to everyday reasoning, such as "My first two therapies were a waste of time, so they're all probably a waste of time." Induction is distinguished from deduction in that a good inductive argument may have true premises yet have a false conclusion. True premises simply increase the probability that the conclusion is true. Errors of induction often take the form of hasty generalizations such as the one arrived at by the head injured patient who, after making two mistakes during a therapy exercise, muttered, "I never get anything right."

Analogical reasoning, sometimes considered a type of inductive reasoning, allows us to draw inferences *indirectly* from experience when known relationships are used to explain or predict different but related phenomena. Analogical reasoning is perhaps the most useful form of reasoning in ordinary problem-solving and decision-making contexts. One common example of analogical reasoning is saying to oneself, "In situations like this in the past I have tried such-and-such a solution and it has generally worked, so it's probably a good idea to try that again now." Problem solving is very often based on tacit analogies, which can be dangerous if one sees too many parallels and draws too few distinctions. Judging the acceptability of analogical reasoning usually means weighing the *relevance* of the analogy. Thus, when a patient says, "If I don't do well in this job, I'll simply get another one with a different company; that's what John did and it worked out well for him," discussion will likely focus on significant similarities and differences between the two individuals and their work.

Evaluative reasoning involves considering the merits of ideas, courses of action, things, or people in relation to explicit or assumed criteria and making judgments of value on the basis of these considerations (e.g., "That's a good idea" or "What he did was wrong" or "It's a great car" or "Tom is a super person"). As in induction, mistakes in evaluative reasoning often result from a failure to gather sufficient information before one makes a value judgment.

From a different perspective, clinicians have found it useful to classify reasoning or abstract thinking as either convergent or divergent. *Convergent thinking* involves the search for main ideas, central themes, or single conclusions. It includes all of the types of reasoning defined above. *Divergent* ("lateral" or flexible) thinking includes creatively exploring possible courses of action, information that may be relevant to a given topic, and alternative interpretations of behavior and events.

Reasoning impairments range from a nearly total inability to think abstractly and inferentially, to the failure to use reasoning abilities when appropriate (impulsive thinking), to the weak exploration of alternative possibilities, to the failure to relate known information to new problems. Stress often contributes to failures in reasoning, such as disorganization or impulsiveness.

PROBLEM SOLVING/JUDGMENT. Psychologists and educators often use the term "problem solving" to stand for virtually all types of cognitive processing or thinking. Problem solving may be more narrowly defined as a complex form of cognitive activity that is engaged in to achieve a goal that cannot be reached directly or automatically. Organized problem solving involves identifying the goal and the problem, gathering and considering information that may be relevant to solving the problem, exploring possible solutions, weighing their merits, choosing the best solution, formulating a plan of action, executing the plan, and evaluating its effectiveness. As such, problem solving includes as components most other types of thinking or reasoning. If a procedure exists that can generate a single correct solution (e.g., problem solving in mathematics), the problem-solving process is regarded as closed-ended. Real-life problem solving, or decision making, is most often open-ended in that no rule or set of rules determines exactly what information is relevant in thinking about a problem or which of the possible solutions is best. *Judgment* is a decision to act based on available information, which includes the prediction of consequences.

Because the cognitive processes that enable organized problem solving and good safety and social judgment are so numerous and varied, impairments in any cognitive process or system can depress problem-solving ability and judgment. Head injured patients who are confused, child-like, and impulsive and who behave inappropriately likely have a combination of various cognitive impairments in problem-solving ability and judgment.

Treatment for impairments of reasoning, problem solving, and decision making is discussed at length in Chapter 4. Patients receiving this treatment often protest that they are being asked to be more careful and deliberate in their thinking than they were before the injury. In response, we often point out that there are three important reasons for training in this area: (a) because of the brain injury, the patient's previously "automatic" reasoning and decision making may no longer be serviceable; (b) the change in the patient's environment and activities may also require more deliberate decision making; and (c) the number and significance of the new problems caused by the injury require greater thoughtfulness than was necessary before the accident. It is crucial that head injured patients have adequate problem-solving skills and sound judgment to succeed at their jobs and to live independently and safely.

Component Systems

WORKING MEMORY. Working memory is the short-term storage, or "holding space" where coding and organizing occur (Deutsch & Deutsch, 1975). Although the structural capacity of working memory is limited (7 plus or 2 minues units in normal adults (Miller, 1956)), it's *functional* capacity can be increased by grouping or "chunking" elements into meaningful units and by making these organizing systems automatic (Chi, 1976). Information is easily lost from working memory unless deliberate action is taken to preserve it (e.g., rehearsing information or coding it for storage). What is done with information in working memory depends in part on an individual's goals.

Although working memory, as measured by a short-term memory span test, is one of the few memory functions *not* typically impaired by closed head injury (Brooks, 1983), in some cases its capacity *is* reduced by the injury, and in others the capacity was limited pre-traumatically. Because information that exceeds an individual's working memory capacity is difficult to process effectively, organizational processes that expand functional working memory are essential to effective processing. If the capacity of a patient's working memory has been reduced *and* if his or her organizational skills are weak, then information must be presented in small quantities and with cues that enable the patient to chunk the information.

LONG-TERM MEMORY (KNOWLEDGE BASE). Long-term memory, sometimes called the knowledge base, is the permanent memory record or store of knowledge. It contains memories of personal experiences (episodes); general information; learned skills or routines; and knowledge of concepts, words, rules, strategies, and procedures; organizational principles; knowledge of frames; abstracted life scripts; goals; and self-concept. The system is thought to be highly organized, with multiple connections among related concepts. How information is stored and organized in semantic memory (e.g., in networks of semantic relations or in feature hierarchies, propositions, and schemes) is currently a matter of debate (Anderson, 1976; Rummelhart, 1984; Smith, 1978).

Professional interest in the integrity of long-term memory is often restricted to retrograde amnesia, the inability to recall events that were experienced during a period before the injury. However, the intactness of the *semantic* knowledge base has greater *functional* significance since this knowledge is involved in virtually every human activity. It is commonly reported that pre-traumatically acquired knowledge and skills return quite completely in all but the most severe cases of head injury (Kinsbourne & Wood, 1982). Our experience with large numbers of moderately and severely injured young adults, however, has been that in-depth academic and language testing reveals some reduction in semantic memory or major gaps in the system in most cases. Many patients continue to evidence a reduction in the pre-traumatically acquired knowledge base after resolution of PTA and the return of functional episodic memory. Furthermore, if the ability of a head injured young person to acquire new knowledge efficiently is also impaired, then the knowledge base will fail to *grow* and the effect of this combination of impairments on academic and vocational functioning becomes cumulative. Locating gaps in knowledge and re-establishing an individual's permanent organized knowledge base is, therefore, a primary target in the treatment of many head injured young adults.

EXECUTIVE SYSTEM. The "executive" system, based in part on an analogy with the role of a corporate executive and in part on the role of a computer's central processor, is involved in setting goals, assessing strengths and weaknesses within the system, planning and directing activity, initiating and inhibiting behavior, monitoring current activity, and evaluating results. Intact executive functioning makes possible the most efficient use of an individual's cognitive potential.

Impairments of executive functions among head injured young adults are common because they are associated with frontal lobe damage which is among the most predictable types of brain injury caused by head trauma (see Chapter 1). Shallow awareness of deficits and of their implications, and the resulting unrealistic goal setting, are among the most debilitating deficits in a vocational rehabilitation context (see Chapters 1, 5, and 6). Initiation and inhibition problems may make patients' social behavior quite inappropriate and may create the impression of greater disability than may in fact be the case. Impaired self-monitoring and self-evaluating of behavior also contribute to social inappropriateness and interfere with those real-life problem-solving activities which buttress independent living and successful employment.

RESPONSE SYSTEM. The response system controls all output, including gross and fine motor activity, speech, and facial expression. Impairments include observable neuromuscular involvement (e.g., weakness, spasticity, tremors), as well as motor planning problems (incoordination). Many patients whose recovery of motor ability is otherwise excellent continue to perform fine motor tasks slowly and to fatigue easily (see Chapter 2). Thorough cognitive assessment should include an investigation of the relationships between the response system and other processes and systems. If, for example, there is a problem in the response system (e.g., incoordination or balance problems), then a portion of "space" in working memory may be occupied by deliberate attempts to control motor functioning that is normally automatic, and the result is reduced *cognitive* effciency. This phenomenon is illustrated by those head injured patients who can converse effectively when seated comfortably but who cannot do so when walking or standing. Conversely, cognitive impairments can negatively affect motor output. Slow processing, for example, can create the appearance of an impaired motor system.

Functional-Integrative Performance

Functional-integrative performance is an individual's interaction with an environment in "real-life" activities (e.g., dressing, preparing meals, conversing, reading for pleasure, studying for a course, playing games, shopping, performing job-related tasks). A focus on functional-integrative performance in cognitive rehabilitation is essential for two reasons. First, it is a common clinical observation that improvements in component processes and systems are not automatically generalized to more functional tasks or to other situations. Second, improved performance in functional social, academic, and vocational settings is the ultimate criterion of the effectiveness of any treatment program.

Systematically tracking variations in performance in complex environmental interactions is not an easy task. Using the performance variables *efficiency, level, scope,* and *manner* has allowed us to maintain a focus on the ultimate value of CRT and to document for patients, family members, and others meaningful changes that have resulted from treatment. *Efficiency* is the *rate* at which performance occurs (which includes receiving and comprehending information), i.e., the *amount* that is accomplished in a *time* period in relation to some standard of quality of the performance. *Level* is the developmental, academic, or vocational level of an activity as it is measured on scales such as: simple to complex; concrete to abstract; low to high language level; early to late grade level. *Scope* refers to the variety of situations in which a performance level can be maintained (e.g., familiar or unfamiliar; structured or unstructured; quiet or noisy). A patient's scope of performance is often restricted following head injury because of problems in generalization. *Manner* refers to the characteristic style or way a task is performed, such as impulsive or reflective, flexible or rigid, dependent (needing cues) or independent, and active or passive. The manner of performance has an effect on the other performance variables; for example, if patients are highly inflexible in the way they perform, then their scope of activity will be restricted. Furthermore, the manner of performance profoundly affects cooperative activity.

The inclusion in this operational definition of cognition of the executive system and the factors that influence functional-integrative performance underscores the extensiveness of the territory covered by the term "cognition" as we are using it and, consequently, the considerable scope of CRT. The widespread use of computer programs and workbooks that are labeled "cognitive rehabilitation" but that focus only on cognitive processes — often basic-level cognitive processes, such as attention, perception, rote memory, simple organizing processes, and speed of basic processing — suggests that our broad concept of cognitive rehabilitation is not the standard approach to intervention. Although involving executive functions in the definition of cognition creates substantial overlap between CRT and psychosocial counseling, cognitive functioning cannot be understood without some explanation of the executive direction of the mechanism and of the cognitive basis of many apparent psychosocial problems. Including functional-integrative performance — and the performance variables efficiency, manner, scope, and level — in the definition as aspects of cognition ensures a programmatic focus on enabling patients to function independently in real-life settings, at meaningful levels of activity, and under real-life forms of stress. The all too common phenomenon of patients showing improved performance on therapy tasks or on neuropsychologic posttesting without being able to use these improvements in their daily lives is a result that a broad definition of cognition and CRT is designed to prevent.

Stages of Cognitive Recovery

Most severely head injured patients move through relatively predictable stages of cognitive recovery. The Rancho Los Amigos (RLA) Levels of Cognitive Recovery (Hagen, 1981) is an eight-stage scale that is widely used in hospitals and rehabilitation centers to track recovery. There are two important reasons to use a scale such as this. First, in cases in which it is possible to place a patient unambiguously at a certain level, clinicians may assume the appropriateness of the general program goals and intervention strategies that have been found to be important for patients at that level of recovery. Second, having a common and well-defined vocabulary of recovery helps clinicians communicate with each other.

There are, however, dangers in using any scale or set of levels, however general or detailed the levels might be. Because of the wide variety of pathophysiologic mechanisms that are involved in closed head injury, varying severity of injury, varying patterns of specific focal brain damage, and varying pre-traumatic characteristics, patients who resemble one another in certain respects may differ dramatically in others. A patient with significant focal right hemisphere damage, for example, whose overall orientation is significantly impaired (Level V or VI on the Rancho Los Amigos Scale) may have regained relatively sophisticated verbal and problem-solving skills. To design a cognitive rehabilitation program for such a patient solely on the basis of his or her gross disorientation and surface confusion would, of course, be a great mistake. It is more common than not for patients to have skills that are significantly scattered among levels of recovery. In addition, the use of general levels of recovery (e.g., the Glasgow Outcome Scale [Jennett, Snoek, Bond & Brooks, 1981]) may inadvertently blind rehabilitation professionals, family members, or third party payers to important functional gains that a patient has made or continues to make despite staying at the same global level of recovery. Finally, sensory and motor impairments may or may not accompany cognitive deficits at any stage of recovery, thereby further complicating unambiguous placement of patients at specific stages of recovery. These considerations suggest the value of an approach to intervention based on careful assessment and individualized treatment plans.

With these qualifications in mind, we have found it useful, from a very general programmatic perspective, to distinguish three broad stages of recovery that correspond to three qualitatively distinct phases of rehabilitation. During the *Early Stage* of recovery (roughly RLA II and III) patients are beginning to "wake up," to respond to some external events without, however, processing much, if any, of the meaning of these events. The principal focus of treatment at this stage is sensory and sensorimotor stimulation which is designed to increase patients' capacity for arousal, to promote recognition of objects or people in the environment, and to prevent the complications that result from sensory deprivation.

During the *Middle Stage* of recovery (roughly RLA V and VI), patients are alert and generally responsive to environmental events, but they are disoriented to some degree, unable to process information in depth, often unable to remember information effectively from day to day, and generally unable to maintain effective and appropriate social interaction. Rehabilitation during this stage focuses on reducing confusion and disorientation through careful environmental structuring, gradually and systematically improving general information processing abilities, and helping patients to regain access to their pre-traumatically acquired knowledge base. Attempts are made to improve patients' organizing abilities and learning efficiency within highly structured situations that promote *involuntary* learning (see Chapter 4).

During the *Late Stage* of recovery (roughly RLA VII, VIII, and beyond), patients are adequately oriented and capable of independent, adaptive behavior, at least in a familiar environment. Although not obviously confused, these patients may be more easily confus*able* than other people in environments that are novel or disorienting. Rehabilitation during this stage focuses on increasing patients' independence and adaptability to varied environments, refining their skills, enabling them to compensate for residual cognitive deficits, and generalizing their treatment gains to functional settings. At this stage attempts to improve most patients' memory and learning efficiency are grounded in the principles of *deliberate* learning which entails an instructional focus on metacognitive abilities (see Chapter 4).

Spontaneous neurologic recovery may slow or cease at any stage of recovery and the patient's response to direct retraining of impaired skills may stabilize at any stage, although the period of recovery following head injury is substantial. As a result, community re-entry decisions and preparations are required for patients at widely separated levels of functioning. Patients in the middle stages of recovery are generally discharged to home or to a facility capable of the intensity of supervision that their degree of confusion and disorientation requires. Vocational options are extremely limited, even when patients have no motor impairment (see Chapter 6). The chief responsibilities of rehabilitation staff in preparing a patient for community re-entry at this stage are (a) training future caretakers to provide the type and amount of environmental structuring and cuing that promote the patient's highest level of functioning and self-direction and (b) helping to create an avocational life for the patient that is as meaningful and satisfying as it can be (see Chapter 8). Re-entry issues for patients at higher levels of cognitive functioning are discussed in Chapters 5, 6, and 7.

Assessment and Diagnostic Therapy

As in any treatment program, assessing strengths and weaknesses is an integral part of cognitive rehabilitation. It is not our goal in this brief section to review tests or test batteries but rather to highlight some of the dangers that accompany the interpretation of formal assessment, and to recommend for rehabilitative planning a broadly focused "detective-work" approach to cognitive assessment that is guided by patient-specific hypotheses rather than by the constraints of fixed test batteries, and that also integrates the results of formal assessment with informal observation, diagnostic therapy, and interviews with patients and their families.

Rehabilitation goals rarely, if ever, flow automatically from formal assessment (Prigatano and others, 1986), which fails to measure many dimensions of functioning that are crucial to rehabilitation. For example, available tests do not formally survey a patient's awareness of cognitive deficits, and they lack standardized procedures that elicit spontaneously used strategies, measure their effects on functional task performance, or measure the effects of strategic suggestions on performance. Formal tests do not measure the efficiency of new learning of significant amounts of information over significant periods of time nor the patient's ability to generalize newly acquired skills to novel contexts. They also do not measure the effects that real-life forms of stress found in a work place or educational or social setting may have on the patient's ability to concentrate, to initiate appropriate problem-solving behavior, to remain oriented to assigned tasks, to flexibly shift orientation from task to task as demanded, or to communicate appropriately. These are exactly the areas in which many head injured individuals have chronic and troublesome problems as they attempt to resume meaningful vocational and social lives. It has often been observed that head injured patients frequently do not perform as well in real-life contexts as their performance in highly structured test situations would predict (Baxter, Cohen & Ylvisaker, 1985; Jennett & Teasdale, 1981; Prigatano and others, 1986). This phenomenon may be explained in part by the fact that although patients have often qute completely recovered pre-traumatically acquired information and skills they still have significant problems with new learning and with those executive functions discussed earlier in this chapter. Alternatively, some patients perform poorly on standardized tests, but are surprisingly effective in familiar, functional settings.

Several of these assessment problems are best addressed by a combination of interview, informal observation, and diagnostic therapy. Family members, teachers, and work supervisors often provide the most useful information regarding the effects of stress (including time pressure, performance expectations, and interpersonal stress) on the patient's functioning. Informally observing patients in a variety of social contexts is often the most important component of assessing communicative and general interactive skills. Diagnostic therapy, including systematic attempts to teach compensatory strategies, is generally the only means by which one can accurately assess (a) the efficiency with which patients learn new information, skills, or strategic procedures; (b) the factors that affect such learning; and (c) the ability to generalize these skills to novel contexts.

INTERVENTION

Forms of Cognitive Intervention

The process of improving cognitive functioning or of improving behavior that is impaired by cognitive deficits may take several forms. The appropriate combination of forms of intervention for a particular patient is often discovered only through a period of trial therapy.

Environmental Compensation

At any stage of recovery, adjustments in a head injured individual's physical or social environment and in the expectations of family, staff, and work supervisors may make the difference between successful adaptive behavior and failure. Clinicians familiar with the cognitive factors that influence the person's functioning may make their most significant contribution by informing and counseling family and staff in techniques of environmental compensation. (This point is discussed in some detail in Chapter 4 in the section entitled "Environmental Considerations".)

Component Retraining

There is some evidence that intensive cognitive retraining, through environmental exercises or drill and practice focused on a particular area of cognitive deficit, can restore to some extent impaired functions that are no longer recovering spontaneously (Ben-Yishay et al., 1982; Gummow et al., 1983). Research in this area is, however, not conclusive (Prigatano and others, 1986), and necessary clinical information is not yet available on the characteristics of good candidates for this type of intervention, specific cognitive processes or systems that are amenable to retraining, the type and amount of training that are optimal, or the generalization of improved underlying functioning brought about in a training environment to activities in a different environment. There appears to be a growing consensus that direct retraining ("mental muscle building") is not particularly effective in restoring complex functions such as memory (Harris, 1984).

Retraining can either be *direct,* that is, focused specifically on the impairment that one wishes to ameliorate, or *indirect,* that is, focused on a cognitive area that is related to the target deficit with the goal of improving functioning in the targeted area through improvements elsewhere in the system. Attempts to improve memory by improving attentional abilities or organizing processes are examples of indirect retraining (see Chapter 4).

Personal Compensation

Compensatory strategies — the procedures or external aids that a person uses deliberately to achieve goals that are difficult to achieve because of cognitive impairments — have received considerable attention in the recent literature on head injury rehabiliation (Haarbauer-Krupa, Henry, Szekeres & Ylvisaker, 1985; Prigatano and others, 1986; Wilson & Moffat, 1984). These strategies may be significant in cases in which a functionally impairing deficit is either not expected to resolve spontaneously, does not respond to retraining, or requires long-term retraining. If an individual's cognitive level supports the learning of new compensatory behavior, these strategies might enable the patient to be more functional than he or she would otherwise be. (Compensatory strategy intervention is dicussed at length in Chapter 4.)

Cognitive Instruction

Instruction that is designed to enhance the awareness and understanding of selected types of cognitive activity or process is an integral component of cognitive rehabilitation for many head injured adults. Most adults live productive and comfortable lives without ever developing this metacognitive awareness. Likewise, before brain injury, most patients never thought directly about such cognitive activities as attending or encoding information or mentally organizing information. Brain injury, however, often requires individuals to learn new information about themselves and the world. Previously automatic patterns of learning, interacting, and solving problems may no longer work. Demonstrating, discussing, and calling attention to these important issues in other ways are necessary elements in teaching a patient to compensate deliberately for a deficit. For some patients, such metacognitive instruction may contribute to improvements in performance even if the goal of instruction is not to teach the patient compensatory strategies. For example, simply understanding what organization is, why we organize things as we do, and the many alternative ways things can be organized has, in some cases, enhanced patients' organizational functioning. For other patients, carefully dissecting and learning the components of conversations (another type of knowledge not needed by non-brain damaged individuals) may be part of the process of improving their conversational skills.

In addition, explicit instruction in brain-behavior relationships, in the types of damage that can occur to the brain and the ways in which they influence thinking and behavior, and in a given patient's particular brain injury is an important component in the often difficult direct process of promoting self-awareness of strengths and weaknesses and in the indirect process of facilitating more realistic goals and more active engagement in treatment.

Functional-Integrative Training

Since brain injured individuals do not automatically transfer skills from a learning task to more complex functional activities which involve integrating many cognitive factors, or from a learning setting to the settings in which these skill will have to be used, attention to both forms of transfer or generalization is essential. Carefully planned functional-integrative training must be a phase of intervention, whether the focus of treatment is retraining or compensation. The specific targets of functional-integrative training are the performance variables (manner, level, scope, and efficiency) as they qualify real-life behaviors that are significant for an individual patient.

In Chapter 4, these forms of cognitive intervention are explored in greater depth, and their application in the treatment of specific cognitive deficits is discussed. For most patients, a combination of these forms of intervention is appropriate. Decisions about relative priorities — such as whether the program should emphasize specific compensatory procedures for functional deficits or concentrate rather on gradual long-term restoration of underlying cognitive processes and systems — depend on several factors, including the patient's profile of strengths and weaknesses, the patient's and family's goals, the severity of the injury and the length of time post-trauma, the patient's response to diagnostic therapy, the demands of the patient's discharge destination, the length of time that rehabilitative treatment is possible, and the economic resources of the family.

The complexity of these factors is illustrated by R.W., who was severely head injured at age 17. He was essentially unresponsive for 6 weeks and was admitted to The Rehabilitation Institute of Pittsburgh 9 months post-injury after a period of rehabilitation at another facility. R.W.'s wide range of physical, cognitive, and personality impairments included very severe memory and learning problems, a near total absence of awareness of his cognitive deficits, and a highly defensive, almost violent reaction to all suggestions that his goal of graduating from college and assuming a professional career was unrealistic. After an extended period of outpatient CRT, along with speech therapy, occupational therapy, physical therapy, and personal counseling, which produced few meaningful improvements in basic cognitive processes, the treatment team decided that its focus must be to convince R.W. and his family that his goal was completely unrealistic, that it was imperative that he consider a more modest and achievable vocational objective, and that he begin working on specific compensatory strategies to achieve that objective. Despite many painful sessions with the rehabilitation team, R.W. adhered resolutely to his own plan. The family purchased a computer for him and hired tutors and, after several failures, he passed his high school equivalency examinations. The family then left the Pittsburgh area. In their new location, R.W. registered for one or two courses per term at a local college, most of which he passed with extraordinary effort on his part, accommodations from teachers, and help from tutors. Two years later, he returned to Pittsburgh for a visit. He reported that he was still taking college courses, was working very hard, and was enjoying his life. Years before, R.W.'s therapists had clearly understood his cognitive deficits, but had inadequately estimated his extraordinary perseverance and commitment to a college experience, and the extent of his family's support for this goal and their willingness to provide whatever resources were necessary to give him a chance to achieve that goal.

Content of Cognitive Intervention

Cognitive rehabilitation is the attempt to improve a patient's functioning in areas of cognitive deficit. Given the broad operational definition of "cognition" that we have presented, the targets of treatment can range from very basic-level attentional and perceptual processes to very high-level reasoning and problem-solving processes, and from narrowly defined components of cognition to functional activities in real-life settings. The goals for a given patient must be based on that patient's profile of strengths and weaknesses, and on a decision as to what improvement would have the greatest impact on his or her life. In our discussion of aspects of cognition, we identified many areas of nonsocial cognitive functioning that are appropriate targets of cognitive remediation. In this section, we will highlight some unique features of social cognition that reveal both its importance and the difficulty of making it a focus of CRT.

Social Cognition

Social cognition may be distinguished from nonsocial cognition in terms of the "objects" of thought that are involved (i.e., what one thinks about). The objects of social thinking include people and their activities, relationships, feelings, intentions, motives, attitudes, institutions, and the like. The distinction between the two types of cognition, however, may not be adequately expressed in terms of differences between the cognitive processes or systems that are involved. "The head that thinks about the social world is the selfsame head that thinks about the nonsocial world" (Flavell, 1977, p. 122). Different areas of problems may thus have an underlying connection. For instance, psychosocial problems following head injury (see Chapter 1) can easily result, in part at least, from cognitive weakness. Cognitive rehabilitation therapists must thus understand similarities and differences that may exist in the processing and representation of social and nonsocial information, and recognize the necessity of integrating cognitive rehabilitation with psychosocial counseling.

Many parallels between social and nonsocial thinking have been proposed in the literature. Isen and Hastorf (1982) point out that nearly every behavior has a cognitive dimension. Shoben (1984) compared the episodic/semantic memory distinction to Hastie and Carlston's (1980) distinction between social event memory (knowledge of specific people and events) and conceptual social memory (general knowledge of social characteristics of situations). Black, Galambos, and Read (1984) drew parallels between the processing of social information and discourse processing. They emphasized that in both types of processing, causally linking events (attribution) is important and is the key to memory.

Although similarities between social and nonsocial processing are impressive and justify a concern for social thinking in CRT, there are some suggestions that social and nonsocial information may be represented differently in long-term memory (Wyer & Gordon, 1984). Holyoak and Gordon (1984) have suggested that social categories are even more "fluid" than nonsocial categories because humans can play a number of different roles and exhibit a variety of traits and characteristics. Social categories are also less formally related in hierarchical fashion. Cantor, Mischel, and Schwartz (1982) found that social categories are also less well defined, more idiosyncratic, and more likely determined by personality factors than nonsocial categories. These factors contribute to the biases that frequently dominate social thinking.

These features of social categories can have powerful treatment implications. For example, staff members, patient, and family members may have fundamentally different concepts of key social categories such as "independent living," "home," and "family." If to the independent living counselor "home" means the lack of autonomy or opportunity for his or her client's personal growth, to the family it means an environment of nurturing and family togetherness, and to the patient it means the chance to be near old friends, then meaningful communication between these parties about independent living goals is unlikely.

The social world also imposes special processing demands (Isen & Hastorf, 1982). For example, social interaction (e.g., a conversation) tends to be variable and unpredictable; one cannot stop to examine social interaction without changing it. Moreover, the factors that dominate social thinking and social interpretation — intentions, feelings, attitudes, and the like — are "hidden" and must be inferred from behaviors that may be subtle. These features of social processing make it especially vulnerable to processing deficits, thereby necessitating careful attention to social cognition in head injury rehabilitation. Treatment issues are further discussed in Chapter 6.

Selecting and Sequencing Treatment Objectives

The complexity of cognition, the variety of cognitive processes and systems, the interrelationships among them, and the number of behaviors affected by cognitive deficits combine to create a genuine problem for cognitive rehabilitation therapists: Where do we start? What do we work on? Where do we go next? When a patient is referred for short-term CRT because of specific cognitive problems that interfere in readily identifiable ways with vocational, academic, or social functioning, the selection of treatment objectives may be relatively straightforward. Cognitive rehabilitation therapists often play an important role in problem solving with patients and their families, employers, or teachers with the goal of overcoming specific obstacles to success through environmental modifications, compensatory strategies, or targeted remedial exercises.

However, when cognitive problems are more pervasive, when specific objectives are not clearly identified in the referral for services, and when there exists the luxury of more time in which to pursue cognitive rehabilitation, then the clinicians' questions are placed in sharp relief: Where do we start? What do we work on? Where do we go next?

Assessment and Brain-Behavior Relationships

The apparently most obvious and straightforward answer to these questions is that treatment should begin with those areas of cognitive functioning which neuropsychological assessment has found to be impaired (Reitan, 1980). To help patients achieve and maintain their most effective thinking, it is necessary to identify those deficits which appear to be blocking effective thinking. Furthermore, with an adequate understanding of brain-behavior relationships, clinicians can look to radiographic, neurologic, and neuropsychological evidence to construct a picture of the relatively intact and relatively damaged parts of the brain. With this information in hand, they then either create training exercises to strengthen functioning in areas of greatest damage or design compensations that are effective precisely because they take greatest advantage of intact cortical areas in compensating for those that are damaged.

Although sensible treatment depends on a thorough assessment of cognitive strengths and weaknesses, formal assessment does not, by itself, dictate the selection and sequencing of treatment objectives or the choice of intervention forms. (See the section earlier in this chapter cautioning against the misuse of formal assessment.) Furthermore, although there is great value in having neuropathologic information and knowing brain-behavior relationships, particularly in the contexts of selecting compensatory strategies and deciding whether to approach a behavioral problem through self-control techniques or through environmental modifications, as with other assessment data this information does not indicate which aspects of cognition are particularly important in effecting meaningful change in a given patient's performance nor does it dictate answers to general intervention questions, such as that of compensation versus restoration.

Cognitive Development

All treatment decisions in CRT should be made with an eye toward the ultimate goal of enabling a patient to engage effectively and independently in meaningful functional-integrative activities in a setting that is as normal as possible. The questions listed above about selecting and sequencing objectives may, thus, be translated initially into the question: What improvements in cognitive functioning will have the greatest effect on the patient's movement toward the ultimate goal of treatment? Since normal cognitive *development* indicates in a general way the kinds of thinking and changes in thinking that move a person from very dependent and ineffective functioning to adult-level cognitive functioning, the research literature on cognitive development suggests a progression that helps to guide clinicians through the largely uncharted territory of cognitive rehabilitation.

The use of patterns of cognitive development as guides for sequencing objectives in cognitive rehabilitation is not meant to suggest that patients systematically regress developmentally after brain injury in all areas of functioning. It is rather to suggest that features of cognitive development reveal relationships among cognitive processes and systems that are important to cognitive growth, whether that growth occurs during normal human development or during rehabilitation following brain injury. Furthermore, in some respects head injured adults *do* exhibit thinking behaviors characteristic of earlier developmental periods. They often have difficulty with abstract concepts, are impulsive, make poor judgments, have difficulty imposing organization, lack ability in strategic thinking and problem solving, have poor self-awareness, and have an egocentric outlook on life. Clinicians face the challenge of using their knowledge of cognitive development in designing tasks that are respectful of adults' self-concept, maturity, and pre-traumatic knowledge while at the same time providing them with optimal learning situations to re-establish cognitive skills.

The extensive literature on cognitive development indicates that virtually every aspect of cognitive functioning has a developmental dimension. Flavell's (1977) categories of cognitive change outline the general flow of cognitive development. By creating tasks that encourage movement along these dimensions, clinicians can systematically encourage more adult-like thinking, recognizing that all of us revert on occasion to thinking that is concrete, superficial, and egocentric. Some of Flavell's categories of cognitive change are:

- *surface to depth:* ranging from attention to superficial characteristics of objects, persons, and events to a focus on underlying causes and inferred meanings.
- *centration to decentration:* ranging from an egocentric concern with the immediate situation and its effects on the self to a perception of more features and an ability to take alternative perspectives. Subcategories include:
  - *time:* ranging from an exclusive concern with the present to an awareness of the past and the future and the ability to understand the causal antecedents and consequences of events;
  - *space:* ranging from perception largely focused on perceptually salient objects and events to the ability to scan an environment for desired information; and
  - *person:* ranging from an absorption with self to the ability to take other peoples' perspectives.
- *qualitative to quantitative:* ranging from gross qualitative judgments about things and people to more precise quantitative judgments that evidence an understanding of proportions, degrees of feelings, and balanced interactions.
- *concrete to abstract/hypothetical:* ranging from an ability to think only about concrete physical things and people and to solve problems only by trial and error with real objects and with out strategies, to thinking about possibilities, reflecting on past

behavior, reasoning hypothetically, experimenting strategically, and comprehending abstract attributes, relationships, and principles.

- *growth of the knowledge base:* including adding information and restructuring or reorganizing knowledge of objects, people, and events which enables individuals to assimilate new information in an increasingly efficient manner.

In recent research more specific aspects of cognitive development have also been isolated:

- *increased efficiency or capacity:* The speed of processing (Gitomer, Pellegrino & Bisanz, 1983; Kail & Bisanz, 1982), the capacity of working memory (Chi, 1978), and the flexibility of the retrieval system (Ceci & Howe, 1978a) have all been found to increase with age, while reaction time decreases (Kail & Siegel, 1977). These changes may result from increases in the amount and organization of knowledge (Chi, 1976, 1978; Gitomer et al., 1983).
- *increased goal directedness:* Deliberateness and persistence in thinking about problems increase with age (Gordon & Flavell, 1977).
- *situational discrimination:* The awareness of the situational appropriateness of engaging in certain activities, including applying strategic procedures, increases with age (Campione, 1980).
- *increased self-monitoring of task performance:* (Pressley, Forrest-Pressley, Elliot-Faust & Miller, 1985).
- *awareness of self and limitations* (Tenney, 1975); *internal memory monitoring* (Lodico, Ghatala, Levin, Pressley & Bell, 1983); *knowledge monitoring* (Markman, 1979); *involuntary to deliberate memory* (Brown, 1975, 1979; Istominia, 1975): Together these constitute much of what is called "metacognition" and explain a great deal about the development of stategic thinking in childhood. The progression involuntary-to-deliberate memory culminates in *automatic* strategic behavior, enabling learners to use strategies without devoting space in working memory to strategic thinking (Pressley et al., 1985).

Clinicians may, then, refer to these fundamental dimensions of cognitive development to understand the extent of a patient's deficit and to determine the general directions, objectives, and activities that might most effectively produce positive changes in the patient's cognitive system. These developmental considerations support a very *general* treatment hierarchy which moves from concrete to abstract thinking tasks and from externally-focused processing to processing that includes self-reflection and deliberate compensation. This general hierarchy is reflected in the cognitive rehabilitation program outlined in Figure 3–1.

It is important to note that component processes and systems (e.g., attention, perception, categorical and sequential organization, memory, reasoning, and executive direction) do not develop in a serial progression, but rather interact throughout childhood development. Each process and system has simple and developmentally very early forms and also complex and developmentally late forms. A 6 month old infant, for example, has growing but still limited selective attention skills, has a developing set of perceptual categories, can anticipate simple repeated sequences, understands certain communicative gestures embedded in a routine context, and is learning at an increasing rate. As the knowledge base grows and as organizational skills improve, the child's ability to maintain attention, to filter out distractions, and to divide attention increases. In a reciprocal fashion, as attentional skills mature, the ability to acquire and organize knowledge likewise matures. A scheme of cognitive development thus cannot be used to justify treatment that is rigidly sequenced from "lower" attentional and psychomotor to "higher" verbal and organizational cognitive processes; it serves rather as an invitation to consider the ways in which a patient's dynamically interacting cognitive processes can be manipulated to make the functioning of the entire system more efficient.

Task Analysis

A third possible answer to the questions which opened this section (Where do we start? What do we work on? Where do we go next?) is to identify those important tasks which the patient may want or need to do but cannot do, analyze the tasks and divide them into components, discover which components obstruct the completion of the task, and then set as an objective the patient's automatic performance of these components so that the tasks can be performed in their entirety with greater facility. One of the most essential and effective tools possessed by clinicians who work with brain injured individuals is the ability to analyze complex tasks, divide them into components, and assess the perceptual, motor, cognitive, psychosocial, and academic demands placed on the individual by the task as a whole and by each part (Table 4–5). Such analysis enables clinicians to determine the points at which breakdowns in processing occur, to fine-tune intervention, and to avoid frustrating patients with unanticipated task difficulties. Using task analysis to select and sequence objectives is particularly useful for those patients who are at a stage of treatment at which their primary goal is performing specific functional-integrative activities, not improving cognitive functioning in general (see Chapter 8).

Although using task analysis and diagnostic therapy to locate breakdowns in a patient's functioning contributes to the process of selecting appropriate objectives, task analysis does *not* by itself yield a sequenced set of treatment objectives or activities for a patient. Having determined, for example, that a patient performs very slowly in a job training context because he or she cannot filter out distracting sights and sounds in the work place, a clinician must choose among the following treatment options (which are not mutually exclusive): (a) engaging the patient in intensive retraining exercises that specifically target selective attention. This option requires another decision: designing the selective attention exercises so that they involve as few cognitive processes and systems as possible, particularly avoiding higher-level thought processes; or designing the exercises so that the focus is selective attention, while making the activities and contexts as much like the work situation as possible; (b) modifying the work environment to reduce distractions; or (c) teaching the patient attention-focusing strategies that he or she can deliberately use to remain on task and improve work speed. In summary, choosing treatment objectives and activities intelligently requires both careful deliberation and a period of investigative diagnostic therapy.

Training/Teaching Procedures

Theories that explain change in cognitive functioning (or learning) are useful sources of cognitive treatment procedures. Although theory is helpful in this respect, selecting teaching or treatment procedures for individual patients is guided primarily by the assumption that instructional strategies, like compensatory strategies, must be adapted to each patient. In this section, we briefly discuss four distinct types of procedures that can be used to promote change in cognitive behavior. The application of these procedures is by no means mutually exclusive, and for most patients there is a stage of recovery or a treatment objective for which each of the procedures is appropriate. These procedures are discussed in terms of the overall perspective on which they are based.

1. *Learning theory,* with its emphasis on contingencies of reinforcement including social, emotional, and informative feedback, has yielded a set of procedures for effecting change and maintaining motivation the effectiveness of which has been documented in a wide variety of treatment areas (Bandura, 1977; Harter 1978; Miller & Dollard, 1941; Skinner, 1969). Change can be produced either directly, through systematic reinforcement of target behaviors, or indirectly, through modeling. For many patients whose motivation is low and whose cognitive skills are weak, it may be necessary to use strict behavior modification techniques including clear instructions to the patient and tangible reinforcement for compliance. Modeling, on the other hand, presupposes a higher level of motivation, attention, memory, and reasoning. Since motivation and initation are often the primary obstacles to progress in therapy, Ben-Yishay and Diller (1983) recommended that a set of inspirational techniques be added to the more standard techniques of behavioral management. These include verbal exhortation, evocative metaphors, the inspirational techniques of a revivalist preacher, psychodrama, and requests that the patient make public assertion of commitment.

2. *Cognitive behavior modification* (Meichenbaum, 1977) adds to traditional learning theory a useful emphasis on self-instruction as a means to control and mediate one's behavior. The techniques of cognitive behavior modification are useful in many areas of cognitive rehabilitation, particularly the teaching of compensatory strategies. Their effective use presupposes on the part of a patient an awareness of deficits, an adequate ability to initiate behavior or at least to use external cues to initiate behavior, a motivation to change, and an understanding of the target behavior. Feuerstein's (1980) techniques of mediated learning, discussed in Chapter 4, have a similar focus on understanding and controlling one's own cognitive behavior.

3. Piaget's explanatory principles, *assimilation* and *accommodation,* provide a somewhat different perspective on learning, somewhat akin to the involuntary learning situation described above. Individuals add to their knowledge and restructure their conceptual framework through interaction with the environment (Piaget, 1970). As they interpret events and objects in terms of what is already known (assimilation) they simultaneously take into account unknown properties and relations (accommodation). Balancing these two adaptive mechanisms gradually modifies schemata of interaction and results in cognitive growth. Cognitive growth can, therefore, be promoted when tasks are presented that have some components that can be easily understood in terms of current knowledge schemata and also other components that require some schematic modification

for the task to be completed. Because learning occurs primarily through discovery, the key to effective treatment is designing tasks that create optimal conditions for discovering targeted information or cognitive schemata. As with modeling, it is unlikely that this approach would be productive with patients who have significant attentional, motivational, or episodic memory problems since it assumes that cognitive growth is driven by a desire to solve problems and requires the storing of experienced episodes from which to extract new principles or procedures.

4. It has been known at least since the time of Aristotle that most people desire understanding for its own sake; Francis Bacon added the insight that one of the fruits of knowledge is power and control over the natural and social environment. The natural inclination to ask "Why?" and to construct causal explanations has been highlighted in recent discussions of social behavior by attribution theorists (Heider, 1958; Jones & Nisbett 1972; Weiner, 1979). We have found it useful in CRT to encourage this disposition to ask "Why?", to ponder ideas and events, to reject gaps in knowledge and understanding, and to persistently question one's own interpretations and explanations of behavior and events.

Individualizing Objectives and Procedures

In designing intervention programs for special populations, it is tempting to identify the central problems of the population, to isolate a sequence of steps that is known or predicted to be effective as treatment for many members of the population, to establish intervention techniques that are similarly effective for many members of the population, and then to construct a "curriculum" that is used for all individuals in the group regardless of the extent of their deviation from group norms. This well-motivated desire to sequence treatment objectives and activities in order to re-establish systematically a patient's cognitive skills following head injury can lead to such a head injury "curriculum."

Our experience with a large number of head injured children and adults suggests that, although careful sequences of objectives are exceedingly important for each individual patient, the sequences used for individual patients can differ quite dramatically for several reasons. The effects of cognitive intervention are ultimately a result of dynamic interactions among the patient (including his or her pretraumatic personality and educational/vocational level and posttraumatic goals, interests, coping style, and cognitive profile), the therapist (including his or her personality, interactive style, clinical skill, and conceptual framework), the treatment tasks (including types of task and duration of treatment), and the environment in which the patient must function (including the family and other support systems and the demands on the patient's abilities).

Difficulty Level

It is an important principle of treatment to engage patients in tasks that have a therapeutic effect, yet are easy enough that overall success at the task is guaranteed. One gains no advantage from frustrating patients, unless the specific objective is to break through a stubborn denial of deficits. However, the relative difficulty of tasks varies from patient to patient, depending upon deficit patterns, background, and interests. For example, a patient with specific right hemisphere damage but well-recovered language and reasoning skills will find purportedly "higher" level verbal and reasoning tasks easier than purportedly "lower" level perceptual scanning tasks. In this instance, adding reading to the patient's scanning training may *decrease* the difficulty of the task (because scanning from far left to right is encouraged by the meaning of the sentence) rather than adding to it, as one might easily infer from most hierarchies of cognitive processes.

The level of difficulty of a task is also intimately related to the specific interests of the patients. Psychomotor tasks, for instance, that are designed to be very simple and to involve few cognitive processes (e.g., reaction time tasks with light stimuli) may, in fact, demand much of a patient's limited attentional resources if the patient perceives no utility in the task and no meaning in the stimuli. A clinician in this case might prefer to work on the patient's speed of processing by using simple arithmetic problems rather than conceptually "simpler" but non-meaningful stimuli. The meaning and utility that certain patients recognize in academic materials may make their task easier and accelerate their improvement in "lower" level attending skills and rate of processing. Other patients may benefit more from tasks that do not confound the attending or speed objective with semantically meaningful stimuli.

Finally, skilled clinicians can use cuing and prompting to simplify tasks that, on the surface, may appear to be too complex and difficult for a patient. For example, a patient who is working on detecting main ideas and integrating information may, with adequate cues, use adult-level reading material for this purpose despite a significant reading impairment. For these reasons, considerations of task difficulty will not support a rigidly "curricular" ordering of treatment objectives and activities, although it is essential that each patient move systematically and gradually from tasks that are simple for that patient to those that are more difficult for him or her.

Patterns of Impairment

Pathophysiologic mechanisms in closed head injury are highly complex (Pang, 1985) and result in cognitive profiles that can be very diverse. Many patients are relatively unaffected in areas addressed by most head injury programs, such as attentional functioning and speed of processing. Others are impaired in these areas, but they have good reasoning and problem-solving skills that can be refined and used in teaching the patient to compensate for the "lower-level" impairments. There are also those who are impaired in these areas and who do not profit from the standard "bottom-up" approach to cognitive remediation. Again, this variety in the population argues against a rigidly applied serial order of retraining tasks within a cognitive rehabilitation program.

Although it is hardly novel, the conclusion to be drawn from these considerations is fundamental: Each head injured patient is unique, and treatment programs must be individualized to reflect this uniqueness.

General Principles of Intervention

The seven principles that are listed here encapsulate several of the themes that we have stressed in this chapter and that underlie the discussion of intervention strategies in Chapter 4. It is our conviction that adherence to these principles in cognitive rehabilitation serves patients' ultimate goal: effective and independent performance of meaningful functional-integrative activities in a setting that is as normal as possible.

Principle 1: Success, which results from controlling the difficulty of tasks, appropriately adjusting performance expectations, and compensating for deficits, both facilitates patient's progress and builds a productive self concept. In designing therapy tasks, clinicians must be respectful of the patient's age and status in the family and community, but must also create an atmosphere that assures the patient that it is both understood and expected that some very basic abilities may be missing and that some very basic knowledge may be inaccessible. Many of our patients have confided that they are troubled when friends and relatives assume they have recovered more of their pre-traumatic knowledge and abilities than they actually have. Patients in this situation tend to be easily embarrassed, and they become reluctant to ask for information or help.

Principle 2: A systematic gradation of activities involving progressive increases in cognitive demands can facilitate cognitive recovery. Demands are gradually increased in the areas of efficiency, level, scope, and manner of performance (see the discussion of these areas above) with the objective of enabling a patient to function independently under conditions of real-life stress. During this process, responsibility for controlling the difficulty level of tasks is moved from clinician to patient.

Principle 3: Habituation and generalization training are necessary for meaningful learning. Many trials are often necessary to make a patient's use of cognitive skills or strategies automatic. It may be necessary to train a patient in a variety of settings and under a variety of conditions to promote generalization. Instructing a patient in how to transfer a skill from one situation to another may also be necessary.

Principle 4: It is essential to patients' motivation and independence that clinicians encourage them to take the initiative in setting goals, planning treatment activities, and solving problems. The ability to see meaningful connections between treatment activities and personal goals presupposes some understanding of current deficits. Patients who fail to see these connections are unlikely to profit from these activities. Patients who become accustomed to yielding control over goals and activities to clinicians, family members, or others reduce their chances for successful community re-entry.

Principle 5: A patient's orientation, learning, and generalization are facilitated when the patient's family and the rehabilitation staff have similar expectations of performance and make consistent and similar demands on the patient. Treatment approaches that are inconsistent or not adequately integrated compound the already sizable generalization problem that brain injured individuals have. This principle is a strong rationale for interdisciplinary programming and for the use of printed forms or diagrams that represent the thinking procedures or strategies that the patient is learning (see Chapter 4). These forms structure not only the patient's thinking but also that of the clinicians.

Principle 6: Chronological age; pre-traumatic social, educational, and vocational status; and current developmental level of cognitive functioning must all be considered in designing tasks. It is possible to design therapy tasks that use interesting or vocationally meaningful adult-level materials and activities, but that make only low-level cognitive demands.

Principle 7: Group therapy is a useful context for developing patients' social cognition and interactive skills and for increasing their understanding of head injury and its consequences. Individual therapy is generally necessary for very specific problems. Head injured patients profit from the support and feedback of peers, from peer modeling, and from peer encouragement. At the same time, a solid relationship with a clinician, which can be developed in individual sessions, is often the foundation patients need to face more threatening social situations.

COGNITIVE REHABILITATION AND SPECIAL EDUCATION

The "community" that a head injured patient re-enters following severe head injury may include work, independent living, recreational pursuits, and home and family. Rehabilitation in relation to these aspects of community re-entry is discussed, respectively, in Chapters 5 through 9. For many head injured adolescents, the community that they re-enter also includes school. Educational programming for head injured patients is rarely addressed in the rehabilitation literature. Since the special education classroom is often a head injured individual's only setting for cognitive rehabilitation, a brief discussion of this important issue is included here.

Presently there are no formal educational programs or classroom categories for this population. A body of literature is developing in which educational programming for head injured individuals is described (Cohen, 1986; Cohen, Joyce, Rhoades & Welks, 1985; National Task Force on Special Education, 1985; Rosen & Gerring, 1986), but research is needed on the effectiveness of varying approaches and techniques. The intensity of services required depends on the individual's level of recovery and the severity of impairments, and may range from a self-contained special education classrooom to a part-time tutor or counselor.

Classroom placement serves a valuable diagnostic purpose. Since academic activities and the classroom environment itself often make greater demands on cognitive functioning and require a higher level of skill integration than individual therapy sessions customarily do, observations of the students' learning rates and styles in this more normal environment usually contribute a more complete body of information than that obtained from formal cognitive assessment and CRT sessions. Therapists and teachers may become aware of previously unobserved behaviors that need to be modified, of impairments that emerge only when stress or learning demands are substantially increased, and of strategies that need to be developed so that students can function more effectively. The information gathered from classroom observations in a rehabilitation center helps the staff make realistic educational recommendations when students are discharged to community schools.

Cognitive Issues

School programs for students with head injuries must emphasize the development of cognitive skills (Cohen, 1986). The goals, principles, content, and techniques of cognitive rehabilitation (discussed in this chapter and in Chapter 4) must thus be incorporated into educational programs in which teachers help students focus on the learning process, develop metacognitive awareness, establish compensatory strategies, and develop and generalize skills.

Teachers often find it difficult *not* to focus directly on academic progress. However, for head injured students it is typically more effective to use academic materials to develop general cognitive skills such as flexible thinking, expressive organization, and on-topic responses than to focus exclusively on academic content. Head injured students must have cognitive abilities in place before significant academic progress can be made. The profiles of head injured students may be extremely varied when higher-level skills that were learned before the accident are combined with much lower-level skills that result from the brain injury. Although in some cases basic reading, writing, spelling, and arithmetic skills are intact or relearned rather easily, in other cases there is a wide scatter among the academic levels. In either case, students' previously learned skills are usually superior to their current abilities to learn and integrate new information. Teachers must be flexible when programming for this population in order to accommodate all levels of functioning. They may have to individualize programs for students within groups, provide one-to-one instruction, change teaching goals and techniques frequently, and develop customized strategies to accommodate students' unique needs. Since head injured students often do not generalize skills, teachers should also relate the development of academic skills to real-life situations, e.g., developing math skills by grocery shopping. Social skills can be role played and then discussed in classroom group activities. Cohen and colleagues (1985) discussed in detail educational programs for students with head injuries and pointed out similarities and differences between these students and other students with learning problems.

Skilled teachers can help these students recognize their present levels of functioning and accept the need to work on academic processes and materials that are significantly less sophisticated than those they used before their injuries. In time, students may realize that they cannot resume their previous academic programs and may then accept as meaningful more functional academic or prevocational programs.

Educational Assessment

Educational assessments have not been developed specifically for the head injured population. Diagnosticians can, however, administer subtests from different levels of standardized instruments to relate students' present abilities to the graded teaching process. Moreover, examiners can use the assessment process to identify behaviors that indicate cognitive strengths and weaknesses, such as attentiveness versus distractibility, organized versus fragmented thinking and expression, flexibility versus perseveration, deliberate versus impulsive manner, and abstract versus concrete thinking. In addition, test instruments can be used to determine if comprehension breaks down when the materials increase in length and complexity (Cohen, 1986).

Great caution must be exercised when predicting classroom performance from test scores. Reasons for interpreting formal test results with caution are discussed earlier in this chapter. Head injured students with generally inconsistent behaviors, impairments in concentrating and organizing information, processing breakdowns with lengthy or complex material, inefficient storage and retrieval, and the inability to generalize may perform better on short, formal test items than they do on longer and more complicated classroom assignments. Teachers should develop educational programs by noting students' performance on specific test items in terms of cognitive strengths and weaknesses as well as academic abilities. Assessment should then continue through the use of prescriptive teaching in the classroom.

ISSUES IN PROGRAM MANAGEMENT

To be effective, a CRT program must have a conceptual framework that staff understand and accept, a well-defined structure, an interdisciplinary scope, careful monitoring of patients' progress, and efficient program direction. These elements of program management are discussed briefly in this section. For a more detailed discussion, see Cohen and Titonis (1985).

CONCEPTUAL FRAMEWORK. A framework of the sort outlined earlier in the chapter provides clinicians with a common set of concepts and a vocabulary that enables them to communicate clearly both with each other and also with patients and families about program goals and patient functioning. Since cognitive rehabilitation is not a formal discipline, key terms such as "cognition," "thought organization," "problem solving," "episodic memory," "executive functions," and many others may not have agreed upon meanings. Furthermore, treatment processes, such as those focusing on the development of metacognitive awareness, are not well established.

PROGRAM STRUCTURE. A clearly defined structure delineates general program goals, aspects of service delivery, and specific treatment approaches and establishes continuity throughout a patient's program. The overall structure of the CRT program at The Rehabilitation Institute of Pittsburgh is outlined in Figure 3–1. Patients receive treatment in both group and individual sessions, but not all patients receive all of the services that are represented in Figure 3–1. Decisions about treatment goals and procedures and about the appropriate mix of individual and group therapies are made by the treatment team on the basis of the patient's specific deficits and needs, and are revised as needed. The overall program is flexible and changes as the staff continues to learn more about head injury and cognition rehabilitation.

The program structure should also create efficient procedures for documenting and reporting a patient's total program and for providing family training. For example, a single team member, the patient's primary therapist, who generally sees that patient for individual

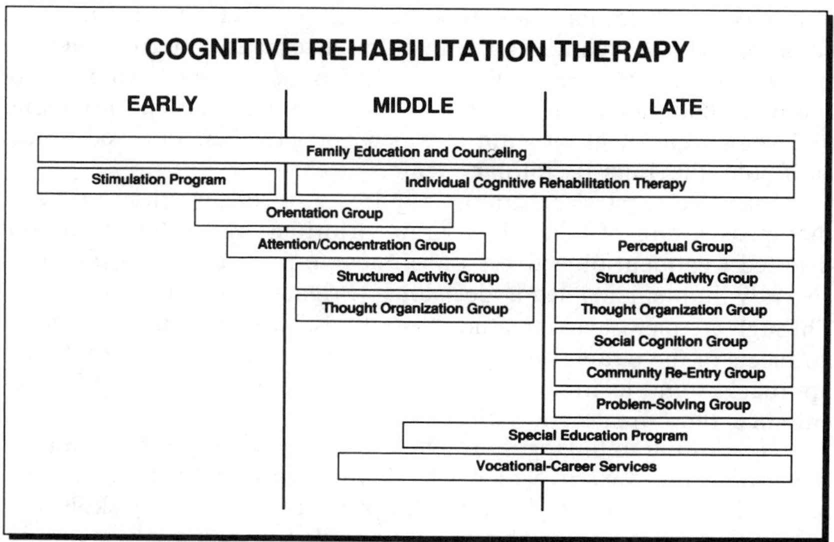

Figure 3–1. A general treatment hierarchy for the cognitive rehabilitation program.

therapy and has the most thorough knowledge of his or her abilities and needs, may assume these documentation and training responsibilities.

The Interdisciplinary Team

Although cognitive rehabilitation is not a formal discipline, it is a service that is provided in many rehabilitation centers (Gianutsos, 1980; McGonagle, Carper & Balicki, 1983; Palmer, 1985; Prigatano & Fordyce, 1986). Because many of the areas of treatment in cognitive rehabilitation have traditionally been the focus of other rehabilitation disciplines, CRT programs are often staffed by therapists from diverse fields, such as psychology, speech-language pathology, occupational therapy, and special education. When therapists from different disciplines treat a head injured patient and do not coordinate their services, programming is inevitably fragmented and can be confusing and detrimental to the patient. Therapists may use different or conflicting approaches to the same problem and their treatment goals may focus on too wide a variety of deficits. Interdisciplinary treatment brings together therapists who have a variety of skills and who understand cognitive functioning and remediation. At The Rehabilitation Institute of Pittsburgh, the interdisciplinary team is composed of speech-language pathologists, occupational therapists, and special educators — all of whom deliver CRT services in consultation with psychologists who administer and interpret neuropsychological assessments. Patients' CRT programs can expand into the more complex environments of the special education classroom and work adjustment program at which point teachers and vocational staff join the interdisciplinary team.

Interdisciplinary programs require clinical direction to keep therapists aware of general program priorities while they focus on detailed treatment objectives, and to ensure that each clinician consistently implements team decisions (Prigatano & Fordyce, 1986). Through frequent team treatment meetings, team members integrate all facets of the patient's program while they also learn one anothers' approaches and techniques, expand their theoretical framework, and enhance their treatment skills.

In addition to having thorough knowledge of the cognitive mechanism and the ways in which it is disrupted by severe brain injury, effective cognitive rehabilitation therapists have certain key skills and personal characteristics. They must be skilled in task analysis and in techniques of retraining and compensation. They must exhibit flexibility when deciding with team members which focus of intervention is appropriate for individual patients. They must be familiar with metacognitive thinking and the role that it plays in cognitive rehabilitation. They must know when to integrate specific treatment objectives into a variety of functional tasks. They must be able to interact effectively and respectfully with adult patients, motivating them to participate in rehabilitation while at the same time heightening their awareness of deficits if necessary. They must be good observers of behavior and be able to use behavior management techniques effectively. They must appreciate individual differences in patients' learning styles, lifestyles, goals, and attitudes. They must be able to teach family members about head injury and cognitive problems and provide the family with training that will enable them to become members of the rehabilitation team. They must maintain objectivity in response to anger and hostility from patients and family members. They must be committed to interdisciplinary team intervention.

Monitoring and Follow-up

Recovery following severe head injury can continue for several years, and spontaneous changes over time, like responses to intervention, are often unpredictable. As a result, treatment goals may need to be revised frequently. In addition, changes in patients' awareness of present levels of functioning influence treatment approaches. For instance, after months of resisting treatment and of frustrating and unsuccessful attempts to resume pre-traumatic activities, a patient may begin to realize the effects of the injury. Consequently, the focus of treatment may change dramatically. Treatment plans are also affected by limitations on programming that are imposed by funding sources or by discharge requests by patients or families. Together, these variables indicate the need for flexible planning, close monitoring of each patient's program, and scheduled follow-up after discharge.

Program Direction

Because cognitive rehabilitation programs address many issues and recovery from head injury can result in rapid or unpredictable changes, CRT programs require intensive direction. Large head injury rehabilitation programs may require two levels of managment: a program coordinator who manages patients' overall rehabilitation program, including admissions, funding, referral for services, discharge plans, and other administrative functions; and a cognitive rehabilitation clinical services facilitator who works with the interdisciplinary treatment team to develop and monitor treatment programs for patients that emphasize continuity of goals and the appropriate integration of services. At The Rehabilitation Institute of Pittsburgh, these two program managers work with a CRT Steering Committee, with representation from each of the departments involved in the program, to update the program as knowledge in the field expands, coordinate training of staff, and ensure interdepartmental cooperation in program development. Cohen and Titonis (1985) discuss management issues in greater detail.

REFERENCES

Anderson, J. (1976). *Language, memory, and thought.* Hillsdale, NJ: Lawrence Erlbaum Assoc.

Anderson, J. & Bower, G. (1972). Recognition and retrieval processes in free recall. *Psychological Review, 79,* 97–123.

Baddeley, A. (1982). Amnesia: A minimal model and interpretation. In L. Cermak (Ed.), *Human memory and amnesia* (pp. 305–335). Hillsdale, NJ: Lawrence Erlbaum Assoc.

Bandura, A. (1977). *Social learning theory.* Englewood Cliffs, NJ:: Prentice-Hall.

Bartlett, F. C. (1932). *Remembering: An experimental and social study.* Cambridge: University Park Press.

Baxter, R., Cohen, S. & Ylvisaker M. (listed alphabetically) (1985). Comprehensive cognitive assessment. In M. Ylvisaker (Ed.), *Head injury rehabilitation: Children and adolescents* (pp. 247–274). San Diego: College-Hill Press.

Ben-Yishay, Y. & Diller, L. (1983). Cognitive remediation. In M. Rosenthal, E. Griffith, M. Bond & J. Miller (Eds.), *Rehabilitation of the head injured adult* (pp. 367–380). Philadelphia: F. A. Davis.

Ben-Yishay, Y., Rattok, J., Ross, B., Lakin, P., Ezrachi, O., Silver, S. & Diller L. (1982). Rehabilitation of cognitive and perceptual deficits in people with traumatic brain damage: A five-year clinical research study. In *Working approaches to remediation of cognitive deficits in brain damaged persons* (Rehabilitation Monograph No. 64). New York University Medical Center: Institute of Rehabilitation Medicine, 127–176.

Black, J., Galambos, J. & Read, S. (1984). Comprehending stories and social situations. In R. Wyer & T. Srull (Eds.) *Handbook of social cognition* (vol. 3, pp. 45–86). Hillsdale, NJ: Lawrence Erlbaum Assoc.

Brooks, D. N. (1975). Long and short term memory in head injured patients. *Cortex, 11,* 329–340.

Brooks, D. N. (1983). Disorders of memory. In M. Rosenthal, E. Griffith, M. Bond & J. D. Miller (Eds.), *Rehabilitation of the head injured adult* (pp. 185–196). Philadelphia: F. A. Davis.

Brooks, D. N. (1984). *Closed head injury: Psychological, social, and family consequences.* New York: Oxford University Press.

Brooks, D. N. & Lincoln, N. (1984). Assessment for rehabilitation. In B. Wilson & N. Moffat (Eds.), *Clinical managment of memory problems.* Rockville, MD: Aspen Systems Corp.

Brouwer, W. & van Wolffelaar, P. C. (1985). Sustained attention and sustained effort after closed head injury: Detection and 0.10 Hz heart rate variability in a low event rate vigilance task. *Cortex, 21,* 111–119.

Brown, A. L. (1975). The development of memory: Knowing, knowing about knowing, and knowing how to know. In H. W. Reese (Ed.), *Advances in child development and behavior* (pp. 104–152). New York: Academic Press.

Brown, A. L. (1979). Theories of memory and the problems of development: Activity, growth, and knowledge. In F. I. M. Craik & L. Cermak (Eds.). *Levels of processing and memory* (pp. 225–258). Hillsdale, NJ: Lawrence Erlbaum Assoc.

Campione, J. C. (1980). Improving memory skills in mentally retarded children: Empirical research and strategies for intervention. Technical Report No. 196. Cambridge: Bolt, Bernak & Newman.

Cantor, N., Mischel, W. & Schwartz, J. (1982). Social knowledge: Structure, content, use, abuse. In A. Hastdorf & A. Ibsen (Eds.), *Cognitive social psychology.* New York: Elsevier North Holland.

Ceci, S. & Howe, M. (1978a). Age-related differences in free recall as a function of retrieval flexibility. *Journal of Experimental Child Psychology, 26,* 432–442.

Ceci, S. & Howe, M. (1978b). Semantic knowledge as a determinant of developmental differences in recall. *Journal of Experimental Child Psychology, 26,* 230–245.

Cermak, L., Butters, N. & Gerrein, J. (1973). The extent of verbal ability in alcoholic Korsakoff patients. *Neuropsychologica, 11,* 85–94.

Cermak, L., Butters, N. & Moreines, J. (1974). Some analysis of the verbal encoding deficit in alcoholic Korsakoff patients. *Brain and Language, 1,* 141–150.

Chi, M. T. H. (1976). Short term memory limitations in children: Capacity or processing deficits? Memory and Cognition, 4, 559–572.

Chi, M. T. H. (1978). Knowledge structures and memory development. In R. S. Siegler (Ed.), *Children's thinking: What develops?* (pp. 73–96). Hillsdale, NJ: Lawrence Erlbaum Assoc.

Chomsky, N. (1968). *Language and thought.* New York: Harcourt, Brace, Jovanovich.

Cofer, C. N. (1977). On the constructive theory of memory. In I. C. Uzgiris & F. Weizmann (Eds.), *The structure of experience* (pp. 319–341). New York: Plenum Press.

Cohen, S. (1986). Educational re-integration and programming for children with head injuries. *Journal of Head Trauma Rehabilitation, 1.*

Cohen, S., Joyce, C., Rhoades, K. & Welks, D. (1985). Educational programming for head injured students. In M. Ylvisaker (Ed.), *Head injury rehabilitation: Children and adolescents* (pp. 383–409). San Diego: College-Hill Press.

Cohen, S. & Titonis, J. (1985). Head injury rehabilitation: Management issues. In M. Ylvisaker (Ed.), *Head injury rehabilitation: Children and adolescents* (pp. 429–443). San Diego: College-Hill Press.

Craik, F. & Lockhart, R. (1972). Levels of processing: A framework for memory research. *Journal of Verbal Learning and Verbal Behavior, 11,* 671-684.

Craik, F. I. M. & Tulving, E. (1975). Depth of processing and the retention of words in episodic memory. *Journal of Experimental Psychology, 104,* 268-294.

Craine, J. F. & Gudeman, H. E. (1981). *The rehabilitation of brain functions: Principles, procedures, and techniques of neurotraining.* Springfield, IL: Charles C. Thomas.

Crowder, R. (1976). *Principles of learning and memory.* Hillsdale, NJ: Lawrence Erlbaum Assoc.

Deutsch, D. & Deutsch, J. A. (1975). *Short-term memory.* New York: Academic Press.

Diller, L. & Gordon, W. (1981). Intervention for cognitive deficits in brain injured adults. *Journal of Consulting and Clinical Psychology, 49,* 822-834.

Dodd, D. & White, R. M., Jr. (1980). *Cognition: Mental structures and processes.* Boston: Allyn & Bacon.

Feuerstein, R. (1980). *Instrumental enrichment: An intervention program for cognitive modifiability.* Glenview, IL: Scott Foresman & Co.

Flavell, J. H. (1977). *Cognitive development.* Englewood Cliffs, NJ: Prentice-Hall.

Gianutsos, R. (1980). What is cognitive rehabilitation? *Journal of Rehabilitation, 46,* 37-40.

Gibson, E. J. (1969). *Principles of perceptual learning and development.* New York: Appleton-Century Crofts.

Gitomer, D., Pellegrino, J. & Bisanz, J. (1983). Developmental change and invariance in semantic processing. *Journal of Experimental Child Psychology, 35,* 56-80.

Gordon, F. & Flavell, J. (1977). The devlopment of intuitions about cognitive cuing. *Child Development, 48,* 1027-1033.

Gronwall, D. & Wrightson, P. (1980). Duration of post traumatic amnesia after mild head injury. *Journal of Clinical Neuropsychology, 2,* 51-60.

Gummow, L., Miller, P. & Dustman, R. (1983). Attention and brain injury: A case for cognitive rehabilitation of attentional deficits. *Clinical Psychology Review, 3,* 255-274.

Haarbauer-Krupa, J., Henry, K., Szekeres, S. & Ylivisaker, M. (listed alphabetically) (1985). Cognitive rehabilitation therapy: Late stages of recovery. In M. Ylvisaker (Ed.), *Head injury rehabilitation: Children and adolescents* (pp. 311-343). San Diego: College-Hill Press.

Hagen, C. (1981). Language disorders secondary to closed head injury: Diagnosis and treatment. *Topics in Language Disorders, 1,* 73-87.

Harris, J. (1984). Methods of improving memory. In B. Wilson & N. Moffat (Eds.), *Clinical management of memory problems.* Rockville, MD: Aspen Systems Corp.

Harter, S. (1978). Effective motivation reconsidered: Toward a developmental model. *Human Development, 21,* 34-64.

Hastie, R. & Carlston, D. (1980). Theoretical issues in person memory. In R. Hastie, T. Ostrom, B. Ebbesen, R. Wyer, D. Hamilton & D. Carlston (Eds.), *Person memory: The cognitive basis of social perception* (pp. 1–53). Hillsdale, NJ: Lawrence Erlbaum Assoc.

Heider, F. (1958). *The psychology of interpersonal relations.* New York: John Wiley & Sons.

Hintzman, D. L. (1978). *The psychology of learning and memory.* New York: W. H. Freeman Co.

Holyoak, K. & Gordon, P. (1984). Information processing and social cognition. In R. Wyler & T. Srull (Eds.), *Handbook of social cognition* (Vol. 1, pp. 39–70). Hillsdale, NJ: Lawrence Erlbaum Assoc.

Huppert, F. & Piercy, M. (1982). In search of the functional locus of amnesic syndromes. In L. Cermak (Ed.), *Human memory and amnesia* (pp. 123–137). Hillsdale, NJ: Lawrence Erlbaum Assoc.

Isen, A. & Hastorf, A. (1982). Some perspectives on cognitive social psychology. In A. Hastorf & A. Isen (Eds.), *Cognitive social psychology* (pp. 1–31). New York: Elsevier North Holland, Inc.

Istominia, Z. (1975). The development of voluntary memory in pre-school age children. *Soviet Psychology, 13*(4), 5–64.

Jennett, B., Snoek, J., Bond, M. R. & Brooks, N. (1981). Disability after severe head injury: Observations on the use of the Glasgow Outcome Scale. *Journal of Neurology, Neurosurgery, and Psychiatry, 44,* 285–293.

Jennett, B. & Teasdale, G. (1981). *Management of head injuries.* Philadelphia: F. A. Davis.

Jones, E. E. & Nisbett, R. E. (1972). The actor and the observer. Divergent perceptions of the causes of behavior. In E. E. Jones, D. E. Kanouse, H. H. Kelley, R. E. Nisbett, S. Valins & B. Weiner (Eds.), *Attribution: Perceiving the causes of behavior.* Morristown, NJ: General Learning Press.

Kail, R. & Bisanz, J. (1982).. Information processing and cognitive development. In H. Reese (Ed.), *Advances in child development and behavior* (Vol. 17, pp. 45–81). New York: Academic Press.

Kail, R. & Siegel, A. (1977). The development of mnemonic encoding in children. In R. Kail & J. Hagen (Eds.), *Perspectives on the development of memory and cognition* (pp. 61–88). Hillsdale, NJ: Lawrence Erlbaum Assoc.

Kausler, D. H. (1974). *Psychology of verbal learning and memory.* New York: Academic Press.

Kavale, K. & Mattson, P. (1983). "One jumped off the balance beam:" Metaanalysis of perceptual-motor training. *Journal of Learning Disabilities, 16,* 165–173.

Kinsbourne, M. & Wood, F. (1975). Short term memory processes and the amnesic syndrome. In D. Deutsch & J. A. Deutsch (Eds.), *Short-term memory* (pp. 257–291). New York: Academic Press.

Kinsbourne, M. & Wood, F. (1982). Theoretical considerations regarding the episodic-semantic memory distinction. In L. Cermak (Ed.), *Human memory and amnesia* (pp. 195–217). Hillsdale, NJ: Lawrence Erlbaum Assoc.

Kintsch, W. (1968). Recognition and free recall of organized lists. *Journal of Experimental Psychology, 78,* 481–487.

Levin, H., Benton, A. & Grossman, R. (1982). *Neurobehavioral consequences of closed head injury.* New York: Oxford University Press.

Lezak, M. (1983). *Neuropsychological assessment* (2nd ed.). New York: Oxford University Press.

Lodico, M., Ghatala, E., Levin, J., Pressley, M. & Bell, J. (1983). The effects of strategy monitoring training on children's selection of effective memory strategies. *Journal of Experimental Child Psychology, 35,* 263–277.

McGonagle, E., Carper, M. & Balicki, M. (1983). Greenery: An integrated approach to cognitive rehabilitation of the head injured patient. *Cognitive Rehabilitation, 1,* 8–12.

Markman, E. M. (1979). Realizing that you don't understand: Elementary school children's awareness of inconsistencies. *Child Development, 50,* 643–655.

Meichenbaum, D. (1977). *Cognitive behavior modification: An integrative approach.* New York: Plenum Press.

Miller, G. A. (1956). The magical number seven, plus or minus two: Some limits on our capacity for processing information. *Psychological Review, 63,* 81–97.

Miller, N. E. & Dollard, J. (1941). *Social learning and imitation.* New Haven: Yale University Press.

Moely, B. E. (1977). Organization of memory. In R. Kail & J. Hagen (Eds.), *Perspectives on the development of memory and cognition* (pp. 203–236). Hillsdale, NJ: Lawrence Erlbaum Assoc.

National Task Force on Special Education. (1985). *An educator's manual.* Framingham, MA: National Head Injury Foundation, Inc.

Norman, D. A. (1976). *Memory and attention: An introduction to human information processing* (2nd ed.). New York: John Wiley & Sons.

Palmer, C. D. (1985). The brain trauma rehabilitation program, Southfield Rehabilitation Center. *Cognitive Rehabilitation, 3,* 4–9.

Pang, D. (1985). Pathophysiologic correlates of neurobehavioral syndromes following closed head injury. In M. Ylvisaker (Ed.), *Head injury rehabilitation: Children and adolescents* (pp. 3–70). San Diego: College-Hill Press.

Parkin, A. (1982). Residual learning capacity in organic amnesia. *Cortex, 18,* 417–440.

Piaget, J. (1970). Piaget's theory. In P. H. Mussen (Ed.), *Carmichael's manual of child psychology* (Vol. 1). New York: John Wiley & Sons.

Piaget, J. & Inhelder, B. (1973). *Memory and intelligence.* New York: Basic Books.

Postman, L. (1964). Short term memory and incidental learning. In A. W. Nelson (Ed.), *Categories of human learning* (pp. 145–201). New York: Academic Press.

Postman, L. & Kruesi, E. (1977). The influence of orienting tasks on the encoding and recall of words. *Journal of Verbal Learning and Verbal Behavior, 2,* 353–369.

Postman, L. & Underwood, B. J. (1973). Critical issues in interference theory. *Memory and Cognition, 1,* 19–40.

Pressley, M., Forrest-Pressley, D., Elliot-Faust, D. & Miller, G. (1985). Children's use of cognitive strategies, how to teach strategies, what to do if they can't be taught. In M. Pressley & C. Brainerd (Eds.), *Cognitive learning and memory in children* (pp. 1–47). New York: Springer-Verlag.

Prigatano, G. & Fordyce, D. (1986). The neuropsychological rehabilitation program at Presbyterian Hospital, Oklahoma City. In G. P. Prigatano & others. *Neuropsychological rehabilitation after brain injury.* Baltimore: Johns Hopkins University Press.

Prigatano, G. P. & others. (1986). *Neuropsychological rehabilitation after brain injury.* Baltimore: Johns Hopkins University Press.

Reitan, R. M. (1980). *REHABIT — Reitan Evaluation of Hemispheric Abilities and Brain Improvement Training.* Neuropsychology Laboratory and the University of Arizona.

Rosen, C. D. & Gerring, J. P. (1986). *Head trauma: Educational reintegration.* San Diego: College-Hill Press.

Rummelhart, D. (1984). Schemata and the cognitive system. In R. Wyer & T. Srull (Eds.), *Handbook of social cognition* (Vol. 1, pp. 161–188). Hillsdale, NJ: Lawrence Erlbaum Assoc.

Sapir, E. (1921). *Language.* New York: Harcourt, Brace, World, Inc.

Schacter, D. & Tulving, E. (1982). Amnesia and memory research. In L. Cermak (Ed.), *Human memory and amnesia* (pp. 21–31). Hillsdale, NJ: Lawrence Erlbaum Assoc.

Shoben, E. (1984). Semantic and episodic memory. In R. Wyer & T. Srull (Eds.), *Handbook of social cognition* (Vol. 2, pp. 213–232). Hillsdale, NJ: Lawrence Erlbaum Assoc.

Siegler, R. S. (1983). Information processing approaches to development. In W. Kessen (Ed.), *Handbook of child psychology* (Vol. 1, pp. 129–131). New York: John Wiley & Sons.

Skinner, B. F. (1969). *Contingencies of reinforcement.* New York: Apple-Century Crofts.

Smirnov, A. (1973). *Problems in psychology and memory.* New York: Plenum Press.

Smirnov, A. & Zinchenko, P. (1969). Problems in the psychology of memory. In M. Cole & I. Maltzman (Eds.), *A handbook of contemporary soviet psychology* (pp. 45–502). New York: Basic Books.

Smith, E. E. (1978). Theories of semantic memory. In W. K. Estes (Ed.), *Handbook of learning and cognitive processes* (Vol. 6). Hillsdale, NJ: Lawrence Erlbaum Assoc.

Szekeres, S., Ylvisaker, M. & Holland, A. (1985). Cognitive rehabilitation therapy: A framework for intervention. In M. Ylvisaker (Ed.), *Head injury rehabilitation: Children and adolescents* (pp. 219–246). San Diego: College-Hill Press.

Tarpy, R. & Mayer, R. (1978). *Foundations of learning and memory.* Glenview, IL: Scott Foresman Co.

Tenney, Y. I. (1975). The child's conception of organization and recall. *Journal of Experimental Child Psychology, 19,* 100–114.

Tomkins, S. (1970). A theory of memory. In J. S. Antrobus (Ed.), *Cognition and affect.* Boston: Little Brown.

Tulving, E. (1972). Episodic and semantic memory. In E. Tulving & W. Donaldson (Eds.), *Organization of memory* (pp. 382–403). New York: Academic Press.

Tulving, E. (1975). Ecphoric processes in recall and recognition. In J. Brown (Ed.), *Recall and recognition* (pp. 37–73). London: John Wiley & Sons.

Tulving, E. & Thompson, D. M. (1973). Encoding specificity and retrieval processes in episodic memory. *Psychological Review, 80,* 352–373.

Vygotsky, L. S. (1962). *Thought and language* (E. Hanfmann & G. Vakan, Trans.). Cambridge, MA: MIT Press.

Weiner, B. (1979). A theory of motivation for some classroom experiences. *Journal of Educational Psychology, 71,* 3–25.

Weisberg, R. W. (1980). *Memory, thought, and behavior.* New York: Oxford University Press.

Wilson, B. & Moffat, N. (Eds.). (1984). *Clinical management of memory problems.* Rockville, MD: Aspen Systems Corp.

Wood, F., Ebert, V. & Kinsbourne, M. (1982). The episodic-semantic memory distinction in amnesia: Clinical and experimental observations. In L. Cermak (Ed.), *Human memory and amnesia* (pp. 167–193). Hillsdale, NJ: Lawrence Erlbaum Assoc.

Wood, R. L. (1984). Management of attention disorders following brain injury. In B. Wilson & N. Moffat (Eds.), *Clinical management of memory problems.* Rockville, MD: Aspen Systems Corp.

Wyer, R. & Gordon, S. (1984). The cognitive representation of social information. In R. Wyer & T. Srull (Eds.), *Handbook of social psychology* (Vol. 2, pp. 73–150). Hillsdale, NJ: Lawrence Erlbaum Assoc.

CHAPTER 4

Topics in Cognitive Rehabilitation Therapy

Mark Ylvisaker
Shirley F. Szekeres
Kevin Henry
Deborah M. Sullivan
Paula Wheeler

In this chapter we discuss selected issues in cognitive rehabilitation therapy (CRT) for head injured patients who are beyond the recovery phase which is characterized by profound confusion and disorientation. This chapter is intended to complement Chapter 3, in which a conceptual framework for CRT services is described. Since the theme of this book is community re-entry, our specific goal is to highlight those aspects of cognitive intervention which in our opinion figure most significantly in a patient's successful return to work, school, or community living. Because the notion remains controversial that retraining in basic-level cognitive processes (e.g., attention, rote memory), systems (e.g., working memory), or pervasive dimensions of cognitive activity (e.g., speed of processing) can effect meaningful improvements in these areas of cognitive functioning (Prigatano and others, 1986), this chapter does not undertake a discussion of such retraining techniques. A useful literature on these dimensions of cognitive rehabilitation already exists and a fair representation of the positions in the debate would extend this chapter beyond its scope (Ben-Yishay et al., 1982; Craine & Gudeman, 1981).

Chapters 1 and 3 describe a large number of cognitive and cognitively based communicative and psychosocial impairments that are common residual sequelae in severely head injured adults. Lists of typical deficits should not, however, blind clinicians to the diversity that exists among head injured patients. Pre-traumatic variation in intelligence, educational and vocational level, and personality creates rich diversity in this population as do the nature and severity of the brain injuries, the patients' coping ability, and the support and rehabilitation services that are available. Patients who receive the types of treatment described in this chapter range from those whose motor, sensory, and cognitive systems are all significantly impaired, who resist rehabilitation efforts, and whose most realistic rehabilitation goal may be an enriched avocational life and a modest degree of independence in daily living to those whose motor and sensory systems are intact, whose cognitive functioning is only mildly depressed, who approach their rehabilitation with enthusiasm, and who ultimately return to their pre-traumatic educational or vocational level. This diversity underscores the importance of rehabilitation programs that are customized to fit the needs and goals of individual patients.

Despite this diversity, there are commonalities that give some unity to this group and that explain the growth of cognitive rehabilitation programs for head injured adults. Even those patients who appear on the surface to have regained their pre-traumatic level of cognitive functioning often give evidence of some combination of the following deficits, particularly under stress:

- Impaired attention, perception, and/or memory
- Inflexibility, impulsivity, and/or disorganized thinking, acting, and/or verbal expression
- Inefficient processing of information (rate, amount, and complexity)
- Difficulty processing abstract information
- Difficulty learning new information, including facts, concepts, rules, and procedures
- Inefficient retrieval of old or stored information and of words
- Ineffective problem solving and judgment
- Inappropriate or unconventional social behavior
- Impaired "executive" functions: self-awareness of strengths and weaknesses, goal setting, planning, self-initiating, self-inhibiting, self-monitoring, self-evaluating

Of course, the specific cognitive profiles of individuals differ and cognitive demands and expectations vary from one discharge destination to another. For these reasons, rehabilitation professionals must determine priorities in CRT for each patient. Although we rely heavily on group CRT, in which a group has its own special focus (see Chapter 3), each patient moves through a set of group and individual CRT sessions with an individualized ranking of cognitive goals. This ranking of goals is based on the patient's profile of strengths and weaknesses, on the functional significance of a given deficit to his or her overall functioning, and on the patient's own vocational, educational, and social goals.

Patients' goals merit separate discussion in a chapter on cognitive rehabilitation. Active engagement in cognitive rehabilitation is largely a product of the perceived utility of the process to one's goals. The question of engagement is particularly acute for head injured patients, who often demonstrate an organically based failure to perceive deficits and their functional implications (see Chapter 1). Furthermore, patients understandably hold onto pre-traumatic goals, aspirations, and expectations. For these reasons, much that is done in cognitive rehabilitation may not relate in an obvious way to their own goals.

Clinicians regularly face a profound dilemma: on the one hand, treatment that is based on an objective evaluation of a patient's functioning and a realistic set of goals may fail to capture the patient's interest and commitment; on the other hand, treatment that is based on a patient's unrealistic self-evaluation and overly optimistic goals will likely be inefficient and unproductive. Resolving this dilemma is complex and time consuming and can frequently constitute the main obstacle to progress. There are several avenues to a solution, any number and combination of which may be useful in a given instance.

- Integrating CRT with psychosocial counseling in the area of self-awareness of deficits and realistic goal setting
- Keeping careful records of a patient's performance, sharing this information with him or her, and if necessary, planning experiences of failure to call attention to areas of cognitive weakness (see Teaching Compensatory Strategies)
- Educating the patient in the area of brain injury and typical sequelae
- Focusing explicitly on the goals of treatment and on the relation between activities in therapy and the patient's goals. Goals are reviewed at the beginning and end of therapy sessions and patients are often required to record in a notebook the purposes, as they see it, of treatment tasks
- Structuring treatment tasks around the patient's current goals,

even if this means some inefficiency in treatment

- Persuading the patient to provisionally accept temporary goals to give meaning to therapy tasks
- Allowing or even encouraging the patient to try to do what he or she most wants to do, even if this is clearly unrealistic. Patients generally learn about their limitations much more effectively through meaningful but unsuccessful attempts to achieve their goals than through feedback from a therapist
- Encouraging the patient not to abandon goals, but to explore other possibilities at the same time
- Designing treatment objectives that relate to pre-traumatic interests and goals, but also accomplish the CRT objectives

TEACHING COMPENSATORY STRATEGIES

Severe head injuries predictably produce various cognitive deficits that do not resolve completely. Ben-Yishay and colleagues (1982) have shown that certain basic-level cognitive processes can be improved with targeted, intensive exercises. (Gummow, Miller & Dustman (1983) reviewed other related studies.) However, full restoration of function is, in most cases, not a reasonable expectation even with the most intensive direct retraining. Recent research has called sharply into question, particularly for such pervasive cognitive functions as memory, the practice of improving a process simply by exercising it (the "mental muscle building" model of rehabilitation) (Harris, 1984; Harris & Sunderland, 1981).

In the face of deficits whose intractibility interferes with a patient's achieving desirable goals, rehabilitation professionals may provide (a) compensations in the environment, including reducing expectations of family members, work supervisors, and others for the patient's performance and offering environmental cues and support to enable the patient to complete a given task, and (b) compensatory strategies which a patient uses deliberately to accomplish a task. Compensatory strategies, which are simply procedures or external aids used deliberately to accomplish a difficult to achieve goal, are in fact staples of daily life for most of us. We use *external aids* (e.g., watches, appointment books, lists, tape recorders) to enhance our orientation and memory and *internal procedures* (e.g., self-instructing and reminding, mental organization of information, rehearsal of responses) to keep ourselves on task, to enhance our comprehension of a subject, and to guarantee appropriate behavior. Brain injured individuals typically reach the limits of their unaided ability to process information more quickly than those who are not brain injured and consequently may need more or perhaps just more systematically applied strategies to successfully negotiate their daily affairs.

Rehabilitation professionals are not, of course, the sole producers of compensatory strategies; most patients fashion for themselves some form of compensation for significant deficits. These self-selected strategies can easily be escapist (e.g., avoiding situations in which an impaired skill is required), may fail to capitalize on a patient's strengths (e.g., using a verbal rehearsal strategy although the patient's visual skills are far superior to his or her verbal skills), or may simply be inefficient in relation to a given goal (e.g., using mnemonics when written reminders would be far more useful). This, therefore, is a second reason to initiate a period of organized strategy intervention.

A third reason to consider compensatory strategies for head injured patients is the finding that, especially in the case of severe bilateral cerebral dysfunction, compensatory training holds greater promise of success than direct retraining of impaired cognitive functions (Prigatano and others, 1986; Zangwill, 1947). Diffuse bilateral damage is a hallmark of severe closed head injury (see Chapter 1).

A carefully designed program of strategy training is thus warranted for many adults in the late stages of recovery from severe head injury. In the sections that follow, we discuss the most important features of such a program. We emphasize at the outset, however, that *training in compensatory strategies can easily be overdone.* It is all too easy for a clinician to recognize a patient's deficit, immediately choose a strategy that may compensate for that deficit, and then attempt to teach the strategy. The processes of choosing appropriate candidates for strategy intervention and appropriate strategies for a given patient are in fact quite complicated. The attentional and processing resources of most head injured patients are restricted to some degree. The value of strategy intervention may thus be compromised if this and other complicating factors are not considered: Adding compensatory procedures to the ordinary demands on these resources can have the effect of making a marginally functional person less functional. Furthermore, in the absence of careful interdisciplinary coordination, a patient who is a good candidate for this intervention may be overwhelmed by a confusing diversity of strategies. Failure to attend adequately to issues of generalization of strategic procedures to functional settings and their maintenance over time equally undermines the effectiveness of strategy intervention. Finally, inadequate attention to patients' awareness of their strengths and deficits and of the functional implications of those deficits, and to their level of personal comfort with compensatory procedures may preclude effective compensation.

We do not wish to suggest by our extensive discussion of compensatory strategies in this chapter that they are the rehabilitation keystone for all patients at this stage of recovery, nor do we recommend neglecting either direct retraining of impaired cognitive functions, when such retraining shows promise of success, or environmental engineering if it can enhance a patient's independence and overall functioning despite residual impairments.

Selecting Candidates for Strategy Training

Table 4–1 lists a large number of variables that must be considered in deciding who should be taught strategic procedures to compensate for residual cognitive deficits and which procedures would be most effective. Each of these variables merits a separate discussion of its relation to strategy intervention. We have selected for brief discussion a few of the variables that in our experience pose stubborn problems for this type of intervention. The type of thinking illustrated here should be extended to the remaining variables before a course of treatment in compensatory strategies is initiated.

1. *General cognitive level:* Patients who remain confused or who exhibit a severely and uniformly depressed cognitive profile are in general not appropriate candidates for strategy intervention. Such patients may, however, be trained to carry and refer to a memory book or schedule card to help them compensate for gross disorders of memory and orientation. It has been shown that, even in the cases of severely amnesic patients, conditioning and procedure learning are possible when they are given an adequate number of trials (Baddeley, 1982). Environmental compensations, however, may be the most effective treatment route for such patients.
2. *Working memory (attentional "space"):* Patients whose working memory (measured by digit span) is significantly restricted may lack the attentional resources to think about both a task at hand and also the compensatory procedures that would facilitate its performance. Filling such a patient's mind with strategies may ultimately interfere with performance. External aids and overlearned procedures may still be useful options.
3. *Awareness of deficits:* Patients who lack an awareness of their deficits or the functional implications of these deficits may, if compliant, go through the motions of rehearsing a strategy but are

Table 4–1. Variables to Consider in the Selection and Training of Compensatory Strategies

1. Developmental Factors
   a. Age
   b. Pre-traumatic intellectual functioning
2. Environmental-Social Factors
   a. Pre-traumatic social-educational-occupational status
   b. Current functional needs and environmental supports
   c. Proposed discharge setting: needs and supports
3. Cognitive Profile: Strengths and Deficits
   a. Sensory-perceptual-perceptual-motor abilities
   b. Attention: span, concentration, flexibility, "space"
   c. Memory: encoding, storage, retrieval
   d. Verbal and nonverbal abilities
   e. Knowledge (level of content and organization)
   f. Organizational abilities
   g. Reasoning and problem-solving abilities
   h. Metacognitive abilities: awareness of cognitive function (e.g., attention, memory, organization), explanation of own strategies, prediction of performance
   i. Strategic intent and spontaneous use of strategies
4. Readiness for New Learning: Degree of Confusion, Disorientation, Attentional Impairment
5. Personality and Social Control
   a. Shy-aggressive; fearful-confident
   b. Attitude toward rehabilitation
6. Motivation
   a. Presence of realistic and meaningful goals
   b. Perceived need to use a strategy
   c. Effective reinforcers
7. Executive Functions
   a. Self-awareness of deficits and their implications
   b. Self-initiation, self-direction, self-monitoring, self-evaluation
8. Cognitive Style (Pre-trauma and Post-trauma): Impulsive-reflective; passive-active; rigid-flexible; indecisive-decisive; easily deterred-persistent
9. Situational Discrimination: Ability to distinguish situations that do or do not require application of a given strategy
10. Medications: Expected positive-negative effects
11. Brain Injury: type, extent, and location

From Cognitive Rehabilitation Therapy. Late Stages of Recovery, by J. Haarbauer-Krupa, K. Henry, S. Szekeres, and M. Ylvisaker, 1985. In M. Ylvisaker (Ed.), *Head Injury Rehabilitation: Children and Adolescents.* San Diego: College-Hill Press.

clearly not engaged in the process. Consequently, the likelihood of the patient's learning or putting the strategy to functional use is minimal. For these patients, treatment that focuses on self-awareness of strengths and weaknesses, emphasizing the relation these have to the patient's goals, is a necessary first stage in the rehabilitation plan (see Table 4–2).

4. *Metacognitive level and "executive" functions* (related to 3): A patient's ability to think abstractly about attending, learning, thinking, problem solving, and other cognitive processes is a fundamental factor in acquiring and using strategies, particularly internal procedures that require the recognition of situations in which a certain type of thinking or mental procedure is appropriate and the ability then to apply that procedure. Again, concrete external aid procedures (such as using a schedule card or memory book) place a lesser demand on metacognitive functioning.
5. *Goals:* Patients whose goals are utterly unrealistic or who simply lack goals are unlikely to acquire strategies, since strategies have significance only in relation to something that one truly wishes to accomplish. A skilled therapist may win a patient's tentative acceptance of provisional goals and thus create a basis for treatment. However, long-term success will depend on the patient's perceiving a relation between a strategic procedure and a genuinely held goal.
6. *Environmental support:* It is not uncommon for a patient to learn a strategic procedure (e.g., requesting repetition or clarification of instructions, or more time to complete a task) and then be discharged to an academic or vocational setting where the procedure is not understood and not honored. This phenomenon underscores the need to solicit the active support of the patient's family members, teachers, and work supervisors in the rehabilitation process.

Additional factors related to strategy intervention are explored in the next section. In cases in which a patient is not clearly a good candidate or a poor candidate for compensatory strategies, there is no substitute for a period of diagnostic therapy with clear objectives and carefully monitored progress.

CASE ILLUSTRATION. J.S. was admitted to The Rehabilitation Institute of Pittsburgh 2 years following a severe head injury which had resulted from a motorcycle accident. Prior to this admission, he had been discharged from a residential program because the staff were unable to manage his behavior. His cognitive profile was dominated by mild to moderate disorientation, marked perseverative behavior, fluctuating attention which, however, was excellent when he was engaged in highly interesting activities, very weak learning and memory, poorly organized behavior, a shallow knowledge base, and poor initiation, inhibition, and self-monitoring. His initial evaluation did not unequivocally endorse his candidacy for compensatory strategies. Consequently, this question was put to the test through a period of diagnostic therapy: (a) J.S. was trained to carry a memory book and to request that staff make a note in his book at the end of each therapy session. Within one month, this practice had become a habit, although several memory books had been lost in the process; (b) In CRT sessions, an attempt was made to teach J.S. to use a four-step task organizing strategy (printed on a card) to improve his initiation, organization, and self-monitoring during the completion of tasks. The treatment included calling J.S.'s attention to the processes of organizing and self-monitoring. The explicit goal of therapy activities was to have J.S. acquire this procedure, not necessarily to complete the concrete task. The same procedure was used daily for 3 weeks, but J.S. did not independently use the procedure, even with the cue card present; and (c) In work adjustment therapy, J.S. was given tasks that were highly motivating because they were clearly related to his preinjury vocational interests. The work adjustment therapist oriented him to the task itself, not to the abstract goal of acquiring a strategy or organizing work more effectively. In this type of "involuntary learning" situation (see section on Memory and Organization), J.S. not only completed tasks more efficiently than in the deliberate learning situation of CRT sessions, but he also habituated a simple procedure for organizing work tasks. From this diagnostic exploration, it was concluded that, although J.S. could be taught to use concrete external aids, like his memory book, he was not a candidate for internal strategies. Indeed, it appeared that the effort involved in thinking about the deliberate strategy actually interfered with completing the task. Thus, it became the job of staff to facilitate learning by providing J.S. with a structrued and relatively distraction free environment and orienting him to interesting and motivating tasks.

Selecting Strategies for Patients

Fitting a patient who is a good candidate for strategy intervention with appropriate strategies also requires careful consideration of the variables listed in Table 4-1. However, in attending to these variables a clinician should be aware of and respect a patient's natural inclinations regarding strategic behavior and his or her level of comfort with the strategies. The deliberation about effective strategies properly involves *negotiating* with the patient and attempting to involve him or her in creative *problem solving,* both of which can result in the patient's self-selection of effective strategies. There is often a tension between a strategy that a patient naturally inclines toward, perhaps due to pre-traumatic learning style, and a clinician's judgment, which is based on careful analysis of the patient's neuropsychological profile.

Spontaneously used strategies — those either observed during the assessment or reported by a patient in response to questioning about what he or she did to complete the assessment task — provide a useful starting point for discussing what strategies are, how they help, and how the patient might put them to use. Other things being equal, a strategy that a patient uses spontaneously, perhaps with modification or expanded application, is more likely to be used and used effectively than a strategy chosen by a clinician. Unfortunately, it is frequently the case that patients evidence little or no strategic behavior or that trial therapy proves the ineffectiveness of procedures that come naturally. In such cases, the decision process ideally involves combining attempts to engage a patient's own problem-solving skills (see Table 4–2) with negotiations with the patient to strike a balance between effective strategies and comfort. The importance of feeling comfortable with strategies is illustrated by the shy and unassertive patient who is unlikely to make effective use of input-control strategies that require him to regularly request repetition or clarification from others. Similarly, patients who, above all, wish not to call attention to their disability predictably reject external aids (e.g., memory books, electronic memo devices), which in their eyes are stigmatizing.

Other factors that figure prominently in the selection of strategies for individual patients are:

1. *Range of applicability of the strategy ("domain specificity"):* Strategic procedures vary considerably in the range of contexts or problems to which they apply. The classical mnemonics, such as using pegwords or deliberately placing words to be remembered in specific places in a mentally constructed scene, may be useful in memorizing lists of words, but these techniques are applicable to very few functional memory or learning tasks of daily life. On the other hand, memory prosthetics (e.g., writing lists or making notes to oneself) and input-control strategies (e.g., requesting that a speaker slow his rate of speech or repeat or explain himself) are applicable to a wide variety of real-life situations. Using visual imagery as a memory strategy appears to fall somewhere between

these two extremes. Other things being equal, the wider the application of a strategy, the more useful it is. It is unfortunate that much of the literature on memory rehabilitation focuses on mnemonic strategies that are of little practical value (Wilson & Moffat, 1984).

2. *Difficulty in using the strategy:* Strategic procedures that are complex or time consuming or in some other way difficult to use are less likely to be acquired than those that are simple. Again, the mnemonics mentioned above tend to be more difficult strategies while verbal repetition, requests for clarification, and, for some, note taking are relatively easy.
3. *Concreteness of the strategy:* Some strategic procedures are extremely concrete (e.g., note taking, consulting a schedule card, using an alarm watch), whereas others are very abstract (e.g., mentally constructing an organizational framework in which to place new information that one is hearing or reading). One can make abstract strategies more concrete by illustrating the thinking procedure on paper (e.g., Figure 4–3). Illustrating procedures is almost always possible and is a very important part of the teaching process. Other things being equal, concrete strategies are preferable to less concrete strategies. For patients returning to an academic setting or a cognitively demanding job, however, relatively abstract organizational and comprehension strategies may be highly useful.
4. *Knowledge presupposed by the strategy:* An organizational strategy that is useful for comprehending and remembering information that is relatively familiar may be ineffective or confusing when applied to information that is entirely novel. For example, patients are often taught to try to organize, or "chunk," incoming information in relation to familiar categories or scripts. This strategy not only makes the processing of information more efficient by virtue of the grouping procedure, but also facilitates recall by having patients associate new information with old information. However, if patients have absolutely no knowledge of a given topic and consequently no idea of the relevant categories or scripts to impose on the information to highlight the main ideas and to filter out irrelevant details, then this organizational strategy may do nothing more than add confusion and complexity to an already difficult learning task. A patient's need for content-specific knowledge in order to use a given strategy is clearly illustrated by the hierarchy of skills required for problem solving in mathematics. Unless basic number facts and arithmetic operations are well known, problem-solving strategies serve no useful purpose. The importance of prior

knowledge to strategic behavior has been underscored in several studies which have been reported in the education and developmental psychology literature (reviewed by Peterson & Swing, 1983).

5. *Extent to which the strategy capitalizes on the patient's cognitive strengths:* Since the purpose of the strategy is to allow a patient to get a job done despite residual cognitive deficits, it is almost a truism that the selected strategy should be based on the patient's strengths. This guideline is often illustrated by the prescription that patients who are weak in auditory-verbal skills should capitalize on visual skills (e.g., should use visual imagery rather than verbal elaboration as a memory aid), whereas patients with visual-perceptual or spatial-organization weaknesses should rely on verbal strategies.
6. *Metacognitive requirements of the strategy:* Many strategic procedures require (a) recognizing one's limitations in a particular area of cognitive functioning, (b) acknowledging the relation between these limitations and achieving one's goals, (c) knowing that a given procedure will compensate for a deficit, (d) recognizing that one is in a situation in which a given cognitive skill is required and to which a given strategy applies, (e) monitoring the effectiveness of one's performance with the strategy, and (f) adapting strategic procedures to changing task demands. Although it is true that extensive practice may make some of this process automatic, it nevertheless is essential that a clinician compare the metacognitive requirements of a strategy with the patient's metacognitive maturity. Strategies that rely on external aids (e.g., memory books, alarm watches) or overt behavior (e.g., requesting repetition or clarification) in general make fewer metacognitive demands than internal procedures. Peterson and Swing (1983) reviewed research evidence linking metacognitive proficiency and the use of strategies.

Appendix 4–1 lists a large number of compensatory strategies under the headings of Attention and Concentration; Orientation; Input Control; Comprehension and Memory Processes; Word Retrieval; Thought Organization and Verbal Expression; Reasoning, Problem Solving, and Judgment; Self-Monitoring; and Task Organization.

Selecting Teaching Procedures

Table 4–2 outlines a program of strategy intervention. The three phases of the program (general strategic thinking, teaching the strategy, generalization and maintenance) are broadly sequential but should

Table 4–2. Teaching Compensatory Strategies

Phase I: General Strategic Thinking

A. Self Awareness

Goals: Patients will discriminate effective from ineffective performance; become aware of deficits; recognize implications of deficits.

Rationale: Patients do not acquire and spontaneously use strategies designed to compensate for deficits that they do not recognize. Given the frequency of frontolimbic involvement in close head injury, self-awareness is a major concern.

Procedures:

1. *Objective:* Improve the patient's perception of successful versus unsuccessful task performance. Show the patient two video tapes (or role-play) illustrating successful and unsuccessful performance of a task. The task should be relevant to the patient's needs and goals. In both cases, analyze the tapes in sufficient detail that the patient can identify the features that account for successful versus unsuccessful performance.
2. *Objective:* Improve the patient's ability to perceive functional impairments. Indivdiually, request the patient to make note of specific deficits of other head injured patients in group therapy. In individual sessions, discuss these observations with the patient. Discuss the effects of head injury on cognitive and social functioning.
3. *Objective:* Improve the patient's awareness of his or her own deficits. Videotape the patient in an activity designed to reveal a weak area of functioning. (Alternatively, use role-play.) Review the tape, first without commentary. This should not be the patient's first self-observation on videotape. Comment on what the patient does well and, if required, on what he or she does poorly. Several sessions of this sort may be required. Gradually turn over to the patient the responsibility of stopping the tape when problems are noted.
4. *Objective:* Improve the patient's understanding of the relation between deficits and long-term goals. Discuss in concrete detail the patient's long-term goals and expectations. Create a list of specific skills needed to achieve those goals. Review with the patient the skills that are present and those that are weak relative to this goal.

B. Value of Strategies

Goal: Patients will agree that strategies are helpful in accomplishing their goals.

Rationale: Head injured patients often lack strategies even when acutely aware of a problem.

Procedures:

1. Show the patient two video tapes: a person (stranger) failing in a functional task without a strategy and then succeeding when a strategy is used. (Alternatively, use role-play.)

(continued)

Table 4–2 (*continued*)

Procedures (continued):

2. In group, have advanced patients demonstrate the value of a strategy or offer a "testimonial."
3. Engage patients in a problem-solving discussion regarding a deficit. Orchestrate the discussion so that a strategy solution is initiated by the patients.
4. Using video tape, have patients evaluate their own success on a task, with and without a strategy. Have the patient keep data over time on his or her performance on a task with and without a strategy.
5. Discuss with patients the widespread use of compensatory strategies (lists, memos, tape recorders, and so forth) by people without head injuries. Find natural occasions to point out to the patient the use of strategies by other people.

Phase II: Teaching the Strategy

Procedures:

1. *Self-Discovery:* Use "product monitoring" procedures as described in I. A. 1. Select tasks that clearly illustrate the value of a strategy (e.g., comprehension of a paragraph when given insufficient reading time versus comprehension when given adequate reading time after making the strategic request, "May I have more time?").
2. *Modeling:* The steps in a strategy can be modeled by the therapist or a peer, by means of video tapes, or other media. Modeling is initially accompanied by overt verbalization of the strategy by the model. The patient then rehearses the strategy with gradually decreasing cues.
3. *Direct Instruction:* Explain clearly the purpose and use of the strategy to the patient. Explain under what conditions the strategy is useful.
4. *Practice:* Extensive practice with the strategy may be necessary for learning. Activities, materials, and other stimulus conditions should be systematically varied.

Visual Aids:

With most patients, the initial use of a strategy should be guided by visual cues: pictures, written instructions, diagrams, outlines, flow charts, game boards, and so forth. This helps to make the strategy procedures more concrete and easier to remember. Patients with significant visual disorganization may not be aided by such concrete visual representations.

Phase III: Generalization and Maintenance

Generalization of a strategy beyond the context of training is a combined consequence of the perceived utility of the strategy for the patient, specific teaching procedures designed to enhance generalization, and the inherent generalizability of the strategy.

1. *Objective:* Improve the patient's discrimination of situations that require or do not require a given strategy.

1. *Objectives (continued)*
   - Use a variety of materials or activities during early strategy training, but require consistent use of the same strategy under these different conditions
   - Use video taped scenes or role playing to illustrate the correct use of a strategy in an appropriate situation, inappropriate use of the strategy, and failure to use the strategy when appropriate. Discuss the conditions that require the strategy and make lists of situations in which the strategy is appropriate.
   - Use short video taped scenes to train the patient in efficient and accurate judgements as to whether a strategy is appropriate.
2. *Objective:* Increase the patient's spontaneous use of the strategy in varied situations.
   - Include family members, teachers, and work supervisors in strategy training to (a) provide varied opportunities for use of the strategy, and (b) reinforce the patient's use of the strategy in varied contexts. Family members and work supervisors may need to prompt strategy use at the outset, and later fade those prompts.
   - Ask patients to keep a log in which they record their successes and failures in strategy use. Make generalization an explicit goal.
3. *Objective:* Increase the patient's awareness of the utility of the strategy.
   - Give explicit feedback regarding the value of the strategy relative to the patient's goals.

From Cognitive Rehabilitation Therapy: Late Stages of Recovery, by J. Haarbauer-Krupa, K. Henry, S. Szekeres, and M. Ylvisaker, 1985. In M. Ylvisaker (Ed.), *Head Injury Rehabilitation: Children and Adolescents.* San Diego: College-Hill Press.

not be thought of as mutually exclusive phases of intervention. For example, although it is necessary that a patient have some awareness of his or her deficits to become actively engaged in learning a strategy, it is not essential that the patient achieve a high level of self-awareness before Phase II.

Our experience with head injured patients has highlighted certain features of this intervention process that deserve special discussion.

Patient initiation and problem solving: Since strategic behaviors may appear to be difficult, unusual, awkward, or stigmatizing, the likelihood that a patient will successfully adopt a strategy is increased if the selection of the strategy is based on the patient's own problem-solving activity. In problem-solving sessions with the patient, the clinician must skillfully manipulate the discussion so that an appropriate strategic soluton is advanced by the patient. (Because the goal of rehabilitation is to turn over to patients the coaching role that clinicians assume at the outset, these problem-solving sessions serve more than the purpose of selecting strategies.)

Limited program goals: Attempting to teach a patient too many procedures at once, particularly if they overlap in their application and all make demands on the patient's limited attentional resources, is one sure way to ensure failure of a program compensatory strategies. This situation occurs almost invariably when interdisciplinary programming is not carefully designed or monitored. Although professionals acting in isolation may all do exemplary jobs of teaching a few compensatory procedures, a patient can easily be overwhelmed by the total amount of information he or she must learn in several different therapies and confused by the various possible applications of strategies to situations.

Engagement with patients' goals: The importance of tying strategy intervention to a patient's goals cannot be overemphasized. With some patients, even unrealistic goals can be the basis for illustrating the value of strategies. Strategy intervention, however, should more often be part of the larger process of counseling and training the patient to be aware of his or her strengths and weaknesses.

Program monitoring: Careful monitoring of a patient's response to treatment will reveal whether or not a strategy is being acquired in the treatment context and is being generalized to other contexts. If not, it is necessary to give further consideration both to the motivational, cognitive, and metacognitive prerequisites for the strategy being taught and to the teaching procedures. In our experience, this deliberation most often results in (a) a simplification of the procedure being taught or a reduction in number of procedures being taught; (b) tighter interdisciplinary coordination of the teaching process; and (c) a problem-solving session with the patient designed to heighten his or her participation in the process.

Support: Since it is not easy for a patient to accept the need to compensate or to learn new ways to do things that used to be automatic and very easy, understanding, encouragement, and support are essential. Treatment groups in which time is alloted for mutual peer support are useful. Kendall (1981) emphasized the need for a strong relationship between therapist and patient in the teaching of self-regulative strategies to children. Our experience suggests that this is equally if not more true of the relationship between the clinician and head injured young adults.

Generalization and maintenance: Little work has been done to document the efficacy of strategy intervention with head injured patients. Of the few reports that have appeared in the literature, many are case studies and in most cases there are no meaningful measures of the durability of treatment gains or of the generalization of strategies from the learning context to other functional settings (Crosson & Buenning, 1984; Crovitz, 1979; Crovitz, Harvey & Horn, 1979; Gianutsos & Gianutsos, 1979; Glasgow, Zeiss, Barbera & Lewinsohn, 1977; Malec & Questad, 1983). Diller and Gordon (1981) and Levin, Benton, and Grossman (1982) reviewed several studies of the effectiveness of strategy intervention with head injured patients. Strategy training has been studied much more thoroughly by researchers in the fields of special education and normal child development. Like the research on strategy intervention with head injured patients, many of these studies are "laboratory bound." There have, however, been systematic attempts to assess the generalization and maintenance of strategies taught to both developmentally normal and learning impaired children (reviewed by Peterson & Swing, 1983). The results are inconclusive, although more recent reports in the special education literature appear to be more optimistic with respect to the functional effectiveness of strategy training. Pressley, Forrest-Pressley, Elliot-Faust, and Miller (1985) reviewed much of this literature and offered valuable suggestions for strategy intervention and for future research. Perhaps the increasing attention of professionals to issues of generalization and maintenance has had the effect of improving intervention in this area, thereby enhancing its ultimate effectiveness.

There is little doubt that the generalization and maintenance of treatment gains are crucial issues in the rehabilitation of brain injured people. Our clinical experience, together with the results of intervention studies in special education, leads us to be cautiously optimistic about the possible usefulness of compensatory strategies for head injured people, but only if: (a) intervention is intensive; (b) candidates are carefully selected; (c) teaching procedures are systematic and involve patients' active participation; (d) strategies are selected that are useful and applicable to the patient's needs, inherently generalizable, and suited to the limitations of patients' cognitive and metacognitive abilities; and (e) generalization and maintenance are explicit targets of the intervention program. Patients who are significantly limited in their ability to generalize may still benefit from training which does not have generalization as its goal; that is, acquiring a specific behavior for use in a specific situation may be an important goal for these patients (Pressley et al., 1985).

Overcoming Resistance to Compensatory Behavior

Head injured adults frequently display resistance to learning compensatory strategies. Even when they are cognitively able to acquire procedures that could well serve their best interests, patients may be reluctant to think seriously about using them. The heightened sensitivity of many patients derives from their seeing strategy use as painfully confirming their impairment or, worse, as indelibly and publicly stigmatizing them as "handicapped." Consequently, they avoid implementing and practicing strategies in order to preserve their threatened self-esteem. With such patients, integrating cognitive rehabilitation therapy with psychotherapy or counseling may be essential.

It is also possible to overcome such resistance by tailoring teaching techniques to the varied thinking styles, interests, and backgrounds of individual patients. The case descriptions that follow illustrate the various modes of communication that may help convey to patients, in ways that are as effective and painless as possible, that using compensatory strategies can be at the same time valuable and natural.

1. *Metaphors:* L.B., 26 years old and formerly a well driller for a natural gas company, was unwilling to use a printed direction form to aid his weak organization and memory skills in attempting tasks he thought should be easy. He insisted that using such a "crutch" was too unlike his pre-traumatic functioning even after he had been given objective evidence that his performance was weak. L.B.'s therapist then suggested that he think of the printed directions as a "backup." Invited to think about "backups" in his own experience, L.B. was able to make the connection: "My gosh . . . The drilling team for the gas company always had a backup truck just in case the equipment being used broke. I even manned those trucks sometimes — just sitting, but getting paid for it because the company couldn't affort to lose the whole day's work if the equipment failed. They had to have a backup system ready to go."

Therapists sensitive to the backgrounds, symbols, and themes that are important to their patients (e.g., sports, cooking, automechanics, theater) may present or help patients to generate metaphors that can be very powerful in promoting understanding of strategies and breaking down resistance to their use.

2. *Personal Images:* J.N., a 29 year old head injured woman, had significant deficits in language processing but would not implement strategies of input control (e.g., requesting repetition, clarification), fearing that others would interpret such behavior as evidence of her being "dull or stupid." When asked whom she considered to be a bright and alert person, she responded "Gloria Steinem." J.N. was asked to close her eyes, to try to imagine Gloria Steinem's asking an interviewer to repeat or rephrase a question, and to note whether Ms.

Steinem could do so with grace, self-respect, and naturalness. J.N. could, and she could also successfully engage in subsequent practice sessions stressing input control, having legitimized the process to herself through a personally meaningful image that served as a powerful role model. J.N. later reported that she had put the image to work for herself when she needed clarification or repetition from speakers.

We occasionally ask patients to interview valued friends or relatives to investigate the strategies they use in circumstances of stress or self-consciousness, and then to explore their applicability to their own situations. These techniques can then be incorporated into a program similar to Meichenbaum's stress inoculation procedures (Meichenbaum, 1977).

3. *Biographical anecdotes:* H.P., 30 year old and herself a former therapist, was reluctant to participate in group discussion with other head injured adults, and resisted straightforward encouragement to speak up. In an individual session, she described her paralyzing fear of "making mistakes" as the chief source of her resistance. She was intrigued, however, by a story her therapist told her about the famous psychiatrist Milton Erickson. Her curiosity was immediately piqued when she learned that Erickson, like herself, was physically disabled, and she was intrigued by Erickson's attitude toward his mistakes. When he was a medical student Erickson was confronted by peers who were annoyed by the veritable glee he expressed when he learned of his own mistakes in mock diagnoses. Erickson responded that if he were invariably correct, he wouldn't learn anything; his errors were opportunities to learn and grow. H.P. spontaneously referred to this story several times in later sessions, alluding to its impact in changing her attitude toward the risk taking that she associated with group discussion.

Stories of how other patients, professionals, or even therapists themselves use strategic procedures to achieve their goals may enhance a patient's willingness to experiment with strategies. Stories are natural, nonthreatening, and engaging, and they can encourage behaviors that may otherwise seem unattractive.

4. *Naturalistic modeling:* We occasionally arrange for a person admired by the patient to "spontaneously" demonstrate a compensatory procedure in a timely, noticeable, and natural fashion. This also can be a more powerful mode of communication than repeated and well-intentioned but ineffective efforts to convince, cajole, or shame a patient into using the procedure.

5. *Attention focusing codes:* Easy-to-remember code words may be helpful for patients who can't remember their strategy or who have trouble discerning the key features of the procedure. For example,

patients whose verbal expression is rambling or tangential may remember their verbal strategy with a code like CBS (clear, brief, and simple), or KISS (keep it simple and sweet), or STP (stop, think, and plan). Such codes and mottos can also be used as written cues that patients can keep handy (e.g., in wallets, on toolboxes or kitchen walls).

In a similiar vein, teaching visually distractible patients to focus their attention on easily accessible objects (e.g., a ring or thumbnail) while organizing thoughts prior to speaking has also been useful in some instances. M.D., 40 years old, claimed that without this strategy she would never have been able to testify coherently at a hearing she had repeatedly delayed because of concerns about her organization and clarity of expression.

MEMORY AND ORGANIZATION

Memory

Residual memory deficits are among the most frequently reported sequelae of severe closed head injury in adults (Brooks, 1984; Kapur & Pearson, 1983; Tabaddor, Mattis, Zazula & Phil, 1984; van Zomeren & van den Burg, 1985). Given the enormous complexity of memory functioning and the strength and variety of the relationships between memory and other aspects of cognition, any treatment program must begin with a precise delineation of the behavioral characteristics of a specific memory problem. The aspects of memory discussed in Chapter 3 (working memory, long-term storage, and memory/learning as a process; episodic and semantic memory; nonverbal and verbal memory; involuntary and deliberate memory; visual and auditory memory), together with the many factors that influence learning, are useful categories for analyzing a memory problem and defining the focus of treatment.

Two approaches to the management of memory disorders have received considerable attention in the literature on head injury rehabilitation: direct retraining and compensation. *Direct retraining* involves the attempt to improve memory functioning by means of repetitive memory exercises (e.g., practicing recalling paragraphs or lists of words, and playing artificial "memory" games). Moffat (1984) reported that the results of such memory "muscle building" exercises have been disappointing. Although in some cases patients working on a specific set of items have improved their performance, this progress was not generalized to any other task. Whereas the value of this kind of mental exercise in the treatment of stable residual memory impairments has not been documented, it may help to build patients' morale which improves when they believe that they are doing something to "improve their memory" (Harris & Sunderland, 1981). Furthermore, memory exercises may have the valuable effects of heightening a person's awareness of a memory problem, promoting improved attention, and causing him or her to begin to think about strategic procedures that could compensate to some degree for impaired memory. Finally, there is some speculation, which is based on analogies with the effects of early physical exercise in brain damaged animals, that memory exercise may in some way enhance recovery during the critical period of neural regeneration (Harris & Sunderland, 1981).

Although repetitive exercise does not appear to improve the overall efficiency of a person's memory or learning, extensive repetition may be necessary to enable amnesic individuals to enter new information into long-term memory (Wood, Ebert, & Kinsbourne, 1982). Such patients can learn facts and procedures through practice, but have no recollection of that practice. We have observed the same phenomenon in the acquisition by amnesic head injured patients of orientation information that is rehearsed daily. This is *not,* however, to say that the memory functioning of these patients has improved.

Compensation, including the deliberate use of internal memory strategies as well as external memory aids, has become a standard part of memory therapy. The use of mnemonics (e.g., creative associations, visual images, and acronyms) has value in the treatment of very specific memory problems, such as inability to remember people's names or difficulty remembering the location of things or lists of things (Moffat, 1984). External aids — a memo book or journal or compact computerized memory aid — are often essential for patients with a significant episodic memory disorder who need a record of events that is permanent and accessible. It is important to select and design such aids carefully and in light of the patient's situational needs and preferences. (See Wilson & Moffat, 1984, for a thorough discussion of compensation for memory disorders by means of mnemonic strategies and external aids.)

Indirect treatment to enhance memory performance involves targeting cognitive processes or systems that are related to memory in such a way that improvements in these areas have the effect of improving memory functioning in a relevant domain of memory. There is some evidence that this more general cognitive approach to treatment of memory problems is productive. Schacter and Tulving (1982) reviewed 2 studies that showed that both amnesic patients and their normal counterparts benefited substantially from "deeper semantic processing" (Cermak, Reale & Baker, 1978) and modifications in context to make it more distinctive (Winocur & Kinsbourne, 1978). Because amnesic patients did not benefit differentially more than control group subjects, however, Schacter and Tulving cautioned against inferring that "shallow semantic processing" or inadequate processing of context were sources of the memory problems of amnesic patients. The significant treatment implication is that the learning of amnesic patients can be improved when the way in which they process information is modified or enhanced. Moffat (1984) reviewed two case studies of head injured individuals whose recall of newspaper articles improved considerably after using an organized study procedure designed to promote deeper, or more elaborate, processing of the material. Gianutsos and Gianutsos (1979) found similarly that the learning performance of four head injured patients who had been taught to use a procedure to enhance semantic processing improved over a range from slight to considerable, with varying stability of gains. Malec and Questad (1983) described a head injured individual who made significant gains in memory performance after training to improve semantic elaboration and organization. A large and growing body of evidence supports the thesis that the memory performance of school-age children with learning disorders improves when they are prompted to actively organize or elaborate information to be learned (Brown, 1979; Feuerstein, 1980; Rohwer, 1973).

Research in the area of learning and memory has clearly established that retention and recall are a function of many interacting variables, including the attention and orientation of the learner (Postman & Kruesi, 1977); depth of processing or degree of elaboration (Craik & Tulving, 1975); the learner's knowledge, organization and degree of integration of the information with existing knowledge (Bartlett, 1932; Brown, 1975, 1979; Moely, 1977; Piaget, 1983); significance (emotional, social, or intellectual) of the information to be learned (Smirnov, 1973); and the context of encoding and retrieval (Jacoby & Craik, 1979; Tulving & Thomson, 1973). Treatment to improve attentional functioning, and derivatively memory, has received considerable attention in recent clinical discussions of head injury rehabilitation (Wood, 1984) and is supported by evidence that memory deficits may be a consequence of attentional problems in patients with frontal lobe damage (Stuss & Benson, 1984; Stuss et al., 1982).

One of the best understood and established relationships that has emerged from decades of research on learning and memory is that which links memory proficiency to knowledge and organization

(Pellegrino & Ingram, 1978). It has consistently been found that when new information is organized in a manner that is congruent with the way in which existing knowledge is already organized, recall is enhanced (Brown, 1975, 1979; Chi, 1978; Schank & Abelson, 1977). In other words, it is relatively easy to learn new information if one already knows a considerable amount about a topic and if one is able to fit new information neatly into the categories that have been used to organize the existing knowledge. This fact explains the ease with which students process and remember a piece of information in an advanced course and the great effort with which they learn the same piece of information in an introductory course. Without an adequately organized knowledge base into which new information can be readily integrated, the learner must either learn the information in a purely rote way, construct a new scheme for organizing the information, or attempt to integrate the information into existing schemes as indirectly related bits of information or as a set of exceptions — all demanding tasks.

Organization is, therefore, a key factor in the type of *active* information processing — involving elaboration and integration — that increases the probability that new information will be efficiently encoded, stored, and subsequently retrieved. Memory therapy for many patients is, then, based on the assumption that memory will improve if they can learn to be more active and effective in the organized processing of new information.

We will focus our discussion of indirect treatment for memory disorders on the relation between organizing processes and memory. The thesis is that by improving a head injured patient's organizational abilities through direct training in organizing, compensatory organizational strategies, and instruction in the concept of organization and how it relates to memory, memory functioning may be improved at least in areas where organizing skills affects learning.

Organization

Most head injured patients evidence organizational problems at some point in their recovery (Hagen, 1981; Szekeres, Ylvisaker & Holland, 1985; Zeigarnik, 1965). Impaired organizing processes may be apparent from formal testing (e.g., from patients' poor performance on tests of semantic associations), rambling, tangential conversation, poorly sequenced daily activities, or general confusion with even simple tasks. In many cases, disorganization remains as a residual deficit that interferes with the efficiency of any activity and creates a distinct disadvantage in encoding, storing, and retrieving information.

A thorough understanding of organization is useful for clinicians in defining intervention targets and also for patients in understanding their own organizational problems. Organization can be understood as a *product,* as an *internal conceptual structure,* and as a *process* (i.e., mental activity). As a *product,* organization exists in a set of objects or events when they are related in a way that is stable and identifiable (Mandler, 1967). Some common organizational principles are perceptual similarity (e.g., organized by color, shape, or size); semantic similarity (e.g., organized by categories or by synonym/antonym relations); part-whole relation; discourse hierarchies (e.g., organized by main ideas and supporting details); functional groups (e.g., organized as things that are all involved in the same activity); and themes or experiential scripts (e.g., organized around consistently structured events such as going to a restaurant).

As a *conceptual structure,* organization is the mental representation of organizational principles or schemes which is hypothesized to explain an individual's organizing of objects, events, or behavior into a pattern; e.g., when he or she recounts an event in sequential order, organizes materials for a task in the order of their use, remembers an organized word list better than a disorganized list, or comprehends an organized story, description, or explanation better than a disorganized one.

As a *process,* organizing is a complex activity that can involve the entire cognitive mechanism. For example, writing a theme, which can be understood as an organizational activity, involves at least the following components: (a) having a goal; (b) scanning the information to be discussed to identify an organization that is inherent in the information; (c) if no inherent organization is found, considering what sort of organization can be imposed; (d) generating a plan to create the appropriate organization (e.g., writing an outline); (e) writing the theme; and (f) monitoring and evaluating the product in terms of the original goal. At the other extreme, organizing can be as simple and automatic as keeping one's clothes consistently in the same drawers or grouping a list of groceries into vegetables, fruits, and meats. Organization can be imposed on information when it is received (input organization), on one's own processes of thinking and retrieving information, and on one's verbal and nonverbal behavior (output organization). What one knows about a given subject, how this knowledge is itself organized, and what one is currently experiencing (including internal emotions) are all involved in the organizing process.

Treatment for Deficits in Memory and Organization

Treating organizational deficits is an important intervention for its own sake, since disorganization can interfere seriously with vocational success and independent living. Because of the strong relationship between organization and memory, organizational deficits are often a primary target in the treatment of memory problems as well. Organization training involves three distinct phases: (a) reestablishing or developing an organized knowledge base; (b) teaching patients to recognize the distinction between organized and disorganized behavior, objects, or events and to appreciate the usefulness of organization; and (c) developing organizing strategies that an individual can differentially impose on appropriate stimuli to facilitate the efficient encoding, storage, and retrieval of information. The first two phases will be discussed under the heading Organization and Involuntary Learning and the third under the heading Organization and Deliberate Learning.

Organization and Involuntary (Incidental) Learning

Patients in a state of post-traumatic confusion and disorientation are not appropriate candidates for learning deliberate strategies to compensate for cognitive deficits. Other patients who are beyond this phase of recovery may nevertheless be so limited in their thinking that it is difficult for them to understand anything more complex than very concrete external aid strategies. Both groups can, however, profit from activities that promote a more organized knowledge base and an appreciation of how better organized behavior can help them to achieve their goals.

The goals of treatment at this stage are to help patients (a) reestablish access to previously acquired knowledge and organizational schemes; (b) develop new knowledge and organizational schemes; (c) develop an awareness of organizational schemes and an appreciation of their value in completing tasks well; (d) think and ponder ideas more deeply; and (e) begin to develop their metacognitive awareness of these processes which they will need later when they learn and deliberately use strategies to compensate for memory or organizational deficits.

At this stage, treatment should take place in a highly structured environment that facilitates learning without the patient making a *deliberate* attempt to learn. The patient's attention is directed toward performing a task effectively and efficiently, rather than toward learning and remembering. The importance of knowledge and the problems that result from knowledge gaps should also be emphasized in relation to the task at hand. The use of reference materials or human resources should be modelled and discussed (e.g., looking up words in a dictionary, consulting an encyclopedia, or asking another person who may know an answer) to underscore the need for adequate knowledge both to do a job well and to increase one's knowledge base. The environmental structure should also include a consistent set of expectations for social behaviors and thinking in all group and individual therapy sessions, such as attending, pondering ideas, thinking before responding, following rules of turn taking (even if a turn is no more than "I don't know"), and producing relevant and concise responses (with prompting as needed).

TREATMENT PROCEDURES. A general instructional strategy for integrating organization and memory treatment includes the following steps:

1. Selecting a functional task that is interesting and meaningful (or at least acceptable) to the patient (e.g., baking a cake; writing a paragraph on an interesting topic)
2. Presenting an organizational scheme as a means to get the job done (e.g., filling out a form that includes the relevant information in outline form)
3. Completing the task using the organizational scheme, with prompting and demonstrating as necessary (e.g., writing the paragraph)
4. Discussing what was done and how it was done, focusing questions on the organizational scheme and how it helped, on whether the job was done well or poorly and what could have been done to improve the "product," on what other tasks could be organized this way, and on activities that require other types of organization

The steps above represent an involuntary memory situation, in which the primary focus is on completing a meaningful task and the target of learning is the means the patient uses to complete it. The organizational scheme then has importance in relation to the individual's concrete goal, a condition which often leads to better retention (Smirnov, 1973). Although metacognitive awareness of cognitive activity is not an explicit objective of treatment, discussing with the patient how tasks are most efficiently completed does introduce thinking about thinking, internal organizing, remembering, and other cognitive processes.

Organization can be explicity introduced as a topic in therapy through either verbal or nonverbal tasks. Feature analysis is a useful verbal activity for discussing organization as a product, conceptual structure, and process. Feature analysis is an organized thinking procedure that is used to promote the reorganization of concepts and an organized search of semantic and episodic memory (Haarbauer-Krupa, Moser, Sullivan & Szekeres, 1985). Basically, it involves considering any familiar concept (representing an object, person, or event) and systematically describing it in terms of predefined categories of description (group, action, use, location, properties, and associations). A feature analysis guide (Fig. 4–1) is used to structure the patient's search through his or her knowledge base. Information is written in the appropriate boxes and evaluated in terms of relevance and completeness. Unfilled or sparsely filled boxes reveal incomplete knowledge and patients are encouraged to fill them in by asking relevant questions or by using appropriate references. When the descriptions are complete, the information and its organization are put to

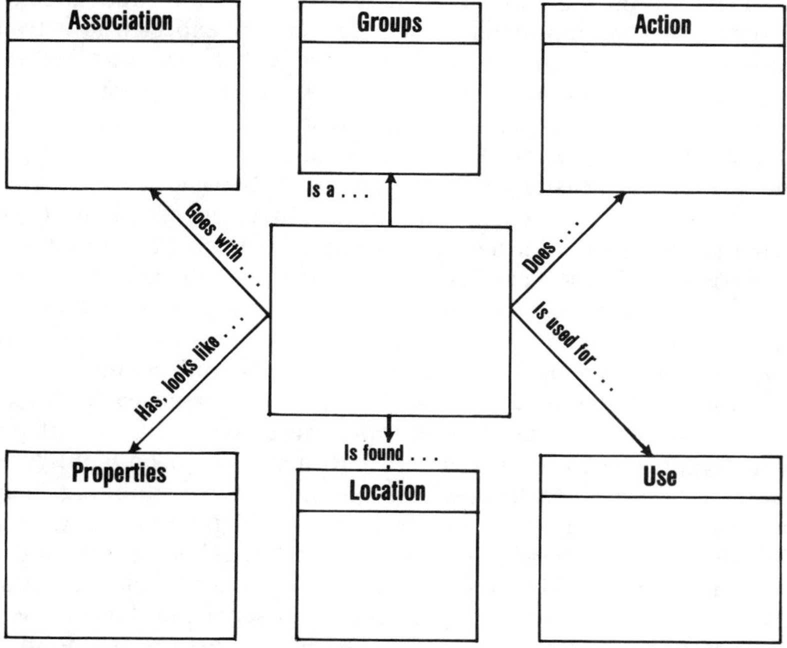

Figure 4–1. Feature analysis guide.

use in a planned functional activity, such as writing a descriptive paragraph or doing a problem-solving exercise involving the concepts that have been analyzed. Subsequent discussion can focus on the organizational scheme (the feature analysis guide) and how it helped to generate a good description; on the product (the descriptive paragraph); and on the patient's process of organizing his or her knowledge about something.

Table 4–3 presents a number of other organizational schemes and treatment activities that are designed to develop schemes. Of equal importance, the activities are designed to promote an understanding of the reasons for organizing in certain ways and of the situations that require one type of organizing rather than another. Table 4–3 also lists questions to prompt reflection, which may result in an adequate degree of metacognitive maturity to move to a deliberate learning condition and the teaching of deliberate compensatory strategies.

Organization and Deliberate Learning

The strong relationship between organization and memory becomes even more apparent when learners are expected to actively integrate new information with what they already know or to elaborate on the new information in order to make it more memorable. Without effective organizing procedures, patients not only forget the information that is presented, but also distort or misinterpret the information very easily. Helping patients to become active learners through the use of organizational schemes involves three goals: (a) an increased *awareness* of a memory deficit, of the relationship between organizing information and remembering it, and of the need to develop effective organizing schemes; (b) the acquisition of effective and reliable *strategies* for organizing information or tasks; and (c) the *generalization* of these strategies to functional contexts and settings.

Since each of these treatment areas is discussed earlier in the Compensatory Strategies section, only those issues that are of particular importance to organization and memory will be highlighted. *Direct metacognitive instruction* in components of thinking helps patients recognize both the role of active organizing in deep thinking and efficient remembering and also their own cognitive style, including both strengths and weaknesses. Figure 4–2, adapted from Feuerstein (1980), illustrates in a highly simplified and schematic form some of the components of thinking and the interrelationships among them. In particular, it highlights the role of "elaboration" (which includes what we have been referring to as "organizing") in thinking. Patients

Table 4-3. Re-establishing Organized Semantic Memory

Organizational Schema (means for attaining the goal)	Task & Goal	Activity	Reflection*
Perceptual Similarity (e.g., Color, Shape, Size, Texture, Rhyme)	"The shop asked us to organize these leftover pieces of sandpaper so they can easily be found. Let's find a good way to do this."	1. Label small boxes for different grains (extra fine, fine, medium, etc.). 2. Sort the pieces according to their "texture" and put them into the labeled boxes. 3. Call out the textures and time how quickly they can be found.	How did you sort? Why this way? Was it "good"? In what other situations might one sort by texture? What would have happened if you had sorted by size? How could this help you remember where your tools or other possessions are kept or at least help you always locate them?
Semantic Similarity (e.g., superordinate category, opposites)	"We got a job to set up the layout of a new department store. We have to make it easy for customers to find what they want."	Make a floor plan specifying the location of departments. Place labeled items into the departments, grouping them by similarity, (e.g.,	How did you arrange the store? Why did you use that arrangement? In what other situations would you group things

continued

Table 4–3 *(continued)*

Organizational Schema	Task & Goal	Activity	Reflection
		TVs, stereos, radios) in one area, but subgrouped within the area. Make display arrangement to entice people to buy (e.g., comfortable chair, flowers, glass of wine and stereo).	this way? When would this arrangement be inconvenient? How could knowing this arrangement help your memory of a visit to a store? How did the display arrangement differ from the floor arrangement?
Function (Use)	"We are moving furniture into a new house. We have to arrange the living room for TV watching and conversation."	Make a floor plan and arrange labeled blocks representing the furniture. Then rearrange them for special occasions, such as a cocktail party, Tupperware party, etc.	How were the items arranged for each activity? Why did you have to change them? How is this different from a department store arrangement?
Main Idea and Topic (Discourse Structure)	"We will present today's news to the orientation group." (Watch a videotaped news items or listen to an audiotaped	Listen to the tape. Fill in a form (see sun diagram, Figure 4–3) answering Who, What, When, Where, Why, and	How did the form help you remember? When wouldn't the form help? How did you stay so

	news item.)	What happened questions and identifying the main idea. Relate the news item to another person using the diagram as notes.	organized and coherent when you related the news item?
Story Schema (Rummehlhart, 1975)	"We will share a short story or TV show with ( ) who was unable to see or hear it."	Watch the video tape of a TV show or listen to an audiotape of a radio show. Fill out a schema diagram, including characters, setting, and episodes. Retell the story using the organizational diagram as a cue.	How did this form help you remember? How is the information arranged? Why is this arrangement good for a story? Would it be good for a math book? Why not?
General Life Scripts (abstracted common life events)	"We will write our autobiographies and present a 'this is your life' program."	Fill out a form with labeled boxes of common life events (birth, school, marriage, job) and uncommon significant events (e.g., head injury). Using the form as a guide, write the autobiography and then present it	How did the form make writing more organized? How could the form help reconstruct the past? How is your autobiorgaphy organized (e.g., chronologically)? How did the written preparation help the oral

continued

Table 4–3 *(continued)*

Organizational Schema	Task & Goal	Activity	Reflection
		formally in a radio program format.	presentation?
Specific Event Scripts (e.g., going to a restaurant, going to the dentist)	"We will explain to (*a small child*) what it will be like when he has to go to the dentist.	Fill in a form with relevant information about the situation to prepare what you are going to say to the child: • Who will be there. • Equipment. • Sequence of expected events and actions. • Expected layout of the room and some variations. Then using the guide, explain to a child or explain in a role-playing situation.	How did this form help you? Why wouldn't a general life script help you? How is your explanation to the child organized? Why would this help you remember what has happened to you?

* Possible probe questions to develop metacognition, understanding, and awareness.

who are highly impulsive (i.e., who seemingly proceed directly from input to output with little thinking) or who seriously distort information because of their emotional or motivational state or who fail to monitor their behavior (i.e., no arrow from output back to elaboration) can easily track their thinking on this diagram and recognize what is missing.

The diagram can be used to highlight several important concepts that are relevant to the cognitive rehabilitation of head injured individuals: (a) there is an intimate relation between emotion and motivation on the one hand and all aspects of information processing on the other; (b) there are sequenced components in thinking, some of which might be strong and others weak; (c) one can isolate weak areas and find ways to compensate for them; and (d) since elaboration (which includes the active organizing of information) is central to thinking, improved elaboration facilitates the retention of information and more effective behavior. In teaching patients to use a schematic diagram of this sort to understand important aspects of their own cognitive functioning, clinicians must clearly explain, with well-

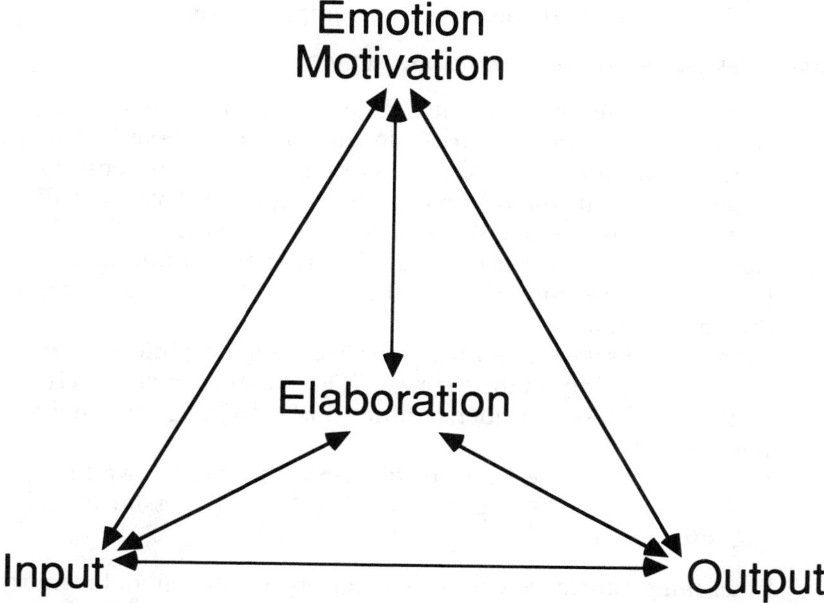

Figure 4–2. Schematic representation of some of the components of thinking, and the interrelationships among them. Adapted from Feuerstein (1980) with permission of the publisher.

chosen examples, the relation of components of the schema to ordinary tasks and experiences.

Strategies for improving memory by enhancing organizational skills can be divided into organizational strategies per se and strategies that help to make organizational activities possible. (Additional compensatory strategies are listed in Appendix 4–1.)

ORGANIZATIONAL STRATEGIES.

- Associating new information with old and making judgments about the importance and usefulness of the new information
- Constructing visual images to associate with the new information (for patients with good visual-perceptual functioning); determining whether novel, comical, and action-based images or more plausible and concrete images are more effective (Crovitz et al., 1979)
- Using special organizing schemes for classifying and arranging new information (e.g., the sun diagram, Fig. 4–3) or for planning and monitoring tasks (e.g., the structured thinking form, Fig. 5–2)
- Taking notes in an organized telegraphic form

STRATEGIES ENABLING ORGANIZATIONAL ACTIVITY.

- Controlling the rate, amount, and level of input by requesting clarification, repetition, or a slowing of the speaker's rate. When information is received too rapidly or is too dense or abstract, the likelihood that a head injured listener will understand and actively organize it is reduced.
- Repeating information subvocally. The retention of information in working memory affords the patient time to organize the information.
- Using active self-questioning when receiving new information (e.g., "Is this important to me?" "Do I know anything else about this?" "Am I understanding this?" "What is the main point of this?").
- Using customized self-cues in situations that are known to be problematic (e.g., "Stay cool — you'll get it" in stressful learning situations).

In teaching patients to compensate for organizational and memory deficits, therapists must give careful consideration to all of the factors listed earlier under Selecting Strategies for Patients. Three of these factors are salient in selecting organization and memory strategies.

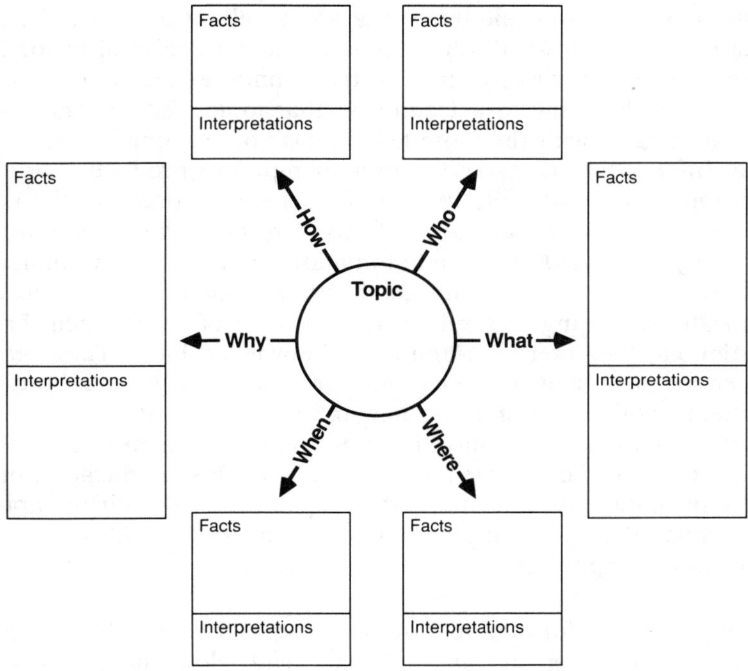

Figure 4-3. "Sun diagram" for classifying and arranging new information.

1. *Range of applicability* ("Domain specificity"): The domain of usefulness of many commonly used mnemonic strategies (e.g., the "peg word" strategy) is severely restricted. Strategies that are known to be useful for memorizing word lists, for instance, may have little usefulness in the academic, vocational, and social lives of adults. In contrast, strategies such as writing important information down or requesting clarification of information that is difficult to understand are broadly applicable.

2. *Difficulty of use:* Strategies that require elaborate mental manipulation of information may be effective and may be used by individuals when the stakes are sufficiently high (e.g., studying for an important exam) but because of simple cost-benefit considerations may not be generalized to more common life situations.

3. *Knowledge requirements:* The ability to organize information presupposes a certain amount of knowledge about a subject. If, for example, one knows absolutely nothing about medieval history, it would be a silly waste of time to try to impose creative organization while listening to a lecture on that topic. Rather, one must either struggle with the more tedious task of learning enough factual information to make the organizing effort productive or ask an appropriate authority for a useful scheme to organize the new information. The implications of this third factor have been insufficiently addressed in the rehabilitation literature. Many patients whose recovery is generally good and who plan to return to an educational setting or a relatively high level of employment have major gaps in their pre-traumatic knowledge base. These gaps interfere with new learning in many ways, including limiting patients' abilities to organize new information. In these cases, we have found that re-eduation is an essential ingredient of cognitive rehabilitation. Comupters are ideal tools for this re-education process since patients can use them independently of their therapists and since there is a large quantity of educational software available for the purpose.

Organizing information requires time and effort. Many head injured patients enter this task with an already slow rate of information processing and with an impulsive manner that resists the effort that is required. *Self-pacing* is thus a crucial dimension of the organizing phase of information processing. Head injured individuals need more time than others to organize, encode, and retrieve information before acting. Helping and encouraging patients to accommodate to this need — for example, teaching a patient to say, comfortably and meaningfully, "Let me think about that for a minute" — may be the clinician's most valuable contribution.

SOCIAL COGNITION

One of the residual deficits of severely head injured patients that is most distressing for family members and friends is impaired social interaction, which frequently deters patients from successfully reentering the community (see Chapter 9). In many cases, interactive problems have an emotional or psychodynamic basis that must be addressed by an appropriately trained professional. It is not uncommon, however, for social awkwardness, impulsiveness, offensive behavior, and unusual interpretations of social events to result from patients' weak social knowledge or shallow and distorted social thinking. This cognitive dimension argues for an interdisciplinary approach to these problems. CRT can facilitate more appropriate social behavior by setting as objectives the patient's reacquisition of social knowledge and an improvement in his or her social thinking. The goal of social-cognitive treatment is to help patients modify the way they process and represent information to enable them to interact more appropriately and effectively. (Chapter 3 includes additional information on the basis for social-cognitive intervention.)

We attempt to achieve this goal in three broadly distinguishable ways. First, we target the patient's social knowledge, which includes an awareness of (a) social events, situations, and routines (i.e., conventional "scripts"), and the rules that apply to each; (b) the conventional meaning of social behaviors and signals; (c) the process of attributing responsibility for behaviors and events, and the ease with which such attribution can be distorted; and (d) objects of social thinking, such as intentions, emotions, attitudes, traits, motives, values, and self-concept.

Second, we attempt to develop a wide variety of the cognitive processes and systems that a patient needs to actively observe, analyze, and interpret behavior and social situations accurately (to "read" behavior and situations), to draw logical conclusions from these interpretations, and to plan action in light of such objective interpretations. This treatment includes practice in "reading" behavior and situations, in drawing inferences, and in questioning the accuracy of these interpretations and inferences. At the same time, we stress the influence of individual biases on this process and practice interpreting behavior from different perspectives.

Third, we attempt to develop the patient's awareness of those situations in which it is particularly essential to interpret behavior or social events accurately (e.g., job interviews, interaction with supervisors), emphasizing the connection between this skill and achieving important life goals.

In this section, we discuss in some detail intervention for conversational deficits and briefly mention the role of CRT in promoting behavioral self-control. These areas are of considerable importance for head injured young adults facing the difficult task of returning to the community, but they do not exhaust the list of social-cognitive issues in rehabilitation.

It is important to distinguish between social-cognitive intervention and social skills training, even though the two overlap in practice. The focus of the former is on knowledge and information processing in relation to social realities and social behavior, while the latter focuses on social skills themselves and does not necessarily approach changing behavior by enhancing social knowledge and processing. The two, of course, converge in their ultimate goal: appropriate and effective behavior in a wide range of social situations. Attention must be given to both in the rehabilitation of head injured adults.

Conversation

Kraut and Higgins (1984) described communication as a "potentially rich intersection of the cognitive and social" (p. 87) and noted that "the construction of communication is the major way that social cognition manifests itself in daily life" (p. 87). Conversation is the primary medium for exchanging social information and maintaining social contact, and is a basic tool for achieving social and vocational goals. As social interaction, conversation involves coordinating and integrating one's plans and intentions with those of others.

Conversation often appears casual and loosely structured; that is, the flow of topics and selection of speakers are not predetermined (Sacks, Schegloff & Jefferson, 1974). There are, however, both general and specific rules governing what is said and where, when, how, and to whom it is said. There are rules ("social conventions") for setting and shifting topics, assigning and taking turns, repairing breakdowns in communication, conveying intention, recognizing status, being polite, and initiating and terminating conversations (Schegloff & Sacks, 1973). At the most general level of analysis, Grice (1967) has identified a central principle of conversation: that speakers and listeners try to cooperate with one another to communicate accurately and efficiently, and in observing this principle try to make their contributions to conversation informative (quantity), truthful (quality), relevant, and clear (manner). Speakers and listeners are highly sensitive to deviations from these conventions and often interpret such deviations as purposeful (Clark & Clark, 1977). Persistent violation of these rules produces unconventional conversation and may profoundly affect social interaction and vocational achievement. Conversations with people who repeatedly violate these rules are often quickly terminated or avoided entirely, as families of head injured individuals have often reported (Bond, 1983).

Successful conversation depends on a number of factors, including knowledge of the rules, knowledge of one's conversation partner, continued monitoring and memory of the topic and other's contributions, comprehension of the meaning of what is said, and, notably, accurate inferences regarding the speaker's intent from overt verbal and non-verbal behavior and contextual cues. This is a complex task indeed. It is not surprising that cognitive problems, such as impaired attention or perception, memory deficits, weak organization of thoughts, impulsiveness, disinhibition, or a reduced knowledge base, can profoundly affect communication and social interaction.

Treatment for conversational deficits varies with a patient's needs. Goals may include (a) developing the patient's knowledge of conversational features and rules (e.g., appropriate openings and closings), (b) developing his or her "listener awareness" and strategies to learn more about listeners during a conversation, and (c) developing the ability to draw accurate inferences about intentions and motives. More generally, treatment may emphasize the importance of correctly interpreting messages and the consequences of unsuccessful conversational interaction. Table 4–4 lists selected goals and procedures that may be included in a social-cognitive program to improve a patient's conversational skills — and, as a consequence, his or her social interaction.

Behavioral Self-Control

Cognitive deficits in the areas of planning, initiating, inhibiting, self-monitoring, reasoning, problem solving, and accessing past knowledge and experience may easily produce inappropriate and poorly controlled social and work behaviors, particularly when a patient is unfamiliar with an environment or is engaged in activities that are not routine.

CRT can contribute to the treatment of those behavioral problems which result from a failure to think about one's actions or from weak or distorted thinking about social realities. Therapy goals might include training the patient (a) to accurately identify and classify inappropriate behavior and to distinguish it from appropriate behavior; (b) to monitor and objectively describe his or her own interactive behavior; (c) to accurately attribute the cause of events to a situation or to the responsible individual, and to examine these inferences for possible bias (e.g., egocentric perspective); and (d) to thoughtfully predict the consequences of behavior from his or her own and from others' perspectives. Finally, training in these areas of social cognition can be incorporated into a program of cognitive behavior modification (CBM), in which patients learn self-instructional strategies to control behavior (Meichenbaum, 1977). Over the past decade, clinicians have evolved a sophisticated technology of behavioral self-control,

Table 4–4. A Program for Improving Conversational Interaction

Goal: Develop awareness of the characteristics of conversation, including conversational rules and conventions

Procedures:

1. Identify the features of conversation (e.g., opening and closing, topics and topic control [setting, maintaining, and shifting], turn taking, speech acts, uses of conversation, appropriate locations and behaviors involved). The Feature Analysis Guide (Figure 4–1) can be used to structure this analysis.
2. Using video or audio-taped conversations, identify and evaluate the features of conversations. Discuss the rules and social conventions that apply to the conversation and explore why those rules may have evolved (e.g., without turn-taking, information would not be transmitted).
3. Role play conversations with varied patterns (e.g., balanced vs. unequal turn-taking patterns). Explore situations in which different patterns may be appropriate.

Goal: Develop awareness of speaker intent and improve ability to interpret speaker intent

Procedures:

1. Using video or audio-taped conversations, discuss the speaker's intent. Consider possible interpretations of the speaker's intent, identifying and evaluating the evidence that supports each interpretation or inference (e.g., "I think that was an insult because of the tone of voice," "I doubt it, because I know that he wouldn't do that and because he was smiling — I think it was good natured teasing.") Discussions should be sufficiently deep to sensitize patients to the complexity of interpretation and the ease with which distorted interpretations are generated. Repeated why-questions are useful to force deeper analysis. If there are patterns to a given patient's distorted interpretations (e.g., regularly inferring negative intent when none was present), this should be pointed out.
2. Role play conversations with a variety of speaker intents (e.g., to console, scare, insult, encourage, threaten, entertain, punish). Identify signals of intent.

Goal: Develop awareness of conversational topics, conventions for setting, maintaining, extending, shifting, or abruptly changing a topic, and methods of conversational control

Procedures:

1. Identify the topic and trace the topic flow in taped TV programs or in group conversation.
2. Practice maintaining the topic in conversation. Write a topic on the board, then analyze a taped conversation to determine the relevance of each contribution.
3. Practice shifting the conversational topic. Determine if the shifts were logical and easy to follow, or might confuse the listener.

4. Practice extending the topic by adding relevant information and seeking information from other interactants by using open-ended questions (e.g., "What do you like about the game?").
5. Practice controlling conversations by using specific techniques for opening, interrupting, shifting topic (e.g., marking abrupt shifts with "Oh, that reminds me."), and closing conversations. Practice using assertions to convey conviction; questions to get more information, confirm information, or transfer a turn; indirect requests to give polite commands (e.g. "Could you please open the window for me?"); and markers such as "Yes, go on" to show that one is listening to the speaker.
6. Make a chart of appropriate topics in relation to situations and conversation partners. This could either be individualized for each patient or identify generic social conventions.

Goal: Develop effective use of varied speech acts

Procedures:

1. Practice techniques for such communicative intents as: giving information, requesting information, directing, demanding, asserting, refusing, warning, threatening, promising, complimenting, criticizing, teasing, joking, and comforting.

Goal: Develop awareness of one's listener

Procedures:

1. Practice "taking readings" and making inferences about the listener's interest in and knowledge of a topic, comprehension of what has been said, emotional reaction to what has been said, and feelings about the speaker. Discuss how best to present information to various types of listener.
2. Role play communication situations with listeners of varying status, age, comprehension abilities, and familiarity. Determine appropriate vocabulary, speech acts, and intonation patterns for each listener.

Goal: Develop effective speaking and listening skills, including compensatory strategies

Procedures:

1. Practice strategies for repairing comprehension or production breakdowns (e.g., "Could you repeat that, please?" "I don't think I'm making myself clear.").
2. Practice strategies for improving speech intelligibility (e.g., self-pacing, using a portable microphone).
3. Practice eye contact, interest postures, and continuation signals.
4. Discuss and rehearse specific rules and social conventions (e.g., use polite phrases, don't say certain things in public, don't talk with your mouth full).
5. Role play conversations that focus on Grice's (1967) conversational maxims: informativeness, truthfulness, relevance, and clarity.

and its effectiveness has been supported in the treatment of several types of inappropriate behavior (Keogh & Glover, 1980).

Having identified the factors that tend to precipitate certain types of behavioral response, individuals can more accurately predict how they will react in certain situations and can formulate a plan to prevent loss of control. For example, if patients are more likely to behave inappropriately or lose control in noisy, stimulating environments or with loved ones, then the goal of therapy may be to create a habit of self-monitoring and self-instructing (e.g., reminding oneself to "Be careful" and "Keep cool") in such situations. In addition, if patients can recognize an internal signal that occurs before they lose control, a self-control strategy may be used to interrupt this sequence.

CRT treatment must be carefully integrated with traditional behavioral approaches and with psychotherapeutic counseling. If inappropriate behavior is strictly attention seeking and not the consequence of cognitive deficits, then the attention that the behavior receives through the cognitive approach may increase rather than decrease its occurrence. Inappropriate behavior is equally beyond the scope of CRT if its source is in the dynamics of interpersonal relationships. When a combination of factors is involved, as is often the case, tight interdisciplinary programming is necessary.

Case illustration: T.R., a head injured adolescent, had a generally poor self-concept and tended to infer negative intent in the behavior of others and to attribute the cause of her own behavior to situational factors. On a community outing, T.R. reacted in an inappropriate and hostile way toward a store clerk. She later explained that the clerk "made her act that way because she was mean." It emerged that she had inferred "meanness" from the clerk's hurried manner, poor eye contact, and failure to smile. T.R. also admitted that she was very anxious about being in the community and had difficulty dealing with any upsetting events.

The goals that were then isolated for T.R. in her social cognition therapy group were: (a) inferring intent (e.g., "meanness") more carefully from overt behavior (e.g., frowning) and considering a variety of possible intents; (b) accepting responsibility for such inferences and for her resulting behavior; (c) identifying those situations in which her behavior was frequently inappropriate; and (d) developing and practicing self-instructional strategies for those situations.

Generalization

Treatment of conversational or self-control deficits is incomplete without a careful plan to generalize treatment gains to functional settings, such as the home, work place, and community. The procedures for promoting generalization and maintenance which are discussed in the section Teaching Compensatory Strategies apply also to social skills and behavioral self-control strategies. Recongizing that individuals do not automatically generalize their use of strategies to nonclinical settings, Meichenbaum (1977) has called upon clinicians to teach generalization directly. This process includes training patients to accurately discriminate situations in which the strategy is appropriate and supervising the patient's practice in increasingly natural settings and situations, including unfamiliar settings and unpredictable activities. Systematic training, essential for effective generalization, requires therapists to gradually increase demands on the patient. Figure 4–4 illustrates this progression from the highly structured clinical setting to less predictable but still relatively "safe" areas of the hospital to unpredictable situations in the community.

In order to ensure success, develop self-confidence, and promote maximum generalization, the clinician should carefully manipulate the control variables of task and environmental complexity, support,

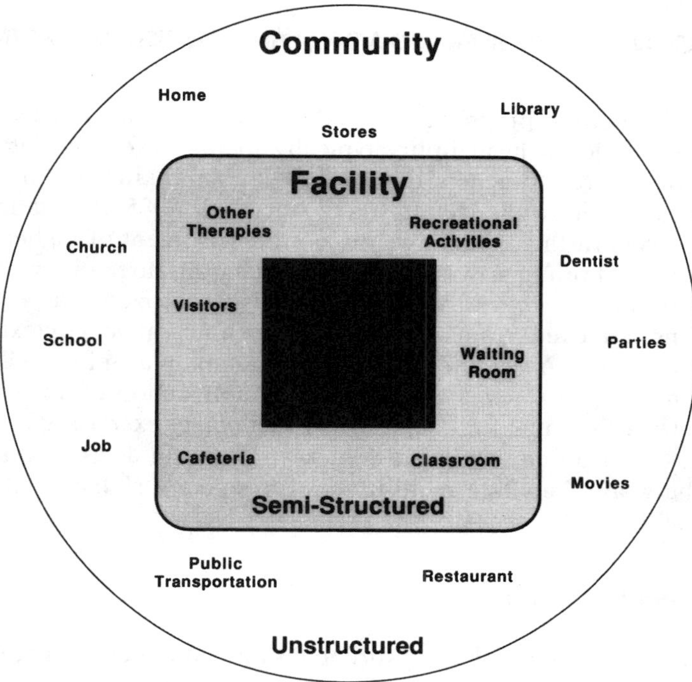

Figure 4–4. Progression for teaching generalization of strategies. Variables to be considered include structure, support, familiarity, task demands, environmental complexity.

and familiarity at each step of this progression. When a patient is able to use a learned skill or strategy with minimal control or cuing in a treatment session, then it is time to move to the next setting, the facility at large, which by its very nature is less structured. Once again, the clinician should provide enough control so that success is ensured, systematically decreasing this control as the patient is able to successfully use and generalize the use of skills and strategies. The same progression from thorough control and cuing to minimal control is repeated when the training moves from the confines of the facility to more unpredictable and stressful community settings. In this way, the patient is required to cope with only one additional stress or change at a time. Success of the intervention is additionally enhanced when the patient's family and other rehabilitation staff members are included in the training, when group sessions are used as a relaxed atmoshpere in which to give and receive feedback on one another's performance, and when only one or two skills or strategies are targeted at one time.

REASONING, PROBLEM SOLVING, AND DECISION MAKING

Rehabilitation programs for adults in the late stages of recovery from severe closed head injury typically include exercises for what are often referred to generally as higher-level thinking or reasoning processes (Adamovitch, Henderson & Auerbach, 1985; Prigatano and others, 1986). In this section, we discuss the treatment of higher-level reasoning and problem-solving impairments from three different perspectives: (a) *Component training:* exercising separate aspects of reasoning removed from a functional or integrative context (see Chapter 3); (b) *Integrative training:* exercising reasoning skills in problem-solving exercises that require the application of all types of higher-level thinking; and, (c) *Functional training:* exercising selected aspects of reasoning within the context of practical decision making, with the goal of making real-life decision-making skills as effective as possible.

Component Training

An increasing number of workbooks and computer programs are available that provide multitrial drill and practice in higher-level thinking and reasoning. The taxonomies of reasoning skills vary from text to text but often include the following categories, which overlap to some extent. These types of thinking are discussed in greater detail in Chapter 3.

Covergent thinking: the ability to discern a central theme or main idea in a set of facts. Clinicians commonly attempt to train patients in this skill with exercises such as: briefly state the main idea in a paragraph read or heard; compose telegrams with a restricted number of words on the basis of given information; identify a common feature in objects or events that are not obviously related; and identify a situation in which each member of a given set of facts may be included.

Divergent thinking: the ability to flexibly explore instances that fall under general concepts, to create varied explanations for events or solutions to problems, and to generate explanations or solutions that differ from standard explanations or solutions. Typical exercises include: give two or more meanings for ambiguous words or sentences; explain both the literal and figurative meaning of metaphors, idioms, or figures of speech; list as many examples of concepts as possible; generate several solutions to given problems or explanations for given events; create several possible endings for incomplete stories; and explain jokes or riddles.

Deductive reasoning: the ability to draw conclusions or make inferences based strictly on the formal logical relationships among propositions (e.g., if all men are mortal and Socrates is a man, then Socrates is mortal). Typical exercises include: evaluate arguments to determine if the conclusion follows necessarily from the premises (the evidence); determine what additional premises must be added to make an argument valid; determine what additional information is needed to solve a mathematical problem; determine what conclusions can validly be drawn from a set of premises; and reconstruct in an explicit way arguments that are embedded in newspaper editorials, political speeches, or other texts.

Inductive reasoning: the ability to generalize from experience; that is, to draw conclusions that are supported by, but do not necessarily follow from personal experience or other empirical evidence. Typical exercises include: generate a hypothesis that would explain a set of observations; evaluate the acceptability of generalizations given the facts on which they are based; and state the likely effects of a given event.

Analogical reasoning: the ability to draw conclusions that are suggested by, but are not directly related to, past experience; to perceive various relationships among sets of words, objects, events, and ideas. Typical exercises include: complete word analogies and give an explanation of the principle of the analogy; and determine if a solution to a problem is reasonable in terms of analogy with similar solutions to similar types of problems.

Evaluative and interpretive thinking: the ability to interpret information objectively, particularly within an emotionally charged context; to weigh the relative merits of alternative solutions and courses of action; and to formulate and defend evaluative opinions about people, objects, events, and beliefs. Typical exercises include: determine which members of a set of sentences are facts and which are opinions; give several reasons for and against an evaluative opinion; rank a set of solutions to a problem in terms of a set of criteria; evaluate the social appropriateness of various behavioral responses to hypothetical solutions; and generate alternative interpretations of behavior within a context and give reasons for and against each interpretation.

Adamovitch, Henderson, and Auerbach (1985) and Burns, Halper, and Mogil (1985) have listed several workbooks that include exercises of this sort.

Integrative Training: Problem Solving

It is doubtless an important goal to restore patients' higher-level thinking processes following head injury to whatever extent possible. There are problems, however, with approaching this goal in a workbook fashion, that is, simply taking a patient through series of exercises that are not embedded in a functional context and may have no perceived relation to the goals that the patient actively espouses. One does not rebuild thinking skills to enable a patient to score well on a test of higher cognitive functions. The goal is ultimately to promote more deliberate, careful, and critical thinking in actual life situations, that is, those requiring problem solving and decision making. To this end, clinicians must actively bridge the gap between cognitive exercises and their functional application to the integrative tasks of daily life. The failure to generalize and functionally apply skills in a novel context is a pervasive consequence of significant brain injury, both congenital and acquired. Furthermore, adults often resist treatment activities whose utility they do not perceive. Without patients' interest and engagement in treatment exercises and plans on the part of therapists to generalize patients' skills to functional contexts, workbook drills run the risk of failure.

Feuerstein (1980) presented a curriculum for teaching thinking skills within the integrative context of problem solving. Training in use of the curriculum includes clear instructions on how teachers or clinicians can create bridges from abstract exercises to functional application. The success of the curriculum with a variety of school children (cognitively capable of formal operational thinking), including mildly retarded and culturally disadvantaged children, has been documented (Feuerstein, 1980). Parts of the curriculum have also been used successfully at our agency with a group of head injured young adults in a work adjustment setting and with a mixed group of learning impaired adolescents, including those with head injuries, in a secondary education classroom.

With selected head injured patients who have good attentional and organizational abilities, we have frequently addressed deficits in higher-level thinking processes in an integrative problem-solving context, but without the formality of an academic curriculum. Systematic, deliberate, and thorough problem solving, the steps of which are outlined below, includes all of the types of thinking and reasoning that we have discussed.

Step 1: *Identifying the problem:* "What exactly is the problem?" (convergent thinking)

Step 2: *Classifying the problem:* "What kind of problem is this?" (convergent thinking)

Step 3: *Identifying the goal:* "What will you gain by solving this problem?" (convergent thinking)

Step 4: *Identifying the information relevant to solving the problem:* "What do you need to know to solve the problem? Have you interpreted the information correctly?" (divergent thinking: sense of relevance; interpretive thinking)

Step 5: *Identifying possible solutions:* "What could you possibly do to solve this problem?" (divergent thinking)

Step 6: *Evaluating the solutions:* "What is good or bad about each of these possibilities?" (evaluative thinking; analogical reasoning; inductive reasoning)
Consider: "Is the solution effective? Do you have enough time to do it? Are you able to do it? Would you like to do it? Does it break any rules? Have solutions like this been useful in the past? What are the effects on yourself? on others? on the environment?"

Step 7: *Determining which solution is best:* "All things considered, what's the smartest thing to do?" (evaluative thinking; deductive reasoning)

Step 8: *Formulating a plan:* "How do you plan to accomplish this?" (executive direction; convergent thinking)

Step 9: *Monitoring and evaluating the results:* "Did it work? Are you satisfied? Do you have any new problems?" (evaluative thinking)

By exercising patients' thinking skills in the context of practical (hypothetical) problem solving, it is possible to highlight for patients the functional significance of these skills in relation to their own goals and daily affairs. Patients can be given targeted, intensive exercises in one or more specific areas of reasoning in which their weakness interferes disproportionately with effective problem solving, but these exercises are always combined with discussions of the usefulness and importance of improved thinking in the weak area to everyday transactions.

When hypothetical rather than real problems are used, these exercises have considerably more value in a group than in an individual setting. For example, each patient may be a weak divergent thinker, but collectively the group may produce excellent divergent thinking. Peer modeling of thinking skills is also a useful teaching medium, and peer testimonials regarding the usefulness of careful and deliberate problem solving may be indispensable.

Functional Training: Decision Making

The purpose of these exercises is ultimately to train patients to be more careful and self-critical in their thinking about problems and to develop a format for dealing effectively with practical real-world decisions. The problem-solving outline presented above, although useful as a source of integrative thinking exercises, is for most patients too elaborate and time consuming to serve as a guide in actual decision-making situations and consequently may not promote independence and self-direction in personal affairs. Furthermore, some patients lack the cognitive prerequisities they need to think in the organized and hypothetical manner of mature problem solving. It is therefore often necessary to create simplified guides for decision making that highlight the types of thinking that a given patient fails to execute well yet needs to develop to make effective decisions.

Figure 4–5 presents one possible decision-making guide that has been simplified to offer a patient a useful and easily remembered sequence of steps. The four fundamental questions that the guide poses require types of thinking in which head injured patients are characteristically weak: careful identification of goals, reflection on how realistic these goals are, careful planning, and ongoing self-monitoring. Depending on the level of a patient's attentional and intellectual resources, more or less attention can be paid to the subquestions listed in the guide. For a patient whose goals are adequately realistic but whose misinterpretations of people and events create difficulties, one of the highlighed questions on a decision-making guide could be, "Could this problem be based on my misinterpretations or distorted thinking?" A useful question to highlight for a patient whose primary obstacle to effective problem solving is an inability to consider alternative solutions may be, "How many reasonable possible solutions can I think of?" Patients whose decision making is dominated by an egocentric perspective may need a guide that highlights the evaluation of possible courses of action in terms of their effects on other people. A seriously impulsive patient who fails to put any thinking procedures to work for himself may have a decision-making guide that consists of nothing but the boldly printed words, **"STOP AND THINK."** In this way, training in decision making can be customized yet remain general enough to be applicable to a diverse array of life situations. In therapy groups, patients who have been given some training in various types of reasoning are expected to actively identify the areas that pose the most serious obstacles to effective decision making for them and, thus, to develop their own decision-making guide.

In the context of group or individual CRT sessions, we combine two types of *education* with these exercises in decision making. First, we explicitly discuss thinking skills under their formal labels (e.g., "divergent thinking" or "evaluative thinking") with the goal of heightening the patients' metacognitive awareness and consequently increasing the likelihood that they will deliberately apply these skills. These discussions focus on the ways weakness in a thinking skill can prevent a patient from achieving his or her own stated goals. Second, we openly discuss the effects of head injury on problem solving, both the typical effects of brain damage in a population of head injured patients and the specific effects of each individual patient's brain injury on these thinking processes.

These discussions emphasize those commonly occurring deficits which impede effective decision making: impulsiveness, compromised judgment and safety awareness, vulnerability to attentional, motivational, or fatigue problems; and frequency of misinterpretation in social spheres. Discussions also highlight:

- those common cognitive distortions which often obscure the accurate identification and assessment of problems; these include overgeneralizations, hasty conclusions, and unrealistic self-expectations (Burns, 1980; Ellis, 1962; Emery, 1981);

What Do I Want? —>

- What is my real goal?
- Is this goal in my own best interest?
- If I have several, which one is most important?
- Are any subgoals correctly prioritized and understood?

Is My Goal Realistic? —>

- Am I able cognitively/physically/emotionally/financially? Enough time?
- Am I creating a problem through distorted thinking?
- Do I need additional information?
- Over which realities do I **have** control?
- Over which realities do I **not have** control?

How Am I Going To Do It? —>

- What effective options do I have?
- Do I have relevant prior experiences?
- What are the positive/negative consequences of each option?
- What's my plan for the option I choose?

Options	Consequences
1.	
2.	
3.	
4.	

Plan:

How's It Turning Out? —>

- Is my plan achieving my goal?
- Do I need to choose another plan?
- Do I need to choose another goal or rethink subgoals?
- Are there now new problems to address?

Figure 4–5. Decision-making guide.

- the importance of flexibility, persistence, and a reflective manner in generating possible solutions and formulating plans;
- sensitivity to the necessity of acquiring relevant information for accurately identifying problems and formulating goals; and
- the utility of perceiving oneself as one's own coach (see below) (Ylvisaker & Holland, 1985).

Case illustration: A.G. was a 32 year old male who pre-traumatically had been a professional with supervisory responsibilities.

In 1981 he suffered a severe head injury which resulted in multiple cortical contusions. Neuropsychological assessment 11 months after the injury revealed A.G.'s motor and surface language functioning were within normal limits, but yet he was having significant difficulty with integrative functions and both semantic and episodic memory. At this stage of recovery, however, A.G.'s most functionally impairing deficits were inappropriate behavior and catastrophic reactions under stress that occasionally produced aggressive outbursts. He repeatedly refused psychiatric and behavioral intervention and would not discuss vocational alternatives.

CRT for A.G. included a variety of cognitive exercises in areas such as speed of processing, integration of information, and compensation for memory deficits. The primary focus, however, was on improving his executive functions (self-awareness of deficits; realistic goal setting; planning and decision making; self-directing; self-monitoring, and self-evaluating behavior). Little improvement was noted until, on his own initiative, A.G. replaced the metaphor of "executive functions," which despite his professional background meant little to him, with "coaching functions," which meant a great deal to him because he was an avid sports fan. With guidance he then created an internalized image of a coach — to make the image as concrete as possible, he used the local university football coach — to teach himself about strengths and weaknesses and to guide himself, particularly under stress.

Shortly before moving from the Pittsburgh area, he related this experience: While cleaning out his apartment with a friend, the friend found and threw out a sports memento that had great sentimental value for A.G. A.G. reported that he felt himself losing control until "the coach" appeared and instructed him to go to the other end of the apartment and do nothing until he cooled down. With considerable pride, A.G. reported that the coach's plan worked, he did nothing that he regretted, and he was ultimately able to retrieve the prized object.

Counseling and CRT

It may appear from this discussion of practical decision making that there is no clear distinction between cognitive rehabilitation therapy and psychological counseling. Were this the case, cognitive rehabilitation therapists would also need to be trained counselors to perform in a professional manner. Although the boundaries between CRT and other types of intervention, including counseling, do overlap to some extent, and although interdisciplinary coordination and communication are vital to the success of any head injury program, intervention aimed at improving cognitive functions should nevertheless not be confused with psychotherapy, counseling, or advice giving.

In practice, this distinction is reinforced in two ways. First, the goal of problem-solving or decision-making exercises in CRT, which we clearly state and review regularly, is to improve a patient's ability to use a variety of thinking skills habitually. Although it is certainly hoped and expected that this training will ultimately affect behavior positively, altering behavior is not the primary objective of CRT. Behavioral changes are, thus, indirect effects. Second, we typically use hypothetical rather than real problems and deliberately avoid basing exercises on problems that we know are personally important to a patient at the time. These personal issues are most properly addressed by a qualified counselor or psychotherapist. The goal of decision-making intervention in CRT is to elicit and reinforce generally useful thinking procedures, rules, and heuristics that enable patients to manage those situations in daily life which, without this training, they might find unmanageable or overwhelming. Using the patient's actual problems is not necessary to this process and may in fact distract patients from the objective of improved thinking. If a therapist, however, artfully selects for treatment sessions those types of problems which a patient is likely to encounter, the patient's ability to generalize problem-solving skills to applicable situations is enhanced.

Executive Functions and Self-Coaching

A.G., the patient described earlier in the case illustration, transformed the popular metaphor of "executive" functions into a personally meaningful image of a coach. This transformation enabled him not only to learn a great deal about functions that are commonly impaired after traumatic brain injury (see Chapter 1) but also to improve his own impaired functions. These "self-coaching" functions include self-awareness of strengths and weaknesses, goal setting, planning and preparing, self-instructing, self-initiating, self-inhibiting, self-monitoring, self-evaluating, and problem solving. If head injured patients are to maintain the progress they have made long after intervention has ended, therapists must turn over to patients the coaching role that they often cherish for themselves.

When they keep this self-coaching goal clearly in focus, cognitive rehabilitation therapists can deal more easily with the frustration they must frequently feel of not being able to accompany patients and train them in the functional and integrative skills they need for each life situation as it arises. Therapists can also transform any cognitive exercise into an occasion to highlight for patients aspects of their cognitive functioning and demonstrate bridges between patients' own goals and cognitive exercises that may seem artificial. Even workbook materials, whose value is questionable at this stage of rehabilitation when they are used merely for drill and practice, may stimulate patients' awareness of their thinking processes and their self-coaching roles. Head injured adults in the late stages of rehabilitation are served by the process of learning about and taking responsibility for their own learning, thinking, and problem solving. Patients have been well served if they leave treatment (a) knowing which of their cognitive skills are strong, which are weak, and thus which skills require special alertness; (b) knowing which approaches or strategies are effective in these areas of weakness; (c) knowing how such approaches will affect their task performance and self-esteem, and how these approaches will impress others; (d) knowing which particular approaches are applicable to a given situation; and (e) knowing that the responsibility of pulling "the team" together to get the job done is their own.

COMPUTER-BASED COGNITIVE RETRAINING

There has been a remarkable fascination over the past decade with the use of electronic retraining devices in attempts to improve certain cognitive functions. Early reports from the experimental head injury rehabilitation program at New York University's Institute of Rehabilitation Medicine supported the effectiveness of custom designed devices in improving basic-level attentional, perceptual, and psychomotor functions (Ben-Yishay et al., 1982). Video games, whose commercial popularity was mushrooming, were subsequently suggested as a medium for enhancing a variety of cognitive, perceptual, and motor skills (Lynch, 1983). More recently, many personal computer software packages have been introduced that provide targeted exercises in areas ranging from basic attentional and perceptual processes to organizing and memorizing processes to higher-level reasoning and problem-solving skills. Computer programs that have been created for use in mainstream and special education contexts target cognitive as well as academic areas. Programs that fall loosely under the general umbrella of "cognitive rehabilitation software" can be grouped under the following categories, which are distinguished by the functional components they address:

- *Basic-level cognitive components:* programs that address, in isolation, attentional functions and speed of processing (e.g., reaction time);

impulse inhibition (e.g., reaction time with a distractor); time estimation; attentional "space" or working memory (e.g., memory span for digits and/or words)
- *Visual-perceptual components:* programs that address visual neglect, systematic scanning, visual discrimination, visual figure-ground relationships, visual-motor integration
- *Cognitive-language organizing processes:* programs that address, with either verbal or nonverbal stimuli, categorizing, sequencing, part-whole relationships, and memory for meaningfully connected material
- *Higher-level cognitive-language components:* programs that address inferential reasoning, problem solving, linguistic abstractions, and multiple meaning
- *Academic/integrative tasks:* programs that address reading comprehension; composition; and curricular content areas such as mathematics, science, social studies, and history

The deficits targeted by cognitive rehabilitation software packages have, of course, been treated for decades by rehabilitation and special education professionals without the assistance of computers or other training devices. In the case of special education populations, attempts to train basic-level perceptual or perceptual-motor functions have, in most cases, either been unsuccessful in improving these components, or have failed to match improvements in basic-level components with improvements in more functional cognitive or academic skills (Kavale & Mattson, 1983). There is, therefore, reason to be cautious and judicious in the use of computer-assisted cognitive retraining if the programs that have been chosen are restricted in focus (as many CRT software packages are) to very basic attentional, perceptual, and organizational (e.g., categorizing, sequencing) processes.

The intoxication that rehabilitation professionals might feel when they perceive high technology solutions to notoriously stubborn problems might be moderated by several sobering considerations: Computers are costly and subject to malfunction; programs often present tasks and cues less flexibly than a skilled therapist who uses more traditional materials; and, finally, most programs explicitly identified as cognitive rehabilitation software fail to address problems of head injured patients that may be most functionally impairing, such as difficulty in integrating various skills, in processing large amounts of information in the performance of complex tasks, and in generalizing treatment gains to functional tasks in natural settings, and weakness in personal interaction and other psychosocial functions.

The key to the productive use of computers in CRT, as with any other clinical procedures and tools, is a careful matching of patients' needs and interests with computer programs and their presentation. There are many clinical advantages to using computers in the treatment of cognitive deficits:

- Computers interest and motivate many, though certinly not all patients.
- Because computers have the capability of endlessly repeating drill and practice exercises, they are very useful to patients with severe learning problems, who need to be patiently instructed.
- Computers make possible the precise, controlled, and consistent presentation of stimuli and, if the program being used includes a record-keeping system, an objective record of performance (e.g., number correct and time).
- Appropriately adapted computers can provide motorically handicapped patients with access to a variety of experiences and training tasks they might not otherwise have.
- Computers can provide immediate and consistent feedback.
- Computers make it possible for patients to *independently* carry out carefully programmed exercises.
- For some patients it is easier to confront deficits when feedback comes from a machine than when it comes from a therapist. Computer exercises therefore can not only exhibit patients' deficits but they can also objectively illustrate the advantages of compensatory strategies.

The tasks facing clinicians, then, are (a) to know what programs are available that are relevant to a given area of cognitive weakness and not to restrict their search to programs labelled "cognitive rehabilitation" software, (b) to be creative in the clinical use of computers, and (c) to make wise decisions about which patients will benefit from computerized therapy tasks and which tasks are most appropriate for each patient. A patient with impaired attentional functioning may, for example, profit from the "contentless" exercises of many attention programs, such as attending to the monitor and pressing a switch when a stimulus light appears. By contrast, a patient who likes arithmetic may "exercise" attentional structures more efficiently when the stimuli are simple math problems and the task is to solve them as quickly as possible when they appear on the screen. Under these circumstances, an exercise can come alive with meaningful and motivating content.

Creative clinicians can also use computer activities as a context for addressing problems in social interaction and in integrating large amounts of information, deficits that computerized intervention does not normally address. Groups of patients can play interesting detective or adventure computer games which require cooperation in problem solving, decision making, and storing of information. Groups of patients can work together to formulate the simplest method to create a design using LOGO programs (Papert, 1980). Programs such as Page Maker, Newsroom, and Print Shop can be used for projects that are as simple or complex as patients want to make them, and they enable therapists to target organizational, planning, and problem-solving skills as well as group cooperation and interaction. Learning to use a word-processing system may not only be vocationally relevant for certain patients, but it can also be a useful context for language organizational activities. Using a spell checker can highlight the process of monitoring one's work for errors. Finally, educational programs that address specific curricular areas (e.g., mathematics, the sciences, history) are also useful for those patients who have significant gaps in their knowledge base following the head injury and who may realistically plan further academic training or higher levels of employment. We have made extensive use of standard educational programs and Scholastic Aptitude Test preparation programs for this purpose. The use of computers for purposes other than those normally grouped under the heading "cognitive rehabilitation" is discussed in a growing number of publications (Behrman, 1985; Hagen, 1984; Schwartz, 1985). Software written for use in educational or special education settings is regularly reviewed in the Sloane Report (Miami, FL; Eydie Sloane, Editor). Kurlycheck and Glang (1984), Bracy (1984), and Skillbeck (1984) reviewed several cognitive rehabilitation software packages.

It is generally accepted that computers *at best* augment other forms of cognitive rehabilitation following head injury. Although there is some evidence that computer assisted cognitive rehabilitation can be effective with carefully selected patients (Imes, 1986), many questions remain unanswered. These include: Who are good candidates for computer assisted retraining? On the basis of what specific characteristics of patients does one select software packages or training tasks? Do improvements result from the training tasks themselves or the skilled clinical coaching that accompanies the computer work? Does a preponderance of computer training tasks promote *passivity* rather than active engagement in rehabilitation? Does improved functioning on computer training tasks generalize to functional social, vocational, academic, or daily living tasks? How does one best promote this generalization? Clearly more research and clinical experience are needed before we can confidently assign a prominent place to computers in cognitive rehabilitation.

VIDEO THERAPY

Video feedback and video modeling are being used increasingly in a wide variety of educational, training, and treatment contexts. The successful use of video technology has been documented in the training of athletes, teachers, psychotherapists, and other professionals and in the psychotherapeutic treatment of a variety of disorders. The use of video feedback techniques has been explored in the cognitive and psychosocial rehabilitation of head injured adults (Helffenstein & Wechsler, 1982; Prigatano and others, 1986) and head injured children (Haarbauer-Krupa, Henry, Szekeres & Ylvisaker, 1985). Applications of video techniques in cognitive rehabilitation fall into three categories: training in self-awareness of deficits, in the use of strategies, and in interactive skills.

Self-Awareness

Difficulty with the self-awareness and self-appraisal of deficits is pervasive following traumatic brain injury (see Chapter 1), and it interferes in important ways with all apsects of intervention. Prigatano and Fordyce (1986) discussed the routine use of videotape feedback in cognitive rehabilitation therapy to objectively draw patients' attention to their own strengths and weaknesses, and to highlight apsects of interactive behavior that might otherwise go unnoticed or be the subject of disputes as to what really happened. In Table 4-2, we propose the use of video tape to improve patients' ability to discriminate between successful and unsuccessful performance of a task, regardless of who the actor is, and to improve their ability to identify their own strengths and weaknesses. Another possible use of videotape technology is serial videotaping, which provides a record of patients' functioning over time and which can encourage and motivate those patients who fail to perceive improvement.

The primary advantage of videotape feedback in heightening self-awareness are the objectivity, immediateness, vividness, and concreteness of the feedback that it provides, and the permanence of its record. Objectivity of feedback means that a patient can be confronted with a deficit without at the same time enduring the stress of interpersonal confrontation. The objectivity of video feedback can, however, be overemphasized. Trower and Kiely (1983) pointed out that using video for self-observation is subject to the same type of selective perception, filtering, and distortion as are involved in other forms of observation. Without guidance, a patient may fail to perceive aspects of behavior that are obvious to other observers. Furthermore, patients with an already reduced self-concept who also negatively distort or exaggerate the quality of their performance on videotape may become more depressed as a result of self-observations, and may become even less functional. Video therapy techniques must, therefore, be used with great caution with patients who are anxious, depressed, or excessively self-conscious, or who have a particularly fragile self-concept. Consultation with the patient's psychotherapist or counselor is mandatory before proceeding with self-observation on videotape, particulary if the therapeutic goal is to confront the patient with a cognitive or interactive weakness.

In our experience, most head injured young adults possess the resources to benefit from carefully introduced self-observation on videotape. When the goals of therapy are self-confrontation and self-awareness of deficits, the following treatment progression is recommended. Patients are first given assignments to observe specific strengths or weaknesses in other patients, either by observing them in therapy groups or by watching former patients on videotape. The goal of these exercises is to equip patients with a vocabulary and relevant categories of description so that when they direct their attention toward themselves, they will understand what to observe and how to observe it. Patients then view themselves, ensuring that the initial viewings illustrate patients' best functioning and that their attention is directed to the illustrated strength. Patients then view themselves engaged in an activity that illustrates a deficit, without commentary from the therapist. Finally, such activities are viewed with commentary from the therapist and with the expectation that patients will identify strengths and weaknessess in their performance, ultimately becoming sufficiently engaged in the task that they can operate the pause and restart switches to highlight relevant features of their own performance.

Strategy Training

In Table 4–2, we list several uses of videotape in strategy training, such as illustrating the value of strategic procedures, engaging patients in the process of selecting strategies for themselves, modeling strategies, and promoting generalization of a learned procedure. It is helpful to develop a library of videotapes, and having tapes in which head injured patients are the actors is ideal. For "product monitoring" activities, one needs paired videotapes, the first illustrating an actor's failure to perform a task successfully without a strategic procedure and the second illustrating successful performance with a strategy. (For example, the first video might portray a person failing to follow rapidly given instructions correctly, while the second might show the same person following the instructions correctly after requesting that the instructions be repeated or written.) After viewing the first video, discussion can focus on why the "actor" failed to do what he intended to do and how he could have succeeded. Discussion following the second video should include an identification of the strategy that the actor used, evaluation of the pros and cons of that procedure in relation to other possibilities, and consideration of situations in which any of these procedures might be of value to the patients.

Video presentation has two primary advantages over role playing as a dramatic basis for discussing strategies. First, videos can be played and replayed as often as necessary to focus patients' attention on the relevant features of an event. Second, video vignettes can be produced that enable patients to observe a variety of situations and settings in which strategic behavior is necessary, a possibility that therapy frequently cannot offer. Both capabilities promote generalization of strategies.

Interactive Skills

Hosford and Mills (1983) reviewed the substantial literature on the use of video modeling and feedback in social skills training. An excellent illustration of this use of the technology is Interpersonal Process Recall (IPR) (Kagan, Schauble & Resnikoff, 1969), a treatment program for improving social and interactive skills that is centered around the systematic use of video feedback. Helffenstein and Wechsler (1982) demonstrated in a controlled study that IPR is effective in improving a variety of interactive skills in head injured young adults. Since video feedback makes possible the microanalysis of several simultaneously occurring behaviors, this medium is particularly appropriate for modeling and training patients in complex interactive behaviors. Hosford and Mills (1983) presented a useful six-step program of video-based social skills training.

Overcoming Resistance to Self-Viewing

Head injured patients, particularly those whose physical appearance or functioning has changed in an easily observable way, often resist self-viewing when it is first proposed. Since video therapy serves several purposes in cognitive rehabilitation, sensitive and well-planned introductions of patients to videotaping are essential. The following techniques are useful:

- Early in treatment, tell the patient that videotaping is routine in head injury rehabilitation and that it will be introduced when the patient is ready.
- Before proceeding to videotape feedback, desensitize the patient by leaving unused video equipment in the therapy room, by exposing the patient to the feedback of mirrors and audiotape, and by having peers and therapists offer objective feedback.
- Have trusted peers offer testimonials to the value of video feedback, while also honestly pointing out that it is embarrassing and threatening at the beginning.
- Have a resistant patient first view other patients on videotape. The first self-viewing should be of the patient doing something exceptionally well.
- Include the therapist in the film with the patient to prevent communicating to the patient that only he or she is on the spot.

The effectiveness of video therapy in a variety of treatment contexts has been reviewed by Sanborn, Pyke, and Sanborn (1975) and by several contributors to *Using Video: Psychological and Social Applications* (Dowrick & Biggs, 1983).

STRUCTURED ACTIVITIES

The goals of cognitive rehabilitation are to improve a patient's functioning in the areas loosely categorized as "cognitive" and to help a patient to compensate for deficits that are not readily improved by remedial exercises. There are several advantages to using meaningful and functional yet highly structured activities to achieve these goals. By splitting a functional activity (e.g., shopping, planning and executing a party, playing a game) into its component parts; throughly analyzing the sensory, motoric, cognitive, academic, and psychosocial demands of the activity; and carefully controlling these components and demands, a clinician can promote a patient's functional improvement of skills and generalization of compensatory strategies. Although the primary focus of the activities in CRT is on relevant cognitive processes (e.g., analyzing, sequencing, organizing, planning, remembering, problem solving, decision making, self-monitoring), by carrying activities out in a group context, therapists promote patients' reacquisition of social knowledge and social skills (e.g., cooperative work, turn taking, and effective interaction). Structured activities can be used to enable patients to achieve cognitive and social goals in the contexts not only of cognitive rehabilitation but also of prevocational/vocational treatment and recreational therapy (see Chapters 5 and 8).

Engaging patients in relatively complex functional activities in a setting that imposes real-life forms of stress also serves an important diagnostic purpose in determining the functional scope of a skill. In these settings, clinicians frequently observe a breakdown of skills that were thought to have been solidly established in a controlled therapy context. Furthermore, they have the opportunity to assess the use of compensatory strategies that patients have learned elsewhere and the effectiveness of these strategies.

Task analysis (i.e., analyzing complex activities and separating them into their component parts) and cognitive analysis (i.e., determining the cognitive demands imposed by each component) are the keys to using structured activities therapeutically (see Chapter 3). If a task is too challenging for a patient, it is likely that it has not been completely analyzed or that the demands of the task are too great in one or more of the areas. Likewise, when an event is planned, it is necessary to divide the task of preparation into its constituent subtasks. It is important for patients to recognize that tasks of this sort include many smaller tasks and that smaller tasks have specific relations to the overall goals. Holidays, for example, are frequently good occasions for members of a structured activity group to plan and host a holiday gathering. The preparation involves many components, each of which requires its own planning and execution. For example, the group members must (a) set a goal and create an overall plan (e.g., determine the type of gathering, the preparations, the schedule of preparation); (b) organize invitations (e.g., create an invitation list; plan, make, and send invitations); and (c) prepare a menu (choose recipes; establish a sequence of steps to prepare the food, including preparing a shopping list and buying the ingredients [which involves a community outing]; prepare the food). This list remains very general. Each task can be broken down still further into a large number of subtasks. Given the possibilities of increasing complexity in task analysis, it should be apparent that the depth of analysis that is appropriate depends upon the patients' level of functioning and specific treatment objectives. (Chapter 8 presents examples of the kind of detailed task analysis that is appropriate for avocational planning.)

At each point at which a patient's deficits interfere with the completion of a subtask, clinicians must decide if it is appropriate to attempt to improve the deficit skill with direct training, to teach a strategy to compensate for the deficit, or simply to assist the patient in completing the task. Shopping for food could, for example, include training in the use of memory aids, in communication skills (asking for information, following directions), in price awareness and money skills, and in organized searching and visual scanning.

In addition to identifying the component parts of a task, it is also necessary to grade each subtask according to its cognitive, content/academic, and psychosocial variables. Table 4–5 lists the major variables and describes ranges of these variables for grading activities for adults in the middle and late stages of recovery. The categories presented in Table 4–5 are to some extent arbitrary; there is, for example, a cognitive dimension in the content/academic and psychosocial variables. These categories are offered merely to serve as guides in the practical process of matching activities with patients' levels of functioning.

In addition to grading activities along the variables listed in Table 4–5, activities must also be adapted to suit patients' sensory (e.g., visual and auditory acuity) and motor functioning. Since cognitive and psychosocial functioning is generally reduced when the demand on patients' physical abilities are great, sensory and motor demands should be decreased when treatment focuses on cognitive or psychosocial areas. The general rule is: adapt an activity to the patient's abilities and place demands on only those few areas which are the focus of treatment.

Activities that we have found useful for achieving cognitive objectives include community and consumer activities (e.g., shopping, banking, and community outings involving public transportation and the use of maps); homemaking activities (e.g., planning meals or parties, cooking, and home maintenance); and leisure activities (e.g., gardening, craft and carpentry projects, science experiments, and playing games).

Since a primary purpose of structured activities is to bridge the gap between therapy exercises and real-life settings, it is important that the activities be meaningful for the patients and that the relationship between a given activity and the patient's goals be clearly established. Arriving at this arrangement often requires that therapists negotiate the choice of an activity with patients and that they discuss very directly with the patient the purpose of the activity, the deficits that it addresses, and the benefits the patient might derive

Table 4–5. Variables for Grading the Difficulty Level of Structured Activities

Variable	Gradation	
Cognitive Variables		
Sensory-integrative requirements	Activities that require the processing of information from only one sensory modality at a time	Activities that require integrated multisensory processing
Visual complexity	Simple visual-perceptual tasks	Activities with complex materials in a distracting setting
Rate of presentation	A slow rate of speech and a stable visual field	A normal rate of speech and rapid presentation of visual stimuli
Environmental distractions	One-on-one treatment in a quiet environment	Group treatment with naturally occurring distractions
Attention span and endurance	Activities that can be completed in one short session	Multicomponent activities that require several sessions to complete
Sequential organization	Activities that involve a small number of steps	Activities that require independent organizing of many sequentially ordered steps
Materials organization	Activities that involve identification of only the salient materials needed for a simple task, given a completed model; no requirement for independent organization of the work space	Activities that require independent analysis of tasks to determine needed materials and equipment, and that require independent organization of the work space to allow for efficient work

continued

Table 4–5 *(continued)*

Variable	**Gradation**	
Analyzing and planning	Activities that involve simple replication of a model	Activities that involve independent analysis of the task into components and planning the execution of the task
Language comprehension	Activities that involve simple instructions along with nonverbal demonstrations, picture cues, and/or completed models	Activities that involve complex or multistep instructions
Memory (storage and retrieval)	Activities that require minimal storage and retrieval of information or instructions	Activities that require efficient storage and retrieval, with the independent use of memory aids or strategies if needed
Integration over time	Activities that are completed in one session	Activities that have many components and require many sessions to complete
Response to time stress	Activities that have no time requirements	Activities that require large amounts of work to be completed within a specific time limit
Cognitive flexibility	Routine and repetitive activities	Activities that involve frequent changes in materials, procedures, personnel, and/or location
Goal setting	Activities with clinician-set goals	Activities with patient-set goals
Initiation	Activities that require little self-initiated action or conversation	Activities that require self-initiated action or conversation with no cueing

Variable	Gradation	
Self-monitoring and evaluating	Activities that require no independent monitoring or evaluating of the success of the process or product	Activities that require independent monitoring and evaluating
Problem solving and decision making	Activities that require minimal independent problem solving or decision making	Activities that require the patient to generate and evaluate varied solutions to problems that arise naturally in the activity and to make independent decisions about a course of action
Safety judgment	Activities that are not dangerous	Activities that require the independent and safe use of potentially dangerous equipment (ranging from scissors and kitchen knives to power tools), take place in a potentially dangerous area, or involve potentially dangerous situations (e.g., electrical appliances near water)
Strategy use	Activities that require no independent use of compensatory strategies	Activities that can be completed efficiently only by using strategies
Content Variables		
Academic: Reading, writing, mathematics, spelling	Activities that do not involve academic skills	Activities that impose significant demands on academic skills

continued

Table 4–5 *(continued)*

Variable	**Gradation**	
Content-specific knowledge	Activities that presuppose little knowledge of tools, factual information, or rules	Activities that presuppose considerable knowledge
Familiarity with the activity	Familiar enjoyable activities	Unfamiliar activities that require new learning
Psychosocial Variables		
Interpersonal relations	Activities that involve little interaction	Activities that require cooperating, conversing, sharing, and turn taking in the planning and execution of the activity
Response to interpersonal stress	Thorough support and encouragement from the clinician and peers	Frequent demands and critical feedback from the clinician and peers
Frustration tolerance	Activities that are designed to guarantee success	Activities that include the possibility of failure

from it. As a general rule, activities should be appropriate to the patient's cultural and educational background and self-concept, including sex roles and family roles. Negative reactions to activities and to feedback from staff are often understandable in light of a patient's background and values. Clinicians must be sensitive to and supportive of such feelings. They must also, however, understand a patient's resistance to therapy tasks and unwillingness to accept instruction or criticism from staff or peers in terms of the patient's emotional adjustment to brain injury. Dealing effectively with these complex emotions often requires the integration of cognitive rehabilitation and psychotherapeutic counseling.

Self-awareness of deficits is an element that is important to patients actively engaging in structured activities. Structured activities, in turn, can promote self-awareness since patients frequently experience considerable frustration when they are unable to complete activities that were once routine. Carefully planned successes and failures on tasks that were unchallenging before the injury can focus patients' attention on their current strengths and weaknesses.

With head injured patients who lack planning and organizing skills, the initial planning stages of an activity may take an unexpectedly large amount of time. Although clinicians might be tempted to hasten this process with frequent cues and suggestions, allowing patients to work at their own pace, to make mistakes, and to experience the frustration that comes from poor planning and organizing enhances the therapeutic effect of the activity. Providing excessive cues, prompts, and suggestions ultimately interferes with clinicians' primary responsibility, which is to promote independence and effective self-coaching.

ENVIRONMENTAL CONSIDERATIONS

When community re-entry becomes the focus of rehabilitation programming, patients are generally beyond the stage of significant confusion and disorientation. However, these patients may become confused relatively easily, and their cognitive abilities and overall functioning may deteriorate as a result (Prigatano and others, 1986). Their confusion is most predictable when they are in a novel or unstructured environment or when their level of stimulation or stress is substantially increased. Environmental factors can promote orientation and efficient functioning or, on the contrary, create confusion and inefficient functioning. The tolerance of head injured people for stress, stimulation, and disorganization is significantly lower than that for persons without brain injury.

Many factors can contribute to patients' cognitive and emotional overload and the reduction in functioning that it causes. These include internal factors (e.g., amount of sleep, types and levels of medication, and interest in the current activity) as well as external environmental factors. External factors include all of the cognitive, perceptual, and psychosocial variables listed in Table 4–5. Other important environmental factors are the predictability of a patient's schedule, the organization of the working/living space, and the style of communication and degree of supportiveness of family, work supervisors, or rehabilitation personnel. These, then, are the factors to be considered when creating an environment that is appropriately controlled to enable a patient to function optimally but that also indicates respect for the patient's need for independence and normal interaction.

The amount and type of environmental structuring that is appropriate vary from individual to individual and from task to task. As task or work demands increase, environmental demands should be decreased. When the efficiency or appropriateness of behavior decreases or when a patient's confusion seems to worsen, environmental demands should be decreased. Attention to the organization and simplicity of an environment is particularly important when a head injured person is new to that environment. Effective environmental structuring requires that family members, care-givers, and professional staff communicate efficiently with each other about the factors that have the greatest influence on a patient's orientation and behavior and the environmental techniques that are most effective. With training, many patients are able to structure their own environments or at least express their needs to professionals or care-givers. M.J., for instance, a mildly disoriented head injured young adult who reacted very negatively to the staff's reminding him of his schedule and responsibilities, prepared with the help of his cognitive rehabilitation therapist audio tapes with instructions and reminders for getting through his day. This relatively simple procedure increased M.J.'s participation in the program and improved his attitude toward rehabilitation.

The following environmental techniques are useful in promoting patients' orientation and adaptive behavior. They are most often productive when the therapist and patient negotiate the most efficient and comfortable structure possible.

Time/schedule related:

- Provide a clear, consistent, and predictable routine; write the day's and/or week's schedule on schedule cards or wall posters; if necessary, remove or reduce time as a factor in task assignments.
- Explain activities in advance and prepare the patient for changes in schedule; introduce changes gradually.
- Provide an alarm watch to keep the patient on schedule.
- Use a journal or log book as a day organizer as well as a reference to information and events.

Space related:

- Organize the patient's living and working space; make it simple; store all important items in a consistent location.
- Decrease environmental distractions (auditory and visual).

Task related:

- Explain tasks carefully in advance; demonstrate the task and use written or pictured instructions as needed to guarantee the patient's understanding of the task.
- Encourage the patient to take notes.

- Use a consistent approach to completing a task; if possible, illustrate this approach with a diagram or flow chart (see Chapter 5, Figure 5–2); use the same organizational strategy in all settings.
- Grade tasks appropriately according to the variables listed in Table 4–5.
- Give the patient extra time to complete the task.
- Help the patient to focus attention on one task at a time.

Other:

- Adjust expectations to the patient's current ability to perform; e.g., allow adequate time for processing of information and completion of tasks.
- Interact in a way that is easy to process and encouraging, but at the same time as natural as possible.

TRAINING FAMILIES

Our experiences and those of others (Diehl, 1983; Prigatano and others, 1986; Rosenthal & Muir, 1983) underscore the importance of involving family members in the rehabilitation of head injured patients. This involvement includes systematic family education and training in addition to family counseling and support (discussed in Chapter 9). To describe family training as systematic is not to suggest a rigid or uniform program for all families, but rather to highlight the importance of planning and organization in a training program that, in fact, is customized to meet the needs of individual families. Including families as members of the assessment and treatment teams benefits family members and, because the approach of clinicians and family members is consistent, also helps to guarantee that patients will respond better to treatment than could be expected otherwise and that they will generalize treatment gains to more natural contexts.

Family education and training programs have the following general goals:

1. *Increasing family support of the patient and the program:* With an understanding of head injury, the strengths and weaknesses of their loved one, and the goals and intervention techniques of the rehabilitation program, family members are better able to support the patient through the recovery process. Family members can offer encouragement, review goals and relate them to the patient's

daily life, and in general support the patient's participation in therapy when he or she feels confused, frustrated, angry, or unmotivated.

2. *Improving communication:* Well-delivered training establishes a rapport and enhances communication between clinicians and family members. With an adequate understanding of the patient's injury and current functioning, family members can follow suggestions better or learn from the modeling that professionals provide. A rapport between clinicians and family members also increases the likelihood that family members will inform the clinician of the effectiveness of specific approaches or strategies as the patient uses them at home and in community settings.
3. *Promoting generalization of the patient's treatment gains:* Generalization of skills and strategies learned in therapy to other settings and maintenance of these skills over time rarely occur spontaneously with head injured patients. Rather, patients require assistance in recognizing similarities among situations and direct teaching and practice in using their skills and strategies in a variety of situations. Trained family members can provide a natural and supportive setting in which the patient can learn to generalize these skills and strategies.
4. *Supporting families during a time of emotional upheaval:* Chapter 9 includes a detailed discussion of the types of intervention that families of head injured patients may appropriately use. It is useful to conceive of family training as part of this supportive intervention. Training brings the entire family and household setting into the treatment context and gives family members an appropriate way to help their loved one while not only permitting but also encouraging them to foster the injured family member's independence.

The content of family training and education programs varies according to a patient's deficits, his or her phase of rehabilitation, the family's readiness to learn, and specific family needs. The topics covered in training programs range from general information about head injury to training in specific intervention techniques. The following topics are often covered, although they should be thought of neither as being necessary for all families nor as exhausting the topics that some families may find important:

1. Understanding brain functioning, brain injury, and the recovery process
2. Relating cognitive and behavioral characteristics to the patient's brain injury

3. Recognizing the patient's strengths and weaknesses and the significance of both; capitalizing on the patient's strengths while providing opportunity to exercise areas of deficit
4. Understanding the goals and techniques of physical and cognitive rehabilitation, the relation of treatment to real-life functioning and to the goals maintained by family members, and the effect of rehabilitation on recovery
5. Communicating most effectively with the patient; promoting natural interactions among family members
6. Structuring the environment and organizing activities to promote the patient's adaptive and independent functioning
7. Encouraging the patient's *active* thinking and problem solving
8. Applying therapeutic techniques and adapting compensatory strategies to use in the home
9. Promoting as much independence as the injured family member's current abilities permit; assisting the patient without being overprotective or robbing him or her of initiative and dignity
10. Engaging the patient in therapeutic activities at home without thereby changing familial roles and becoming a professional helper
11. Training and supporting other family members

Family training ideally begins on the day a patient is admitted to the rehabilitation facility. Initially, it is important that clinicians and family members develop a relationship of mutual respect and trust and that clinicians make family members aware that the treatment team needs their special expertise and understanding of the patient. If family members are enrolled in a counseling program, their counselor should work closely with the other clinicians who are involved in family training. The counselor can be a liaison between the family and other clinicians and can help the clinicians understand the family and address their concerns at an appropriate level. Table 4-6 presents a list of suggestions for training families of head injured patients.

SUMMARY

In this chapter, we have presented a treatment perspective on several issues central to cognitive rehabilitation. We have focused on themes that are particularly important at the stage of recovery

Table 4–6. Guidelines for Training Families

A. *Content of Training*

- Ask family members what they need to know and what they want to be able to do; follow their lead — be a good listener; negotiate training priorities with the family, recognizing that these priorities will change over time. Home visits are often helpful for gathering concrete information about the problems and needs of patients and family members alike in the home environment. (For a useful home visit evaluation form, see Diehl, 1983).
- Once training is underway, regularly request information from families regarding the techniques and strategies they find most useful; acknowledge and respect their expertise; remember that family members observe at home both the patient's optimal functioning and also his or her most severe and chronic problems under the stress of daily life.
- If family members are not ready to accept training or suggestions, inform them that you are available when they are ready; periodically explore their readiness; be sensitive to the stage of their own response to the injury; be respectful of the limitations that their situation might impose on their ability to respond or to accept training or suggestions.
- Remember that it is most important that family members retain their roles as family members and not try to assume the role of the therapist; give family members ways to help the patient without interfering with their primary roles.
- Begin with the basic information and suggestions; remain respectful, but make no assumptions about what families know about head injury, physical or cognitive deficits, or head injury rehabilitation.

B. *Training Methods*

- Include family members in the patient's treatment sessions.
- When teaching a skill or technique, use a systematic approach; explain the technique and its purpose, demonstrate it, and then coach the family member as he or she practices; when giving important information, give it several times and in several ways; follow up on a periodic basis.
- If appropriate, use videotape as well as live models for demonstration.
- Provide simple written or pictured training materials that family members may use as a reference.
- Coordinate the training that family members are receiving among all members of the treatment team.

C. *Communication*

- Use ordinary language; avoid professional jargon, yet teach family members the meaning of those professional terms that they may encounter or need to know.
- Avoid giving too much information at once; divide information into appropriately small units; repeat information as needed.
- Be understanding; avoid defensiveness; recognize that it is natural for families to direct anger at the professional community.
- Establish a relationship of mutual respect, understanding, and acceptance; avoid creating an "expert-novice" or "teacher-student" relationship; promote active communication by providing training in a private and relaxed setting; help family members to relax; provide refreshments.
- Create a supportive environment; make family members aware that many aspects of the rehabilitation process often do not work out as planned; try to create realistic expectations, and be understanding when family members are unsuccessful or fail to carry out assignments.

D. *Follow-up*

- Look for objective evidence that family members have maintained the skills or knowledge that they learned in training; periodically meet with and talk to family members to determine how effective their training has been or how useful the techniques or strategies are.

---

at which head injured young adults face the challenge of re-entering a social, academic, and/or vocational community. The discussion in this chapter certainly does not exhaust the important issues in CRT. Furthermore, since much that is included in cognitive rehabilitation is relatively new in its application to individuals with severe head injury, major research efforts are needed to determine what works and what does not work. Our fundamental conviction, which we have attempted to express in this and the previous chapter, is that these questions must be raised anew with each unique head injured individual who needs services. The effects of intervention are ultimately a result of dynamic interactions among the patient (including pretraumatic personality and educational/vocational level and post-traumatic goals, coping style, and cognitive profile), the therapist (including personality, interactive style, clinical skill, and conceptual framework), the treatment tasks (including type and duration of treatment), and the characteristics of the environment in which the patient must function (including the family and other support systems and the demands on the patient's ability).

REFERENCES

Adamovitch, B., Henderson, J. & Auerbach, S. (1985). *Cognitive rehabilitation of closed head injured patients.* San Diego: College-Hill Press.

Baddeley, A. (1982). Amnesia: A minimal model and interpretation. In L. Cermak (Ed.), *Human memory and amnesia* (pp. 305–335.). Hillsdale, NJ: Lawrence Erlbaum Assoc.

Bartlett, F. C. (1932). *Remembering: An experimental and social study.* Cambridge: University Park Press.

Behrman, M. (Ed.) (1985). *Handbook of microcomputers in special education.* San Diego: College-Hill Press.

Ben-Yishay, Y., Rattok, J., Ross, B., Lakin, P., Ezrachi, O., Silver, S. & Diller, L (1982). Rehabilitation of cognitive and perceptual deficits in people with traumatic brain damage: A five-year clinical research study. In *Working approaches to remediation of cognitive deficits in brain damaged persons* (Rehabilitation Monograph No. 64). New York University Medical Center: Institute of Rehabilitation Medicine, 127–176.

Bond, M. (1983). Effects on the family system. In M. Rosenthal, E. Griffith, M. Bond & J. D. Miller (Eds.), *Rehabilitation of the head injured adult* (pp. 209–217). Philadelphia: F. A. Davis Co.

Bracy, O. L. (1984). Using computers in neuropsychology. In M. D. Schwartz (Ed.), *Using computers in clinical practice* (pp. 245–256). New York: Haworth Press.

Brooks, N. (1984). *Closed head injury: Psychological, social, and family consequences.* New York: Oxford University Press.

Brown, A. L. (1975). The development of memory: Knowing, knowing about knowing, and knowing how to know. In H. W. Reese (Ed.), *Advances in child development and behavior* (pp. 104–152). New York: Academic Press.

Brown, A. L. (1979). Theories of memory and the problems of development: Activity, growth, and knowledge. In L. Cermak and F. I. M. Craik (Eds.), *Levels of processing and memory* (pp. 225–258). Hillsdale, NJ: Lawrence Erlbaum Assoc.

Burns, D. (1980). *Feeling good.* New York: New American Library.

Burns, M. S., Halper, A. S. & Mogil, S. I. (1985). *Clinical managememt of right hemisphere dysfunction.* Rockville, MD: Aspen Systems Corp.

Cermak, L., Reale, L & Baker, E. (1978). Alcoholic Korsakoff patients' retrieval from semantic memory. *Brain and Language, 5,* 215–226.

Chi, M. T. H. (1978). Knowledge structures and memory development. In R. S. Siegler (Ed.), *Children's thinking: What develops?* (pp. 73–96). Hillsdale, NJ: Lawrence Erlbaum Assoc.

Clark, H. & Clark, E. (1977). *Psychology and language.* New York: Harcourt Brace Jovanovich, Inc.

Craik, F. I. M. & Tulving, E. (1975). Depth of processing and the retention of words in episodic memory. *Journal of Experimental Psychology, 104,* 268–294.

Craine, J. F. & Gudeman, H. E. (1981). *The rehabilitation of brain functions: Principles, procedures, and techniques of neurotraining.* Springfield, IL: Charles C. Thomas.

Crosson, B. & Buenning, W. (1984). An individualized memory retraining program after closed head injury. A single-case study. *Journal of Clinical Neuropsychology, 6*(3), 287–301.

Crovitz, H. (1979). Memory retraining in brain damaged patients: The airplane list. *Cortex, 15,* 131–134.

Crovitz, H. F., Harvey, M. T. & Horn, R. W. (1979). Problems in the acquisition of imagery mnemonics: Three brain-damaged cases. *Cortex, 15,* 225–234.

Diehl, L. N. (1983). Patient-family education. In M. Rosenthal, E. Griffith, M. Bond & J. D. Miller (Eds.), *Rehabilitation of the head injured adult* (pp. 395–406). Philadelphia: F. A. Davis.

Diller, L. & Gordon, W. (1981). Interventions for cognitive deficits in brain-injured adults. *Journal of Consulting and Clinical Psychology, 49,* 822–834.

Dowrick, P. W. & Biggs, S. J. (1983). *Using video: Psychological and social applications.* New York: John Wiley & Sons.

Ellis, A. (1962). *Reason and emotion in psychotherapy.* New York: Lyle Stuart.

Emery, G. (1981). *A new beginning.* New York: Simon & Schuster.

Feuerstein, R. (1980). *Instrumental enrichment: An intervention program for cognitive modifiability.* Glenview, IL: Scott Foresman & Co.

Gianutsos, R. & Gianutsos, R. (1979). Rehabilitating the verbal recall of brain injured patients by mnemonic training. An experimental demonstration using single case study methodology. *Journal of Clinical Neuropsychology, 1,* 117.

Glasgow, R. E., Zeiss, R. A., Barbera, M. & Lewinsohn, P. M. (1977). Case studies on remediating memory deficits in brain-damaged individuals. *Journal of Clinical Psychology, 33,* 1049–1054.

Grice, H. (1967). William James Lectures, Harvard University. Published in part as Logic and Conversation. In P. Cole & J. Morgan (Eds.), *Syntax and semantics: Speech acts* (Vol. 3, pp. 41–58). New York: Seminar Press, 1975.

Gummow, L., Miller, P. & Dustman, R. (1983). Attention and brain injury: A case for cognitive rehabilitation of attentional deficits. *Clinical Psychology Review, 3,* 255–274.

Haarbauer-Krupa, J., Henry, K., Szekeres, S. & Ylvisaker, M. (1985). Cognitive rehabilitation therapy: Late stages of recovery. In M. Ylvisaker (Ed.), *Head injury rehabilitation: Children and adolescents* (pp. 311–343). San Diego: College-Hill Press.

Haarbauer-Krupa, J., Moser, L., Sullivan, D. & Szekeres, S. (1985). Cognitive rehabilitation therapy: Middle stages of recovery. In M. Ylvisaker (Ed.), *Head injury rehabilitation: Children and adolescents.* San Diego: College-Hill Press.

Hagen, C. (1981). Language disorders secondary to closed head injury: Diagnosis and treatment. *Topics in Language Disorders, 1,* 73–87.

Hagen, D. (1984). *Microcomputer resource book for special education.* Reston, VA: Reston Publishing Co.

Harris, J. (1984). Methods of improving memory. In B. Wilson & N. Moffat (Eds.), *Clinical management of memory problems* (pp. 46–62). Rockville, MD: Aspen Systems Corp.

Harris, J. E. & Sunderland, A. (1981). A brief survey of the management of memory disorders in rehabilitation units in Britain. *International Rehabilitation Medicine, 3,* 206–209.

Helffenstein, D. & Wechsler, F. (1982). The use of interpersonal process recall (IPR) in the remediation of interpersonal and communication skill deficits in the newly brain injured. *Clinical Neuropsychology, 4,* 139–143.

Hosford, R. E. & Mills, M. E. (1983). Video in social skills training. In P. W. Dowrick & S. J. Biggs (Eds.), *Using video: Psychological and social applications* (pp. 123–150). New York: John Wiley & Sons.

Imes, C. (1986). The effect of computer assisted cognitive rehabilitation on neuropsychological functioning in brain damaged patients. Master's Thesis. Indiana University.

Jacoby, L. & Craik, F. (1979). Effects of elaboration of processing at encoding and retrieval: Trace distinctiveness and recovery of initial context. In L. S. Cermak & F. I. M. Craik (Eds.), *Levels of processing and human memory* (pp. 1–20). Hillsdale, NJ: Lawrence Erlbaum Assoc.

Kagan, N., Schauble, P. & Resnikoff, D. (1969). Interpersonal process recall. *Journal of Nervous and Mental Diseases, 148,* 365–374.

Kapur, N. & Pearson, D. (1983). Memory symptoms and memory performance of neurological patients. *British Journal of Psychology, 74,* 409–415.

Kavale, K. & Mattson, P. (1983). "One jumped off the balance beam": Meta-analysis of perceptual-motor training. *Journal of Learning Disabilities, 16,* 165–173.

Kendall, P. C. (1981). Cognitive-behavioral interventions with children. In B. Lahey & A. Kazdin (Eds.), *Advances in child psychology* (Vol. 4). New York: Plenum Press.

Keogh, B. K. & Glover, A. T. (1980). The generality and durability of cognitive training effects. *Exceptional Education Quarterly, 1,* 75–82.

Kraut, R. & Higgins, E. (1984). Communication and social cognition. In R. Wyer & T. Srull (Eds.), *Handbook of social cognition* (Vol. 3). Hillsdale, NJ: Lawrence Erlbaum Assoc.

Kurlycheck, R. T. & Glang, A. E. (1984). The use of microcomputers in the cognitive rehabilitation of brain-injured persons. In M. D. Schwartz (Ed.), *Using computers in clinical practice* (pp. 245–256). New York: Haworth Press.

Levin, H., Benton, A. & Grossman, R. (1982). *Neurobehavioral consequences of closed head injury.* New York: Oxford University Press.

Lynch, W. J. (1983). Cognitive retraining using microcomputer games and commercially available software. *Cognitive Rehabilitation, 1,* 19–22.

Malec, J. & Questad, K. (1983). Rehabilitation of memory after craniocerebral trauma. *Archives of Physical Rehabilitation, 64,* 436–438.

Mandler, G. (1967). Organization and memory. In K. W. Spence & J. T. Spence (Eds.), *The psychology of learning and motivation* (Vol. 1). New York: Academic Press.

Meichenbaum, D. (1977). *Cognitive behavior modification: An integrative approach.* New York: Plenum Press.

Moely, B. E. (1977). Organization of memory. In R. Kail & J. Hagen (Eds.), *Perspectives on the development of memory and cognition* (pp. 203–236). Hillsdale, NJ: Lawrence Erlbaum Assoc.

Moffat, N. (1984). Strategies of memory therapy. In B. Wilson & N. Moffat (Eds.), *Clinical management of memory problems* (pp. 63–88). Rockville, MD: Aspen Systems Corp.

Papert, S. (1980). *Mindstorms: Children, computers, and powerful ideas.* New York: Basic Books.

Pellegrino, J. & Ingram, A. (1978). Processes, products, and measures of memory organization (Learning Research & Development Report). Pittsburgh: University of Pittsburgh.

Peterson, P. L. & Swing, S. R. (1983). Problems in classroom implementation of cognitive strategy instruction. In M. Pressley & J. R. Levin (Eds.), *Cognitive strategy research* (pp. 267–287). New York: Springer Verlag.

Piaget, J. (1983). Piaget's theory. In W. Kessen (Ed.), *Handbook of child psychology: History, theory and methods* (Vol. 1, pp. 103–128). New York: John Wiley & Sons.

Postman, L. & Kruesi, E. (1977). The influence of orienting tasks on the encoding and recall of words. *Journal of Verbal Learning and Verbal Behavior, 16,* 353–369.

Pressley, M., Forrest-Pressley, D., Elliot-Faust, D. & Miller, G. (1985). Children's use of cognitive strategies, how to teach strategies, what to do if they can't be taught. In M. Pressley & C. Brainerd (Eds.), *Cognitive learning and memory in children* (pp. 1–47). New York: Springer-Verlag.

Prigatano, G. P. & Fordyce, D. (1986). The neuropsychological rehabilitation program at Presbyterian Hospital, Oklahoma City. In G. P. Prigatano and others, *Neuropsychological rehabilitation after brain injury.* Baltimore: The Johns Hopkins University Press.

Prigatano, G. P., and others. (1986). *Neuropsychological rehabilitation after brain injury.* Baltimore: The Johns Hopkins University Press.

Rohwer, W. D. (1973). Elaboration and learning in childhood and adolescence. In H. W. Reese (Ed.), *Advances in child development and behavior* (Vol. 8, pp. 1–57). New York: Academic Press.

Rosenthal, M. & Muir, C. (1983). Methods of family intervention. In M. Rosenthal, E. Griffith, M. Bond & J. D. Miller (Eds.), *Rehabilitation of the head injured adult.* Philadelphia: F. A. Davis Co.

Rummelhart, D. (1975). Notes on a schema for stories. in D. Brown & A. Collins (Eds.), *Representation and understanding: Studies in cognitive science* (pp. 237–272). New York: Academic Press.

Sacks, H., Schegloff, E. & Jefferson, G. (1974). A simplest systematics for the organization of turntaking for conversation. *Language, 50,* 696–735.

Sanborn, D. E., Pyke, H. F. & Sanborn, C. J. (1975). Videotape playback and psychotherapy: A review. *Psychotherapy: Theory, Research, and Practice, 12,* 179–186.

Schacter, D. & Tulving, E. (1982). Amnesia and memory research. In L. Cermak (Ed.), *Human memory and amnesia* (pp. 21–31). Hillsdale, NJ: Lawrence Erlbaum Assoc.

Schank, R. & Abelson, R. (1977). Scripts, plans, and knowledge. In P. N. Johnson-Laird & P. C. Wason (Eds.), *Thinking: Readings in cognitive science* (pp. 421–432). New York: Cambridge University Press.

Schegloff, E. & Sacks, H. (1973). Opening up closings. *Semiotica, 8,* 289–327.

Schwartz, A. H. (Ed.) (1985). *Handbook of microcomputer applications in communication disorders.* San Diego: College-Hill Press.

Skillbeck, C. (1984). Computer assistance in the management of memory and cognitive impairment. In B. A. Wilson & N. Moffat (Eds.), *Clinical management of memory problems.* Rockville, MD: Aspen Systems Corp.

Smirnov, A. (1973). *Problems in psychology and memory.* New York: Plenum Press.

Stuss, D. T. & Benson, D. F. (1984). Neuropsychological studies of the frontal lobes. *Psychological Bulletin, 95*(1), 3–28.

Stuss, D. T., Kaplan, E. F., Benson, D. F., Weir, W. S., Chiulli, S. & Sarazin, F. F. (1982). Evidence for the involvement of orbitofrontal cortex in memory functioning: An interference effect. *Journal of Comparative and Physiological Psychology, 6,* 913–925.

Szekeres, S., Ylvisaker, M. & Holland, A. (1985). Cognitive rehabilitation therapy: A framework for intervention, In M. Ylvisaker (Ed.), *Head injury rehabilitation: Children and adolescents* (pp. 219–246). San Diego: College-Hill Press.

Tabaddor, K., Mattis, S., Zazula, T. & Phil, M. (1984). Cognitive sequelae and recovery course after moderate and severe head injury. *Neurosurgery, 14*(6), 701–708.

Trower, P. & Kiely, B. (1983). Video feedback: Help or hindrance? A review and analysis. In P. W. Dowrick & S. J. Biggs (Eds.), *Using video: Psychological and social applications.* New York: John Wiley & Sons.

Tulving, E. & Thompson, D. M. (1973). Encoding specificity and retrieval processes in episodic memory. *Psychological Review, 80,* 352–373.

van Zomeren, A. & van den Burg, W. (1985). Residual complaints of patients two years after severe head injury. *Journal of Neurology, Neurosurgery, and Psychiatry, 48,* 21–28.

Wilson, B. & Moffat, N. (Eds.) (1984). *Clinical management of memory problems.* Rockville, MD: Aspen Systems Corp.

Winocur, G. & Kinsbourne, M. (1978). Contectual cuing as an aid to Korsakoff amnesics. *Neuropsychologia, 16,* 671–682.

Wood, F., Ebert, V. & Kinsbourne, M. (1982). The episodic-semantic memory distinction in amnesia: Clinical and experimental observations. In L. Cermak (Ed.), *Human memory and amnesia* (pp. 167–193). Hillsdale, NJ: Lawrence Erlbaum Assoc.

Wood, R. L. (1984). Management of attention disorders following head injury. In B. Wilson & N. Moffat (Eds.), *Clinical management of memory problems.* Rockville, MD: Aspen Systems Corp.

Ylvisaker, M. & Holland, A. (1985). Coaching, self-coaching, and the rehabilitation of head injury. In D. Johns (Ed.), *Clinical management of neurogenic communication disorders,* 2nd ed. Boston: Little, Brown & Co.

Zangwill, O. L. (1947). Psychological aspects of rehabilitation in cases of brain injury. *British Journal of Psychology, 37,* 60–69.

Zeigarnik, B. V. (1965). *The pathology of thinking.* B. Haigh (Trans.). New York: Consultants Bureau, International Behavioral Sciences Series, J. Wortis (Ed.).

APPENDIX 4-1.
EXAMPLES OF COMPENSATORY STRATEGIES FOR PATIENTS WITH COGNITIVE IMPAIRMENTS

Attention and Concentration

A. External Aids

1. Use a timer or alarm watch to focus attention for a specific period.
2. Organize the work environment and eliminate distractions.
3. Use a written or pictorial task plan with built-in rest periods and reinforcement; move a marker along to show progress.
4. Place a symbol or picture card in an obvious place in the work areas as a reminder to maintain attention.

B. Internal Procedures

1. Set increasingly demanding goals for self, including sustained work time.
2. Self-instruct (e.g., "Am I wandering? What am I supposed to do? What should I be doing now?"). (Written cue cards may be needed for these during training period.)

Orientation (to time, place, person, and event)

A. External Aids

1. Use a log or journal book or tape recorder to record significant information and events of the day.
2. Refer to pictures of persons who are not readily identified (carry pictures attached to logbook).
3. Use appointment book or daily schedule sheet.
4. Use alarm watch set for regular intervals.
5. Refer to maps or pictures for spatial orientation; make maps with landmarks.

B. Internal Procedures

1. Select anchor points or events during the week and then attempt to reconstruct either previous or subsequent points in time (e.g., "My birthday was on Wednesday and that was yesterday, so this must be Thursday").
2. Request time, date, and similar information from others, when necessary.
3. Scan environment for landmarks.

Input Control (amount, duration, complexity, rate, and interference)

A. Auditory

1. Give feedback to speaker (e.g., "Please slow down; speed up; break information into smaller 'chunks' ").
2. Request repetition in another form (e.g., "Would you please write that down for me?").

B. Visual

1. Request longer viewing time or repeated viewings; request extra time for reading.
2. Cover parts of a page and look at exposed areas systematically, as in a "clockwise direction" or "left to right."
3. Use finger or index card to assist scanning and to maintain place.
4. Use symbol to mark right and left margins of written material or top and bottom segments as anchors in space.
5. Use large print books or talking books.
6. Request a verbal description.
7. Remove an object from its setting to examine it; then return it to the original setting and view it again.
8. Place items in best visual field and eliminate visual distractors.
9. Turn head to compensate for field cut.

Comprehension and Memory Processes

A. Use self-question (e.g., "Do I understand? Do I need to ask a question? How is this meaningful to me? How does this fit with what I know?"). Periodically look for GMC's (gaps, misconceptions, or confusion) by summarizing or explaining and checking back with speaker, a written source, or reference material.

B. Build "frames" or background for new information that is of particular significance or interest. Read summaries, general textbooks, and ask knowledgeable persons about topic of special interest (a procedure in building frames).

C. Use a study guide for extended discourse material (e.g., SQ 3R procedure — survey, question, read, recite, review).

D. Make charts and graphs of important relationships in textual material.

E. Use external memory aids (e.g., tape recorder, logbook, notes, memos, written or pictured time lines).

F. Rehearse: Covert or overt; auditory-vocal or motor (pantomime).

G. Organization: Scan for or impose some order on incoming information.

H. Mnemonics: Methods of loci, rhymes, imagery (meaningful and novel associations).

I. Use diagrams of forms that facilitate deeper encoding of information and its subsequent retrieval (e.g., sun diagram, Fig. 4–3).

J. Relate the information to personal life experiences and current knowledge. Use semantic knowledge of basic scripts (e.g., going to a restaurant, buying groceries) to help reconstruct previous events.

K. Project and describe situations in which target information will be needed or used.

L. At retrieval, reconstruct environment in which information was received.

M. Verbalize visual-spatial information (e.g., "X is to the left of Y"). Visualize verbal information in graphs, pictures, cartoons, or action-based imagery.

N. Keep items in designated places.

Word Retrieval

A. Search lexical memory according to various categories and subcategories (e.g., person: family).

B. Describe the concept; circumlocute freely (talk about or around subject).

C. Use gestures or signs.

D. Attempt to generate a sentence or use a carrier phrase.

E. Search letters or sounds of the alphabet (more effective in retrieving members of a limited category, such as names).

F. Describe perceptual attributes and semantic features of the concept.

G. Draw the item.

H. Attempt to write the word.

I. Create an image of the object in a scene; then attempt to describe the scene.

J. Attempt to retrieve the overlearned opposite.

K. Free associate with image in mind.

L. Associate persons' names with physical characteristics or a known person of the same name.

Thought Organization and Verbal Expression

A. Use a structured thinking procedure (e.g., feature analysis guide, Fig. 4–1, or sun diagram, Fig. 4–3).

B. Use knowledge of scripts to generate real or imagined descriptions of experiences (narratives).

C. Construct a time line to maintain appropriate sequence of events.

D. Note topic in any conversation; self-question about the main point of expression; alert others before shifting a topic abruptly.

E. Watch others for feedback as to whether your words are confusing. Watch facial expression, and so forth, or directly ask listeners, "Am I being clear?"

F. Rehearse important comments or questions and listen to self.

G. Set limits of time or allowable number of sentences in any one turn.

Reasoning, Problem Solving, Judgment

A. Use a problem-solving guide (see Figure 4–5).

B. Use self-questioning for alternatives or consequences. ("What else could I do?", "What would happen if I did that?").

C. Look at possible solutions from at least two different perspectives.

D. Scan environment for cues as to appropriateness or inappropriateness of behavior (e.g., facial expression of others; signs like "No Smoking;" formality verses informality of setting).

E. Set specific times or places for behaviors that are appropriate only in specified situations.

F. Actively envision situations to which successful procedures can be generalized.

Self-Monitoring

A. Use symbols or signs, placed in obvious places, or alarms that mean: "pause" or "stop" or "Am I doing what I should be doing?"

B. Use book or notebook with cards inserted at selected places with self-monitoring cues (e.g., "Summarize what you read").

C. Pair specific self-instruction with the associated emotion (e.g., "Calm-down" when angry).

Task Organization

A. Use task organization checklist: materials, sequenced steps, timeline, evaluation of results. Check each when completed.

B. Prepare work space and assign space as task demands.

From Cognitive Rehabilitation Therapy: Late Stages of Recovery by J. Haarbauer-Krupa, K. Henry, S. Szekeres, and M. Ylvisaker (1985). In M. Ylvisaker (Ed.), *Head Injury Rehabilitation: Children and Adolescents.* San Diego: College-Hill Press.

CHAPTER 5

Work Adjustment Services

Eva Marie R. Gobble
Kevin Henry
James C. Pfahl
Gloria J. Smith

The rehabilitation of head injured adults often requires the integration of a variety of services and treatment approaches to address the multiplicity of physical, cognitive, emotional, and social problems found in this population. Cognitive and psychosocial disturbances are the most commonly cited residual deficits and are the major cause of long-term disability following traumatic brain injury (Bond, 1975; Dikman & Reitan, 1977; Glenn & Rosenthal, 1985; Levin, 1979; Levin, Benton & Grossman, 1982). Although patterns of cognitive and psychosocial problems differ from client to client, they often reduce the individual's potential for vocational activity (Bruckner & Randle, 1972; Humphrey & Oddy, 1980; Thomsen, 1984). These problems include difficulty concentrating, poor memory and inefficient learning, irritability, restlessness, apathy, and depression (Bond, 1975; Brooks, 1984; Lezak, 1978b; Lishman, 1973; Prigatano and others, 1986). With or without concomitant physical problems, these symptoms often lead to chronic unemployment and social isolation (Bond, 1984; Gilchrist & Wilkinson, 1979; Lezak, 1978a; Rimel, Giordani, Barth, Boll & Jane, 1981).

A major responsibility of the rehabilitation team is to help the client achieve the highest possible level of vocational independence. This chapter's focus is on intensive work adjustment treatment, often a necessary component of the vocational rehabilitation process for head injured individauls. Chapter 6 discusses vocational evaluation, including ongoing treatment for cognitive and psychosocial problems, and work placement. Throughout these discussions, it should be remembered that interdisciplinary teamwork is essential to promote the most effective reintegration of the client into family, work, and social settings (Glenn & Rosenthal, 1985).

WORK ADJUSTMENT SERVICES

Employment is often the primary community re-entry goal for clients, families, and funding sources. The general skills that are critical to achieving this goal include:

- adaptability to work demands
- self-direction and motivation
- effective interpersonal and communication skills
- ability to apply academic knowledge
- ability to manage personal and self-care needs
- self-reliance in transportation and mobility in the community

The development of these critical vocational skills in head injured clients requires a systematic delivery of vocational rehabilitation services. There are four major components of the process: work adjustment, vocational evaluation, job training, and job placement (Cull & Hardy, 1972; Hardy & Cull, 1973; McGowan & Porter, 1967; Sankovsky, Arthur & Mann, 1971). Vocational rehabilitation involves the comprehensive integration of these components over time (see Figure 5–1). The intensity of programming and level of integration of the four components depends on the needs of the client. The order of services can also vary; it is, for example, often preferable to provide job training in the form of "on the job training" *after* job placement has occured rather than before (see Chapter 6). Adequate work adjustment forms a solid basis for the other three components. Vocational evaluation, training, and placement are all seriously limited in their effectiveness if work adjustment problems are still present.

Work adjustment is the process through which handicapped individuals develop work-related skills which facilitate increased productivity and the ability to handle the day-to-day demands of employment. In addition to the critical vocational skills listed above, successful work adjustment promotes self-confidence, self-control,

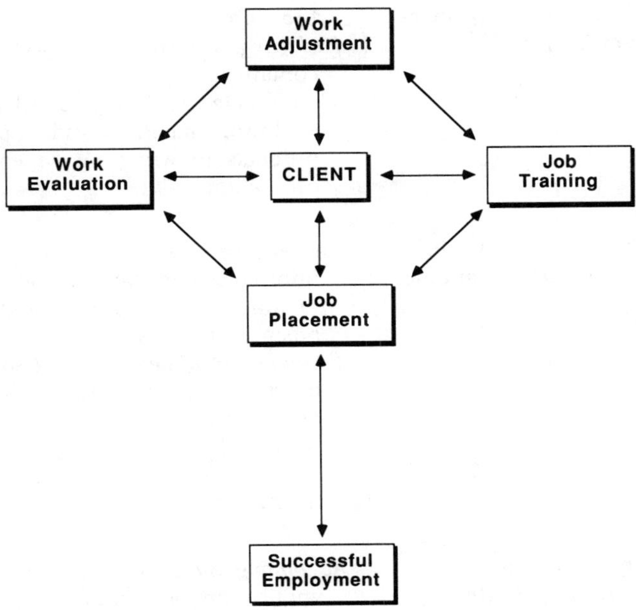

Figure 5–1. Integration of vocational rehabilitation services.

work tolerance, interpersonal skills, and an understanding of work (Cowood, 1975). A useful breakdown of specific abilities that may be required of a worker in a specific job is included in *A Guide to Job Analysis* (1982) and in the *Classification of Jobs According to Worker Trait Factors,* (Field & Field, 1982). These work abilities (originally referred to as work "situations") are described in Table 5–1.

Four methods used to meet the goals of work adjustment are:

- diagnostic assessment
- vocational therapy
- work conditioning
- counseling

The mix of services offered to a client must be adjusted to meet individual needs. Within a work adjustment setting, these services are

Table 5-1. Abilities needed for specific work situations

Situational Work Abilities	Examples of Work Situations Requiring the Ability
1. Ability to maintain attention on a repetitive short-cycle job	*Clerical Work:* e.g., addressing brochures or envelopes for mailing *Packaging:* e.g., putting objects into containers *Machine Operation:* e.g., enveloping and enclosing materials and paper products in wrapping paper or cellophane
2. Ability to move flexibly from one task to another	*Clerical Work:* e.g., scheduling, giving information to callers, and attending to minor administrative and business matters *Equipment Maintenance or Testing:* e.g., overhauling, repairing, modifying, and testing equipment; following work orders; diagnosing malfunctions; engraving new instruments
3. Ability to accept responsibility for the direction or control of an activity	*Accounting Supervision:* involving the application of accounting procedures to manage fiscal data and supervision of subordinates in bookkeeping activities *Maintenance Supervision:* involving the planning and directing of the activities of maintenance workers
4. Ability to reflect original ideas or feelings in work	*Dance Instruction:* involving the creation and demonstration of original dances *Journalistic Activities:* e.g., writing syndicated columns
5. Ability to influence people's opinions, attitudes, or judgments about ideas or things	*Advertising or Public Relations Work:* e.g., writing promotional advertisements for newspapers *Fundraising:* seeking support from individuals or firms

Situational Work Abilities	Examples of Work Situations Requiring the Ability
6. Ability to make generalizations, evaluations, or decisions based on subjective or objective criteria	*Quality Control:* e.g. testing and inspecting products at various stages of production *Real Estate Appraisal:* involving the determination of property values for sales or loans
7. Ability to interact with people beyond simply giving and receiving instructions	*Nursing:* involving patient care activities *Sales Clerk:* e.g., assisting customers in selecting clothes
8. Ability to perform under stress when confronted with emergency, unusual, or dangerous circumstances, or in situations in which speed and attention are critical aspects of the job	*Power Line Maintenance and Repair:* involving service delivered under hazardous circumstances *Firefighting:* involving the use of proper techniques in controlling and extinguishing dangerous fires; requires speed and quick judgment in carrying out techniques
9. Ability to meet precise standards or requirements on the job using precision measuring instruments, tools, or machines	*Machinist:* requires the calibration of equipment to perform operations to requested specifications *Pharmaceutical Dispensing Activities:* requires accurate weighing, measuring, and mixing of drugs and accurate counting of tablets
10. Ability to work continuously under specific instructions in oral, written, or diagrammatic form	*Inspecting:* requires inspection of materials and products for conformity to specifications using fixed or preset measuring instruments *Assembling:* e.g., interlacing and joining parts, such as boards or precut and fabricated wood or metal units
11. Ability to work alone, either in isolation or simply independently of others	*Forest Ranger:* involves the locating and reporting of forest fires and weather phenomena from remote lookout stations *Overland Truck Driver:* involves long distance driving to transport products

provided by a vocational rehabilitation professional as defined by the Vocational Evaluation and Work Adjustment Association (Meers, 1985; Sax, 1981). If a rehabilitation facility offers only work adjustment services, it is important to provide continuity of care by establishing an affiliation with a facility or agency that offers vocational evaluation and placement services. Job training could, then, be included throughout the work adjustment and vocational evaluation processes. In Pittsburgh, The Rehabilitation Institute of Pittsburgh and the Vocational Rehabilitation Center have formed such a networking agreement in order to provide intensive cognitive and vocational programs for head injured adults (see Chapter 10).

The goals of work adjustment are to help the client:

- understand the impact of the injury on vocational functioning;
- set realistic work goals;
- develop effective interpersonal and social skills for the work environment;
- develop motor skills, endurance, and stamina;
- develop competencies in the critical vocational skills; and
- develop adequate competency in at least two of the basic work abilities listed in Table 5–1.

Interdisciplinary team work: To prevent duplication and fragmentation in programming, to promote more efficient acquisition and generalization of skills, and to facilitate revisions and refinements in the intervention program, the number of goals for a patient at any one time should be limited, intervention approaches and strategies should be consistent among the therapies involved, and information about the client's response to treatment should be regularly shared. This interdisciplinary framework is illustrated by our team's approach to J.P., a 32 year old head injured male whose goal was to return to work in a dairy product processing company. By reviewing the results of the multidisciplinary assessment and carefully analyzing J.P.'s job, the vocational rehabilitation specialist identified for the team the key cognitive and physical skills that the client would have to acquire to resume the job. With this information, the team jointly agreed upon a small set of goals and a distribution of responsibilities:

1. The occupational therapist focused on developing eye-hand coordination and improved fine motor speed, both required by conveyer line assembly work.

2. The physical therapist attempted to improve J.P.'s balance since he would be required to climb several platforms to retrieve work materials.
3. The cognitive therapist devised a task direction form to help keep J.P. organized and oriented to his task.
4. The vocational rehabilitation specialist coached J.P. through work trials to help him generalize skills learned elsewhere to a functional setting and to help him integrate his skills within complex vocational tasks.

Methods of Work Adjustment

Prigatano and Ben-Yishay have demonstrated that intensive treatment that includes cognitive and psychosocial components can improve employment outcome for head injured adults (Prigatano and others, 1986; Silver et al., 1983). Prigatano stressed, as a result of his experience, that head injury programs should additionally include a specific vocational component. Since severely head injured people are known to have difficulty generalizing skills or strategies from one setting to another (Zahara & Cuvo, 1984), there is reason to believe that training in real or simulated work activities enhances the positive effects of traditional physical rehabilitation when combined with cognitive and psychosocial intervention. In the remainder of the chapter, we discuss four methods of work adjustment: diagnostic assessment, vocational therapy, work conditioning, and counseling.

Diagnostic Assessment

The purpose of diagnostic assessment in the work adjustment process is to identify areas for therapeutic intervention by carefully examining components of the client's ability to perform work-related tasks. Critical vocational skills and work abilities can be functionally analyzed by examining the client's work proficiency. A proficient worker is one who has the ability to:

- understand the task and the procedures used in performing the task;
- organize and plan the task;
- complete the task in a systematic fashion; and
- evaluate the results and, if necessary, make adjustments.

The assessment in this phase of vocational rehabilitation differs from the formal vocational evaluation. In work adjustment, diagnostic assessment is used to identify work-related problems for remediation (Cohen, 1985). The vocational evaluation incorporates the results of this assessment and further evaluates the client to determine vocational ranges (e.g., competitive employment, semi-sheltered work) and possible goals (e.g., food service worker, accountant).

The vocational specialist should observe and record those parts of a task which are performed correctly and incorrectly and efficiently and inefficiently. Tentative hypotheses are then generated to account for the client's performance. Subsequent tasks can be designed to answer questions that remain regarding the specific reasons for a breakdown in task performance. Factors that frequently interfere with efficient work performance include:

- language impairments which affect comprehension of instructions and explanations, and which affect clear expression of ideas; language processing impairments are frequently related to the amount or complexity of the information to be processed or to the rate at which it is delivered;
- cognitive deficits (e.g., attention and concentration problems, memory problems, organizational problems, impulsiveness, poor self-monitoring);
- perceptual difficulties (e.g., diplopia, hemianopsia, decreased proprioception/kinesthesia);
- behavioral problems;
- fatigue or problems with endurance;
- general slowness;
- pain;
- effects of medication;
- stress reactions to particular situations; and
- disincentives to work (e.g., worker's compensation benefits).

Organized lists of factors that affect task performance, such as that presented in Table 4–5, are useful in attempting to identify precisely where breakdowns in performance occur. Furthermore, performance on several tasks must be measured in relation to the situational work abilities listed in Table 5–1. Finally, techniques of task analysis can be used to break a task down into a large number of subtasks, thereby facilitating the identification of work-related deficits. The need for more than one task in the assessment of situational work abilities is illustrated by R.E., a head injured client who had expressed interest in a job that required the ability to meet precise standards. R.E. was first asked to locate zip codes for a number of addressed envelopes. Because he could read well and had adequate clerical skills, he performed well on this task. A subsequent task, simulated electrical assembly, required refined perceptual and fine motor skills in order to meet precise standards. R.E.'s rather subtle impairments in these areas were magnified by the demands of the task, and consequently he was unable to perform adequately.

Tasks that are useful in the assessment of work abilities should be carefully designed to systematically highlight those abilities and should simulate specific job situations. Botterbusch (1980) comprehensively reviewed commercially available work evaluation systems that can be used for this purpose. These work samples are time efficient, standardized, offer normative information, and have "face validity" (i.e., are clearly related to work) for the client. The Microtower Work Evaluation system [ICD Rehabilitation and Research Center]) has the added advantage of incorporating a learning component in the assessment process. For these reasons, a commercial system is desirable, particularly if in-house tasks are limited.

During the assessment, the vocational rehabilitation specialist should pay particular attention to the following components of task competence: work rate, work quality, endurance, and behavioral skills.

Work Rate: Work rate is the speed at which a client can perform a task or components of the task. Since both cognitive and psychomotor skills can affect work rate, an attempt should be made to measure their effects separately and also in combination. Assessment questions include:

1. How long does it take a client to understand the task?
2. How long does it take the client to organize and plan the task?
3. How long does it take the client to complete the task? What is the difference in time between familiar and novel tasks?
4. How efficiently does the client monitor work performance and products, and correct work errors?
5. What factors have the greatest effect on the client's rate of work (e.g., motor impairments, perceptual impairments, cognitive impairments, reduced initiative, pain)?

Work Quality: The quality of a client's work can be assessed both objectively and subjectively. For example, a typing sample can be evaluated objectively in terms of number of typing errors and inclusion of all of the information specified on the rough draft. Subjective evaluation would include overall appearance of the letter (e.g., visible erasures and centering of the text). Work that is of poor quality suggests either an inability to self-monitor one's performance or a failure to fully comprehend the nature of the assignment.

Endurance: Endurance refers to stamina or the ability to maintain a uniform level of productivity for an expected period of time. Following prolonged hospitalization and consequent inactivity, head injured clients are often unable to sustain high levels of work activity even in the absence of specific motor impairments or medical conditions that would predict reduced endurance. Assessment of endurance should include adequately long work assignments in a variety of work settings. It is not uncommon for patients to demonstrate the ability to do sedentary work for 2 to 3 consecutive hours at a productive rate, but tolerate no more than 30 consecutive minutes of moderately strenuous activity. When clients lack work stamina, the stress created by prolonged activity can cause cognitive breakdowns (e.g., inattention to task, disorientation, disorganization, inability to follow multistep directions), physical complaints (exhaustion, headaches, reduced coordination), or irritability and interpersonal problems. Movement disorders can also negatively affect endurance. The effect depends on the type (e.g., hyper/hypotonicity, tremor, ataxia), extent (e.g., one limb, one side of the body), and severity (e.g., mild, moderate, severe) of the motoric involvement. Persistent headaches are a common complaint following head injury and can be a major factor in endurance. Rimel, et al. (1981) reported that 79 percent of the mildly head injured clients they surveyed had persistent headaches. Conditions such as asthma, diabetes, and chronic pain can also reduce the client's work endurance.

Behavioral Skills: The client's behavioral repertoire should be analyzed during work activities to identify behaviors that interfere with vocational functioning as well as behaviors that contribute positively to vocational functioning. This analysis should also determine what environmental contingencies maintain inappropriate or maladaptive behavior (Goldstein & Ruthven, 1983). Interviews with family members, rehabilitation team members, and work supervisors help to identify behaviors that need to be monitored in the work setting. Subsequent observation, then, is used to determine

- inappropriate or maladaptive behavior;
- antecedents of inappropriate or maladaptive behavior; and
- functional consequences of inappropriate or maladaptive behavior.

Several behaviors that interfere significantly with vocational functioning are frequently observed in head injured clients. These include distractibility or inattention to task, chronic tardiness, inappropriate communication with peers and supervisors, and defensive responses to supervision or constructive feedback.

It is essential to determine, especially in the case of head injured clients, whether or not an observed behavior is a direct consequence of the brain injury. If so, the appropriate solution may be to explore means of compensation for the deficit. If it is an operant behavior under the control of environmental contingencies, consistent behavior management techniques are indicated, possibly combined with training in compensatory strategies.

Case illustration: C.M. was observed to have an attention span for work tasks of approximately 30 minutes, much shorter than would be required in competitive employment. After 30 minutes of work, he either left the work area or disrupted the other clients in the area. Initially, it was not known if this behavior was the result of a skill deficiency (e.g., inability to tell time, inability to comprehend his assignment, or primary attention span disorder) or was somehow reinforced and maintained by environmental contingencies. It was first learned that he could tell time. Then, by presenting very simple and interesting tasks and observing the same 30-minute limit, it was learned that the reduced attention to task was not a result of noncomprehension or disinterest. During an interdisciplinary team treatment meeting, the occupational therapist told the team that she had used a smoke break as a reward for successful completion of 30-minute treatment sessions. This powerful environmental contingency had apparently generalized to the vocational setting, creating the same expectation in that setting. By rescheduling smoke breaks and carefully explaining to the client the vocational importance of longer work periods, he was able to maintain attention for an adequate length of time.

Behavioral assessment should also focus on the client's ability to respond in an appropriate and discriminating way to nonverbal social cues (e.g., a frown of disapproval on the supervisor's face when examining a task). Within a noninjured population of people, there is wide variation in the ability to "read" such social cues. Given the cognitive and perceptual deficits that are frequent consequences of closed head injury combined with psychosocial adjustment problems, it is understandable that many head injured clients lack this discriminative ability and may easily either miss or misread nonverbal cues (Zahara & Cuvo, 1984). They may need either training in social cognition (see Chapter 4), less subtle cues, or fully explicit verbal feedback (Gajar, Schloss, Schloss & Thompson, 1984) that does not rely on the nonverbal communication of information.

The vocational specialist needs to be alert to the subtlety of the patient's manifested behavior and thoroughly explore areas of strength and weakness. A written plan of action is helpful in systematically analyzing specific components (e.g., work rate, work quality, endurance). This plan should specify the objectives of the assessment and the procedures that will be used to examine the client's performance. Each plan should be individually developed, taking into account the unique circumstances of the client's vocational background and current level of functioning.

Information gathered during the assessment of the client's work abilities is used (a) to target areas for intensive work adjustment therapy, (b) to assign goals to each member of the interdisciplinary team and to coordinate the treatment provided, and (c) to measure progress in vocational therapy.

Vocational Therapy

The goal of vocational therapy is to improve a client's work-related skills and behaviors within a therapeutic environment by utilizing simulated work activities. Effectively guiding this process of learning and behavior change in clients with varying degrees of brain damage requires the vocational rehabilitation specialist to be acquainted with relevant theories of learning, techniques of instruction and behavior modification, and principles of vocational rehabilitation. Techniques that have been useful in the vocational therapy setting and that can be combined to promote learning and behavior change include:

1. mediated learning that includes an explicit focus on learning and problem-solving processes themselves and on cognitive deficits that block effective learning (Feuerstein, 1980) (See Acquisition Phase)
2. the acquisition of strategies that are deliberately applied to compensate for cognitive weakness (see Chapter 4)
3. behavior modification techniques that effect changes in behavior by controlling antecedent events that elicit the behavior or consequent events that reinforce and maintain the behavior and by attaining behavioral goals in small steps through successive approximation or shaping (Mercer & Snell, 1977)
4. repeated practice to promote proficiency in skills and strategies, and thus increase the likelihood of generalization to work settings
5. step-by-step chaining, forward or backward
6. task analysis and systematic sequencing of skill learning (Mercer & Snell, 1977)

PROGRESSION OF VOCATIONAL THERAPY. Whichever methods of instruction, or combination of methods, is used, vocational therapy should proceed systematically from (a) diagnostic exploration of skills, strategies, and intervention techniques to (b) acquisition of skills and strategies to (c) development of proficiency in skills and strategies to (d) generalization of skills and strategies. We will refer to these as "phases" of vocational therapy. Since the goal of vocational therapy is effective and independent vocational functioning, therapists should give clients only that amount of cuing and prompting that is necessary to elicit a target behavior. When a behavior needs to be cued, therapists should begin with a verbal cue; if that is insufficient, then a model or gestural prompt is added to the verbal cue; if that is insufficient, a physical prompt is added (Wehman, 1981).

Vocational therapy using the four phases (exploration, acquisition, proficiency, and generalization) provides more comprehensive services than what is typically afforded in traditional programs that include counseling plus partial acquisition of skills (Salamone, 1971; Stokes & Baer, 1977). The acquisition, proficiency, and generalization stages, essential to successful vocational therapy for head injured individuals, require additional training time for the client, increased flexibility and creativity among staff and administrators, and more clinical skills on the part of the vocational rehabilitation specialist than are required by traditional programs.

Diagnostic Exploration Phase: The goal of this phase is to determine:

1. the rate at which the client can acquire work-related skills and behaviors;
2. the most effective instructional methods; this includes the client's ability to benefit from feedback (charting of performance, video feedback, time studies, quality checks, and anecdotal summaries) and from a mediated or metacognitive approach to learning;
3. the client's ability to acquire and functionally use compensatory strategies;
4. the client's ability to learn and functionally use problem-solving procedures;
5. the client's ability to behave in a socially appropriate manner when given cues;
6. the client's ability to handle work materials through ergonomic redesign and rehabilitation technology; and
7. the client's ability to recognize, understand, and respond to expectations inherent in a formal work environment.

Based on the results of the assessment and this diagnostic exploration, the team decides that a client is or is not appropriate for vocational programming. Clients who exhibit severe cognitive, physical, and/or emotional limitations may be encouraged to pursue avocational options (see Chapter 8). If a client is found to have vocational potential, the vocational rehabilitation specialist works with other members of the rehabilitation team to identify the best treatment approach and to create an individualized treatment plan for the acquisition, proficiency, and generalization stages of treatment.

Acquisition Phase. With the overall goal of maximum vocational independence, the vocational specialist designs activities to teach skills and strategies, and to shape behaviors that will enhance employability. Objectives for individual clients are selected from the lists of critical vocational skills and situational work abilities (discussed earlier in this chapter) on the basis of that client's profile of work-related strengths and weaknesses. Of equal importance, the vocational rehabilitation specialist uses counseling techniques to help the client understand the relevance of treatment objectives and activities, and the relationship between therapy and possible vocational goals. It is very common for head injured clients at this stage of their vocational rehabilitation to resist work adjustment therapy either because they fail to recognize that they have deficits that will interfere with their return to work or they fail to see any connection between the therapy activities and their own goals. R.C. was a head injured young adult who had lost his job. One of the problems, it was learned, was his consistent interpretation of most of his former employer's requests and directives to be unfair attempts to single him out for extra work. His response to therapy was similar; he frequently complained that his work in therapy had no purpose and was too demanding. Treatment at this stage, therefore, focused on helping R.C. to understand the purpose — in relation to his own goals — of therapy tasks, the role of work supervisors in a work setting, and the vocational consequences of noncompliance.

The development of compensatory strategies and the use of a "mediated learning" approach often begins at this phase. Mediated learning (Feuerstein, 1980) is an instructional technique that promotes more efficient learning by mobilizing clients' own problem-solving skills. Central to mediated learning is the clients' understanding of their own active role in learning and of the cognitive processes involved. In a work adjustment setting, this technique allows clients to understand, organize, and interpret the demands of work tasks with heightened self-awareness and to problem solve in a creative way so that their performance improves despite possible residual cognitive and perceptual problems. Since even non-brain damaged adults rarely have words like "cognitive organization," "information processing," and "self-monitoring" in their active vocabulary, it is necessary to teach the vocabulary that is used to describe cognitive processes and systems (see Chapter 3). This facilitates comprehension of cognitive strengths and weaknesses, and consequently makes clients more receptive to compensatory strategies as a means of improving task performance.

Mediated Learning: A Case Illustration: J.M., a 36 year old head injured male, had difficulty following directions correctly, particularly when those directions were not fully explicit. This problem was judged to be a significant work impediment since J.M. appeared to lack initiative and self-directedness on jobs to which he was assigned. The vocational specialist addressed this problem by guiding J.M. through several mediated learning exercises in which the goal was to determine the implicit directions of the task.

One such exercise involved a task sheet which presented a series of picture frames each of which contained a set of dots that could be connnected to create geometric figures (e.g., square, triangle). The first picture frame illustrated how the dots might be connected to make two geometric shapes. The client's goal was to determine the implicit directions of the task (i.e., connect the dots in the remaining picture frames to make similar shapes), to write down the task directions, and, finally, to complete the task. Some of the frames contained thickened dots that aided in the projection of a particular shape. However, no verbal information was presented on the worksheet.

The vocational specialist's goal was to highlight for J.M. the cognitive activity (successful and unsuccessful) that he engaged in to complete this task. The session was also videotaped for later review by J.M. and the clinician. During the review session, J.M. was presented with a written list of the cognitive activity he had engaged in to determine the directions. These processes are summarized below along with the mediation that was used to facilitate completion of the task and to promote self-awareness of J.M.'s cognitive functioning.

I. *Input Stage* (gathering information):

A. J.M. impulsively wrote names of geometric shapes in each frame.

Mediation: J.M. was simply asked if these were the directions to the task. He said that he was unsure. He was then cued to look at the worksheet and to see if he could determine the directions.

B. J.M. looked only at the first frame, failing to scan all of the relevant information (inefficient scanning); he stated that he was to find two shapes.
Mediation: J.M. was cued to look at each frame; he had not been aware that several of the dots were thickened in some of the frames. The clinician suggested that he scan the entire sheet for relevant information, pointing out the importance of complete information.

C. J.M. searched the entire sheet systematically to gather relevant information.
Mediation: The clinician praised J.M. for his effective search and his ability to avoid impulsive responses.

D. J.M. asked relevant questions to gather additional information.
Mediation: In response to J.M.'s question as to whether the work should be done in pen or pencil, the clinician simply asked him to consider the consequences of each. J.M. stated that if he used pen, he would have difficulty erasing mistakes.

II. *Elaboration Stage* (mental formulation of the principle or rule and a plan of action):

A. J.M. searched for and drew only the squares.
Mediation: J.M. was reminded that he needed to state the directions to the task and to make sure that he had accounted for all of the information he had. With this cue, J.M. realized that he could not account for the drawing of the triangles.

B. J.M. formulated and wrote directions to the task (not entirely correct).
Mediation: The clinician reviewed the directions with J.M. and clarified several points.

III. *Output Stage* (carrying out the plan):

A. J.M. performed the activity based on the written directions.
Mediation: J.M. made one mistake. The clinician asked him to monitor his work before turning in the worksheet.

B. J.M. checked his work thoroughly.
Mediation: The clinician praised J.M. for checking his work, finding the mistake, and making the necessary correction.

In the review session, J.M. was asked to judge the effectiveness of each step in his completion of this task. Those cognitive behaviors which were judged to be ineffective (e.g., impulsive responding, inefficient searching) were eliminated from the list. Finally, J.M. was encouraged to "bridge" each of the successful behaviors to a work activity — that is, to describe their potential usefulness in job settings that were realistic possibilities for him. He suggested, for example, that systematic searching would be essential in jobs such as mailroom distribution and that asking questions might be a necessary means to clarify job instructions in almost any work setting. Bridging is used within mediated learning exercises to help the learner apply effective cognitive behavior to broader areas of everyday functioning. Later, during a simulated work activity, J.M. was required to put to use the insights that he had gained from these mediated learning exercises and identify their role in his performance and in his subsequent problem-solving efforts.

Since clients often have their own unique vocabulary to refer to their prominent cognitive deficits, it is essential that the client and the therapist negotiate a mutually acceptable and consistently used set of terms. Failure to establish clear meanings for the words used during the mediated learning process, and the consequent communication breakdown, are illustrated by D.J., a head injured client who had difficulty processing information efficiently. He had tried to return to work as an assistant manager in a fast food operation, but his supervisor reported that, despite excellent effort, he did not complete his assignments efficiently and never seemed to get the whole picture of what needed to be done. To some degree, D.J. was aware of his difficulty and described it as a "speed" problem, but was unable to elaborate beyond that. The vocational therapist and cognitive rehabilitation therapist designed organizational strategies and language comprehension strategies that they felt would help D.J. function more effectively in the work environment despite generally inefficient information processing skills. D.J. did not see the relevance of these strategies and therapy activities, and requested instead "speed" activities. When the therapists showed D.J. simulated and videotaped examples of what they meant by inefficiency in processing information, it quickly became clear to D.J. that what he meant by "speed" problem was part of what they meant by "processing" problem and that his resistance to therapy was based on a communication breakdown. D.J. also recognized that he had problems in other areas of processing (e.g., comprehending instructions and following conversations) and that these problems were related to what he had thought of simply as a "speed" problem. The clarification resulted for D.J. in an increased commitment to treatment.

For some clients, the mediated learning approach is inappropriate. Generally, these are individuals who remain somewhat confused and disoriented, are very concrete in their thinking, are severely limited in their ability to generalize skills or information, or learn better in an incidental learning situation than in a deliberate learning situation (see Chapter 4). Good descriptions of alternative methods of vocational instruction are provided in Bellamy, Horner, and Inman, 1979; Rusch and Mithaug, 1980; Wehman, 1981; and Wehman and McLaughlin, 1980.

The vocational specialist and cognitive therapist should work closely to design strategies that capitalize on the client's strengths, that are relevant to specific vocational objectives, and that can be combined to form standard procedures. These standard procedures, if practiced until firmly habituated, can often help client's perform specific work tasks. For example, the "structured thinking form" (Figure 5-2) is used in a variety of work settings by clients who are disorganized and impulsive. The procedure combines several individual strategies (telegraphic note taking [part 1], visualization of steps [part 2], and self-talk [part 3] and has been successfully used to improve planning, decrease impulsiveness, and increase production in vocational settings. The teaching of compensatory strategies is discussed at length in Chapter 4.

Throughout the acquisition stage, the vocational specialist carefully monitors both the effects of strategic procedures on the client's work performance and also the client's acceptance of the strategies. Chapter 4 includes a list of features of strategies that are relevant to their effectiveness and also to the acceptance. We have, for example, worked with several head injured individuals with significant memory impairments who refused to carry large notebooks to serve as a memory aid, but did effectively use pocket-size memo books for the same purpose. Since the small discrete memory aid drew less attention to the client's memory deficit, it was more acceptable to them and was also consistent with Wolfensberger's (1972) principles of normalization.

When the acquisition of skills, strategies, and work-related behaviors has reached a point at which it is meaningful to begin to consider realistic vocational goals, the vocational rehabilitation team should meet to make plans for a vocational evaluation and subsequent training or placement services. Identification of possible vocational areas for the client remains very tentative at this stage, but this discussion gives the vocational evaluation/placement team an opportunity to prepare their phase of the client's vocational rehabilitation and helps the work adjustment specialist to modify the client's treatment plan so that the most essential issues are addressed during the proficiency and generalization stages of work adjustment.

1. Task: Directions/Notes

- Are there time limits?
- Do I understand what I'm to do?
- Do I have all the information I need?

2. Plan

Steps:

Materials Needed:

3. Review

- Are my steps and materials accurate?

Yes → DO IT

No → Rethink steps and materials → Ask for additional information if necessary → DO IT

4. Final Evaluation

- Does my work look acceptable?
- Is it done on time?
- Any special concerns:

Figure 5–2. Structured thinking form.

Proficiency Phase. For brain injured individuals, proficiency in a skill or behavior, or habituation of that skill or behavior, often requires numerous repetitions, or rehearsals. This process must be carefully monitored and alternative instructional techniques should be explored if progress is not evident. To avoid creating "splinter skills" or skills that are firmly bound to the conditions of training, it is important to build into the training tasks a range of discriminative stimuli and response requirements (Wilcox & Bellamy, 1982). This lays the foundation for subsequent generalization training. Work activities selected for training the target skills should range from simple to complex and contain components of the situational work abilities listed in Table 5–1. Simple tasks are those that have low demands in the areas of *amount* of work required, *rate* at which it is to be done, *duration* of the task, and level of environmental *distraction.* By providing the client with simple tasks initially, emphasis is placed on proficiency in specific target behaviors. Later the client's ability to demonstrate a given behavior is challenged by more complex tasks and higher expectations for quality of performance.

The use of varied work activities also begins the difficult process of helping clients accept realistic work goals (see Chapter 6). Guided success and failure with these work activities promotes the client's openness to comprehensive vocational evaluation and, later, to the consideration of alternative work placements. To facilitate this process, clients are asked at this stage to evaluate their own performance. This self-evaluation uses performance criteria similar to those used by the vocational rehabilitation specialist during the assessment. The criteria are given to the client with the explanation that these are the standards that must be met if competitive employment is to be considered a realistic option. A gradual introduction of self-evaluation requirements and skilled counseling are necessary to help the client accept the feedback and begin to draw appropriate conclusions about vocational potential.

Generalization Phase. The goal of this stage of work adjustment therapy is to have the client independently use newly acquired skills, strategies, or other work-related behaviors in a guided work trial. In our facility, these work trials are realistic work experiences within the hospital setting in such departments as housekeeping, food service, and office services. It is important that the client demonstrate basic behavioral competencies in this setting before proceeding with further vocational training or placement. It is unlikely that a client who cannot generalize work adjustment skills to these work trails will do so in a more demanding vocational training or actual job setting.

Generalization involved the transfer of stimulus control over a given behavior from specific instructions and prompts in a treatment setting to naturally occurring stimuli in a work setting. This process can be facilitated in a variety of ways, including (a) systematic variation in the treatment environment; (b) gradual fading of cues; and (c) time delay techniques.

During the *proficiency stage,* training should include systematic changes in the place of training, the activities, the staff, and the specific verbal or nonverbal cues used to elicit a behavior. The types of settings, activities, and cues selected for this process should be based, to whatever extent possible, on the types of setting, activities, and cues that will be present in the projected work environment (Stokes & Baer, 1977). This begins the process of transferring stimulus control (Zahara & Cuvo, 1984).

During the *acquisition and proficiency stages,* the client's behaviors are elicited by specific instructions. In most work settings, workers are expected to perform their jobs without explicit and repeated instructions. Fading is a technique for transferring stimulus control that involves substituting systematically less intense cues for the cues that originally established the behavior (Mercer & Snell, 1977). Ultimately, the client must be able to maintain the behavior when only naturally occurring prompts in the work environment are operative. For selected clients, it is possible to transfer control over a behavior from the clinician's instructions to the client's own covert self-instructions (Meichenbaum, 1977).

Time delay involves the pairing of a controlling stimulus with a second stimulus (which should be present in the natural work environment) to which control is to be transferred (Mercer & Snell, 1977). The technique requires progressively longer delays between the presentation of the new stimulus (e.g., the supervisor's instruction) and the original controlling stimulus (e.g., the therapist telling the client to record information on a task direction sheet).

Monitoring of the client's progress during this stage helps to refine plans for vocational education, for further training, and for ultimate placement. Some clients demonstrate very little ability to generalize skills, despite their possession of genuine work potential. These individuals may be candidates for work placements that include on-the-job coaching or training (see Chapter 6). Some client's may be able to generalize skills to some settings but not to others. This knowledge will help to define the focus for vocational evaluation. As always, the factors that influence task competence (discussed in the Assessment section of this chapter) should be examined to determine the causes of poor performance.

In this section, we have discussed stages and techniques of vocational therapy that are a means of overcoming work adjustment difficulties. It certainly is naive to assume that work adjustment problems are completely resolved before vocational evaluation, training, and placement are initiated. The goals and techniques of work adjustment intervention, in most cases, must be integrated into the evaluation, training, and placement phases. This important theme in head injury rehabilitation is highlighted in Chapter 6.

Work Conditioning

Work conditioning services are often necessary to improve a client's work tolerance, which is the ability to sustain work performance over a specified time period (Smith & McFarlane, 1984). Due to complications associated with the head injury, including motor problems (Berroll, 1983), forced inactivity, depleted nutritional status (Newmark, Sublett, Black & Geller, 1981), and cognitive deficits (e.g., reduced initiation), many head injured individuals have difficulty resuming former levels of physical activity. Fatigue and reduced endurance have been identified as major problems following head injury (Glenn & Rosenthal, 1985; Gronwall & Wrightson, 1974; Lynch & Mauss, 1981; Rutherford, Merrett & McDonald, 1977) and contribute to this inability to resume former activity levels. As a consequence of these factors, many clients have little work tolerance during the initial phases of vocational rehabilitation. Clinically, we have noted that decreased stamina and fatigue appear to depress the clients ability to function cognitively.

A client's work tolerance is related in part to the physical and psychomotor activities that are basic to work output, including lifting, carrying, sitting, kneeling, reaching, climbing, walking, balancing, running, stooping, coordinating eye-hand movements, and coordinating finger movements (May, 1985). The goals of work conditioning services are:

1. initially to improve the client's ability to work productively at a sedentary to light job for 2 hours with minimal breaks and to progress to higher activity levels (e.g., longer periods of time or more physically demanding work) when indicated. (This may require consultation with the client's physician.);
2. to improve the client's ability to sit, stand, walk, or stoop (within individual guidelines) for specified periods without undue fatigue;
3. to help the client meet specific physical requirements for a possible job area; and
4. to improve the client's overall body mechanics while handling objects.

A professional with training in work conditioning (e.g., an exercise physiologist, physical therapist, or vocational rehabilitation specialist with certification in work hardening) should oversee the work conditioning program under the guidance of a physiatrist or other appropriate physician. Exercise activities can be chosen on the basis of their usefulness in meeting specific fitness goals (e.g., cardiovascular activities to promote tolerance for long periods of work) and also on the basis of their interest and perceived relevance for the client. High interest activities, identified through client or family interview, will increase the likelihood that the client will continue the exercise program after discharge. Using work-related materials and work activities in the exercise program helps the client see the relevance of the activity to vocational rehabilitation. An individual exercise program is, then, prescribed on the basis of physiological needs, motor abilities, interests, and projected vocational placement. Exercise may have the noteworthy side benefits of reducing some forms of depression and generally elevating the client's spirits.

A description of the client's performance in the work conditioning program is shared with the vocational evaluation team and possibly also with prospective employers so that realistic expectations for and limitations on work performance may be established. Work conditioning is further described in Chapter 2.

Counseling

Severe closed head injury often results in an organically based failure to perceive deficits and their implications for vocational and social functioning (Ben-Yishay & Diller, 1981; Humphrey & Oddy, 1980; Prigatano et al., 1986; Silver et al., 1983). The predictable consequence of this impaired self-awareness is resistance to considering alternatives to pre-traumatic goals and aspirations and, derivatively, resistance to the vocational program that is not specifically directed toward those pre-traumatically held goals. For those who do have an adequate awareness of what they cannot do, the resulting inability to reconcile past and present levels of performance can be a constant source of sorrow, frustration, and helplessness (Lezak, 1978a; Prigatano et al., 1986). The injury often places the individual in a marginal position, caught between a role that is desirable but not achievable and a role that is available but not acceptable (Shontz, 1975). These psychodynamic issues may be interrelated in a highly complex way with cognitive and physical deficits.

If weak self-awareness or psychoreactive problems are at a level of severity at which they significantly impede progress in work adjustment therapy, then they must be addressed by vocational specialists. Clients may, at the same time, be engaged in individual counseling or psychotherapy with a social worker, clinical psychologist, or psychiatrist. Communication among counseling professionals is essential for establishing a consistent approach to treatment. Given the focus on work-related issues, the vocational rehabilitation professional has the opportunity to confront resistance and denial, or promote a more realistic self-appraisal of strengths and weaknesses, in a context that is concrete and meaningful for the client. Vocational counseling, when integrated with vocational therapy and work conditioning, can, then, be both an effective method of improving work adjustment and also an essential component of effective personal counseling (Lynch, 1983; Super, 1980).

The goals of the vocational counseling process are:

- to assist the client in developing realistic self-perceptions relative to vocational skills, aptitudes, performance, and potential;
- to assist the client in adjusting to these changes in self-perception;
- to assist the client in developing realistic occupational choices; and
- to assist the client in developing an action plan for reaching the desired goals.

Due to impaired cognitive functioning, head injured clients tend to benefit more from directive counseling techniques that are instructional in nature than from "insight" therapies (Ben-Yishay & Diller, 1983). Three counseling approaches that we have found useful are rational emotive therapy (Ellis, 1962), cognitive behavior modification (Meichenbaum, 1977), and reality therapy (Glasser, 1965). Ben-Yishay found that head injured individuals often lack the understanding and will to benefit from traditional psychotherapy. Effective intervention for head injured clients, therefore, requires that the therapist establish intervention priorities and clearly state to the client the rationale for the needed behavioral changes (Ben-Yishay & Diller, 1983). Okun (1982) also reported that directive techniques are beneficial for clients who have cognitive problems.

In the process of helping clients improve their self-awareness of strengths and deficits, understand the vocational impact of deficits, and accept more realistic vocational goals, vocational counselors often uncover a fundamental dilemma: while clients are driven by the reality of unemployment, they also resist changes in their behavior and domain of acceptable job options. This dilemma is, of course, not unique to head injured clients. It is a predictable response when individuals find that they must give up old behavior patterns because they are no longer adequate to cope with new stresses. For example, it is the type of dilemma that faces older women who re-enter the work force and discover that previously habituated patterns of nonassertiveness are no longer effective for job mobility (Goldstein, Heller & Sechrest, 1966). Counselors must be sensitive to the fact that change in behavior patterns and change in self-concept are threatening challenges for the client, particularly when it is the client who must become the agent of the change (Goldstein et al., 1966). The counselor must artfully provide a certain measure of comfort, reassurance, and advice, while persistently encouraging the client to consider changes in existing behavior patterns and goals.

When individuals begin a counseling process that will require behavioral change, it is often helpful to organize the experience for them by giving them information about the nature and goals of counseling (Glasser, 1965; Goldstein et al., 1966; Holland, 1966; Okun, 1982). The absence of such structure and information may produce anxiety (Kelly, 1955), while providing such structure is known to facilitate learning and improved performance (Ausubel, 1960; Woodworth & Schlosberg, 1954). A useful method of organizing the counseling process for head injured individuals is to present, at the outset, information on the nature and consequences of traumatic brain injury and on the career development process, and how these relate to the goals of the counseling process. The categories of brain dysfunction and the stages of career development can then be applied to the client's own case as resistance abates and cognitive awareness improves.

The purpose of presenting information about brain functioning is to help head injured clients understand their own deficits and see the relevance of rehabilitation. It is useful to present this information in a group counseling setting (Ben-Yishay et al., 1983; Prigatano et al., 1986). We present information about traumatic brain injury in several different formats, including lecture, videotape, handouts, roleplays, client's own descriptions, and testimonials of former clients.

To make this relatively abstract and difficult-to-process information more concrete and personally meaningful, we encourage clients to create their own labels for brain functions and areas of the brain, and to create metaphors that help them organize the information and make it applicable to their own life. Clients who have difficulty understanding the complex functions of the frontal lobes may gain insight into some of these functions by using metaphors like "switchboard operator," "coach," "executive," or "guide." The client who used the image of a switchboard operator to understand certain frontal functions had no difficulty understanding the concept of a catastrophic reaction, i.e., the circuits are all full and the switchboard operator cannot handle the pressure. Clear and simplified three-dimensional models of the brain and visual illustrations are also helpful for instruction.

The vocational rehabilitation counselor, working with a psychologist, can also help the client to become more aware of the impact of specific cognitive deficits on vocational performance. Information about cognitive and cognitive deficits is initially presented objectively, without discussing individual client's cognitive impairments. In our experience, it has been helpful for clients to acquire the ability to describe cognitive functioning and deficits objectively before attempting to identify their own cognitive strengths and weaknesses. After introducing the terms that can be used to describe cognitive functioning, clients may be asked to identify cognitive strengths and weaknesses in videotaped performances of models. Also clients are encouraged in group discussion to share personal insights regarding their own situation. Prigatano and colleagues (1986) have used this type of informational approach successfully in their work with head injured adults.

Career development theory (Ginzberg, 1972; Holland, 1966; Osipow, 1968; Super, 1957) is presented in simplified form to clients to help them understand the process by which individuals achieve vocational status, to help them explore vocational identity, and, most importantly, to help them identify and accept the effects of brain injury on their career development and on the vocational identity. Examples from other illnesses or disabilities are used (e.g., the effects of heart disease on vocational options) to illustrate important principles in a nonthreatening way and to help clients see that their problems are not unique.

Presenting this organizing information early in the counseling process often, though certainly not always, makes the client a more willing participant in rehabilitation and a more active agent of behavioral change. We encourage clients to understand the vocational counseling process as a way of developing a plan to achieve acceptable vocational status. Throughout the process, we ask clients to ask themselves four questions (see Figure 4–5):

1. What is my goal?
2. How realistic is my goal?
3. What is my plan for achieving my goal?
4. Is my plan working?

These questions not only focus the counseling process, they also help to reduce natural resistance to change. Video feedback and goal setting are counseling techniques that are useful in the process of promoting a more accurate self-perception of deficits and more realistic vocational goals.

Video Feedback: Video feedback can be a source of powerful, but nonpersonal, confrontation. While the feedback is not fully "objective," since the client's affective and perceptual set can easily distort the image that is seen, it is much more objective and less easy to dispute than observations of performance made by a clinician. For this reason, clients achieve a clearer and more accurate perception of their performance than by means of other forms of feedback. Video feedback is best suited for those clients who are simply unaware of their current functioning. Those clients who are aware of their limitations and are struggling with or are depressed about the implications of those limitations are not good candidates for video feedback since the vividness of the moving image of oneself can exacerbate depression or anxiety. (Chapter 4 includes other considerations that are important in using video therapy techniques.)

Videotaping must always be done with the client's permission. Furthermore, clients should be given time to become comfortable seeing themselves on the screen before they are videotaped performing challenging tasks. During her first several self-viewings, one young woman commented continuously on the appearance of her hair and make-up and hence was unable to attend to the quality of her performance or any other aspect of the event. The initial taping sessions should, therefore, be designed to show clients at their highest level of performance and the counselor should highlight these positive points during the tape review. Furthermore, it is often important to include the vocational counselor on the screen to avoid communicating the impression that clients are being singled out for humiliation. For similar reasons, it is preferable to begin videotaping in individual sessions and only later use the medium in group sessions.

When video feedback is used to improve the client's perception of deficits and to train specific behaviors, it is essential that the behaviors to be monitored be understood in advance and explicitly labeled. If, for example, the focus is the client's weak attending behaviors during conversations, then the client should be alerted to specific behaviors such as eye contact and maintaining the topic of conversation. Using clear behavioral terms helps to avoid the impression that the client's character is under attack and also helps to identify those specific skills that need to be improved.

It is not uncommon for clients to respond to a videotape self-observation by overgeneralizing a specific behavior to their overall performance (e.g., "I can never do anything right; I will always be a failure!"). Using techniques developed by Ellis (1962) and Burns (1980), the counselor can confront such irrational thinking patterns and help to replace them with more productive patterns. Irrational thinking patterns are illustrated by the following statements (Ellis, 1962):

1. It is a necessity for me to be loved and approved by everyone for everything I do.

2. Certain acts are wrong and evil, and I feel people who perform these acts should be severely punished.
3. It is terrible and catastrophic when things are not the way I would like them to be.
4. Much human unhappiness is externally caused and is forced on me by outside people and events.
5. Dangerous and fearsome things cause me great concern and I must continually consider their impact.
6. I must be perfectly competent, adequate, and achieving to be considered worthwhile.
7. I find it easier to avoid certain difficulties and responsibilities than to face them.
8. I am dependent on others and need to rely on someone stronger.
9. My past experiences and events are the determinants of present behavior and the influences of the past cannot be eradicated.
10. I need to be upset over other people's problems and disturbances.
11. I need to always have a right and perfect solution and it must be found or the results will be catastrophic.

When a client expresses one of these ideas, the counselor encourages him or her to consider the irrational components and the self-defeating cycle that this expression causes. The client is encouraged to take charge of what he can and to make deliberate self-statements to counter the negative aspects of an irrational idea. For the client who says that he or she can never do anything right and will therefore be a failure, counseling focuses on deliberately charting "right" things that he or she does. The client is told that persisting in letting irrational ideas govern behavior only results in frustration and depression. The client is encouraged to make a commitment to "beat" this self-defeating cycle. He or she can be taught to use positive self-talk when a failure occurs (e.g., instead of "I have done it again, I will never get it right," the client is encouraged to say, "How might I solve this problem").

Interpersonal Process Recall (IPR) is a technique for improving social interactive behavior by targeting specific aspects of interaction, practicing these behaviors in conversation, and then reviewing the interactions on video with a "coach" present to highlight the target behaviors and suggest alternatives to those that are socially inappropriate or simply ineffective (Kagan, 1969). Helffenstein and Wechsler (1982) found this technique to be effective in improving interactive behavior in head injured adults and in maintaining those improvements over time.

In the work adjustment setting, target behaviors are identified and taped for subsequent review. Work-related behaviors that lend themselves to this technique include interaction with peers and supervisors, and job interviews. Later, the counselor carefully guides the client through the review of the tape. Using directive counseling techniques such as those developed by Glasser (1965), the counselor and client identify the problems that are associated with the key behavior being reviewed. The key steps in reality therapy are:

1. Focus on present behaviors rather than on the past.
2. Stimulate self-evaluation of problem behaviors with the questions, "Is what I did appropriate?" and "Is it helping me?"
3. Develop a plan to change behavior. The client is asked to specify what behaviors should be changed; the counselor offers suggestions about behaviors to be changed and procedures to be used.
4. Make a contract to seal the plan. The plan specifies what course of action should be taken.
5. Review progress toward the goal. Excuses for failure in achieving the goals are redirected into positive action (e.g., "When will you do this?" rather than "Why didn't you do this?"). The plan is modified if necessary.

It is important for the counselor and client to jointly engage in problem solving to identify ways in which a behavior can be changed and plans for changing the behavior. This plan is then transferred to the vocational therapy setting where, through the use of coaching, prompting, and reinforcement, the client is helped to develop more appropriate and effective work-related behaviors.

Deliberate goal setting (Glasser, 1965) is a counseling technique that can help clients to learn new skills and increase productivity (Gardner & Warren, 1978). A key to adult rehabilitation is the development of a partnership between clinicians and clients in most areas of their program. Gazzaniga (1985) warned of the dangers of doing otherwise: "Studies show that a behavior has to be strongly perceived as freely willed in order for the behavior to be powerful in participating in a belief change. Behaviors easily dismissed as carried out because of external forces do not engage in the dissonance reduction process, and as a result the belief system remains unthreatened" (p. 141).

It is essential that clients understand why a particular goal has been established and that they are reasonably committed to the behavior change process (Glasser, 1965). Counselors must be alert to signs of frustration with goals and be flexible in renegotiating goals with the client. This helps to maintain the individual's feeling of control over behavior change and thereby promotes commitment to the rehabilitation process. Goal setting as a counseling technique includes the following sequence:

1. The client and counselor together establish a specific goal (e.g., improving typing speed) that is clearly related to more general goals (e.g., obtaining clerical work).
2. The client and counselor together identify factors that impede progress toward the specific goal (e.g., impaired attention; off-task behavior). Videotape review of performance may help to facilitate this awareness.
3. The client and counselor together establish objectives to reach the desired goal. The counselor's role in this problem-solving process is to encourage the setting of realistic goals and objectives, and to suggest possible routes to achieve the goal.
4. The client systematically and regularly documents progress toward the established goals. If progress does not occur, then the entire goal-setting process may need to be repeated.

This process of deliberate goal setting and monitoring of progress facilitates the client's awareness of goals and the relation between goals and ability to perform. In addition, it heightens the client's engagement in the treatment process. Other techniques that are useful in the counseling process include role playing, modeling, imaging, and role reversal (Patterson, 1980). Ben-Yishay and Diller (1983) proposed the use of various motivational techniques in remedial training of head injured clients. These included exhortatory techniques (e.g., "Show me your stuff"), evocative metaphors (e.g., "Remain cool and calm like an ice cube"), inspirational techniques (e.g., "What a pleasure to watch a mind at work"), psychodrama with role reversals, and encouragment to facilitate the client's assertions of intent to comply with the task demands and of the importance of therapy. Group treatment has a number of advantages: (a) it makes available a support system for the client; (b) it makes possible peer modeling, teaching, and testimonials; and (c) it creates a natural context for training in social skills. Ben-Yishay et al. (1983) and Prigatano et al. (1986) have both found group counseling to be effective in the rehabilitation of head injured adults.

Case Study: R.J. was 24 years old and 2 years post-injury when he was admitted to The Rehabilitation Institute of Pittsburgh's outpatient head injury program. At age 22 he had suffered a severe brain injury as a result of a motor vehicle accident. Neuropsychological assessment revealed significant right hemisphere damage. R.J. had deficits in spatial relations, concept formation, problem solving, and abstract thinking. He had left college after 2 years because of disinterest in his studies and problems related to alcohol abuse. At the time of his accident, he worked as a manager-trainee in a local fast food restaurant. Six months after the accident, he returned to this job without the benefit of rehabilitative services. He was dismissed, however, for "poor work speed" and other "unsatisfactory performances" which included repeated attempts to date other employees, a behavior strictly prohibited by restaurant policy for manager-trainees.

After his dismissal from work, R.J. entered the rehabilitation program, largely at his parents' urging. He insisted that his dismissal from the restaurant was unjustified, adding that "everybody breaks the rules sometimes." He actively resisted his treatment and had again become involved in substance abuse. Midway through his rehabilitation program, he announced to staff that he had found another manager-trainee job. Against the advice of the staff and his family, he left the program and refused all supportive services. After 2 weeks on the new job, he was again dismissed.

R.J. returned willingly to the Institute for continued rehabilitation. He explained to the work adjustment specialist that he had experienced "minor difficulties" on the job. With pride he described his excellent relationship with his new work supervisor. In support of this, he said that on one occasion he had bet his supervisor that his memory for procedures on how to prepare hamburgers would be more accurate than the supervisor's. Ironically, this incident, which R.J. cited in support of his good relationship with his supervisor, was the major reason cited by his employer for dismissal.

R.J.'s rehabilitation program included occupational therapy, cognitive rehabilitation therapy, vocational therapy, and vocational counseling. The program emphasized motor speed, finger dexterity, balance, general information processing skills, problem-solving skills, comprehension of social phenomena, and social skills. In addition, counseling sessions focused on self-awareness and self-monitoring of social interaction in the work setting, impulse control, ability to discriminate among situations that require different types of interaction, and accurate perception of the impact of his comments and nonverbal communication on his listeners. Social service counseling specifically addressed substance abuse.

Given the reasons for both of R.J.'s dismissals from work, treatment in the areas of social cognition (see Chapters 3 and 4), social judgment, and social skills took on special urgency. The following program components were emphasized:

1. R.J. was taught to identify cognitive distortions that operated in his social interactions. Through systematic examination of his responses to people, he was correctly able to identify "overgeneralizations" (e.g., assuming that all women wanted to date him), "being right" (e.g., always having the correct solution), and "jumping to conclusions" (e.g., assuming that the supervisor wanted to hear a "better" way to do the job) as prominent themes that shaped his belief system and consequently affected his behavior in unwanted ways.
2. Video therapy sessions were used to sensitize R.J. to the impact of inadvertent facial expressions and intonation patterns on his conversation partners. R.J. did come to agree that he often communicated condescension when he did not intend to do so.
3. To enhance problem-solving and decision-making skills, R.J. did exercises with the "Decision Making Guide" (Figure 4–5). The hypothetical situations selected for practice most often involved interpersonal issues in job-related contexts. We particularly emphasized the primacy of simple, clear vocational goals (e.g., keeping a job and communicating a sense of cooperation as opposed to defying company rules and initiating arguments with supervisors simply to prove a point).
4. R.J. kept a special journal in which he recorded events, information, of thoughts related to the issues that were the focus of his treatment. Journal entries would subsequently be raised for discussion in treatment sessions. He was advised to pay particular attention to those actual situations in which the reactions of his communication partners indicated a need to re-assess the clarity of his verbal and nonverbal messages, and make the necessary adjustments.
5. R.J. practiced compensatory strategies, such as covert self-coaching with rehearsed statements like, "Get the big picture, . . . don't distort things" and "Remember, keeping the job and giving a good impression are the important things."
6. With encouragement, R.J. developed his own action plan to achieve his vocational goals. In problem-solving sessions with his counselor, he was able to identify his treatment needs and appropriately revise his vocational aspirations.

This program was implemented during a 5-month period of outpatient treatment that also included a comprehensive vocational evaluation at the Vocational Rehabilitation Center of Allegheny County.

R.J. demonstrated significant progress in social cognition and social skills, both in specific treatment sessions and also in a variety of trial work placements. His progress was sufficient to warrant community placement, and volunteer work in the local Science Exhibit Center was arranged.

R.J.'s duties included several that required skill in communication and social judgment: (a) escorting visitors to and from exhibits while engaging them in conversation; (b) setting up exhibits while being observed by supervisors and patrons; (c) seating audiences for demonstrations and chatting pleasantly about the demonstrations; and (d) occasionally giving 10 to 15 minute presentations that included answering questions from the audience.

Follow-up reports from the supervisors at the Science Center were consistently favorable and indicated exemplary efficiency and cooperation in all areas of R.J.'s work. He was subsequently hired to work at the Science Center performing duties similar to those of his volunteer work. Concurrently, he became active in his local Narcotics Anonymous organization and accepted an invitation to volunteer in the group counseling sessions of that organization. Ongoing follow-up contacts have documented continued success one year following placement in this job.

CONCLUSION

Vocational rehabilitation of head injured adults is often a lengthy and difficult process that requires flexibility in treatment decisions, consistency in the application of treatment methods, and perseverance from clients and clinicians alike. Work adjustment is a key component in the vocational rehabilitation process and is often a prerequisite to vocational evaluation, placement, and training. Our goal in this chapter has been to describe a framework for delivering work adjustment services to head injured clients and to present selected techniques that facilitate the development of critical vocational skills. Chapter 6 addresses selected issues in vocational evaluation and job placement that are particularly important for head injured clients.

REFERENCES

Ausubel, D. P. (1960). The use of advance organizers in the learning and retention of meaningful verbal material. *Journal of Educational Psychology, 51,* 267–272.

Bellamy, G. T., Horner, R. H. & Inman, D. P. (1979). *Vocational habilitation of severely retarded adults: A direct service technology.* Baltimore: University Park Press.

Ben-Yisay, Y. & Diller, L. (1981). Rehabilitation of cognitive and perceptual defects in people with traumatic brain damage. *International Journal of Rehabilitation Research, 4,* 208–210.

Ben-Yishay, Y. & Diller, L. (1983). Cognitive remediation. In M. Rosenthal, E. R. Griffith, M. R. Bond & J. D. Miller (Eds.), *Rehabilitation of the head injured adult.* Philadelphia: F. A. Davis.

Ben-Yishay, Y., Lakin, P., Ross, B., Rattok, J., Piasetsky, E. B. & Diller, L. (1983). Psychotherapy following severe brain injury — Issues and answers. In *Working approaches to remediation of cognitive deficits in brain damaged persons* (Rehabilitation Monograph No. 66, pp. 127–148). New York: New York University Medical Center, Institute of Rehabilitation Medicine.

Berroll, S. (1983). Medical assessment. In M. Rosenthal, E. R. Griffith, M. R. Bond & J. D. Miller (Eds.), *Rehabilitation of the head injured adult* (pp. 231–239). Philadelphia: F. A. Davis.

Bond, M. R. (1975). Assessment of the psychological outcome after severe head injury. *Outcome of severe damage to the central nervous system: Ciba Foundation Symposium* (Vol. 34, pp. 141–190). Amsterdam: Elsevier.

Bond, M. (1984). The psychiatry of closed head injury. In N. Brooks (Ed.), *Closed head injury: Psychological, social, and family consequences* (pp. 148–178). Oxford: Oxford University Press.

Botterbusch, K. (1980). *A comparison of commerical vocational evaluation systems.* Menomonie, WI: Materials Development Center, University of Wisconsin-Stout, Stout Vocational Rehabilitation Institute.

Brooks, N. (1984). Head injury and the family. In N. Brooks (Ed.), *Closed head injury: Psychological, social, and family consequences.* Oxford: Oxford University Press.

Bruckner, F. E. & Randle, A. P. H. (1972). Return to work after severe head injuries. *Rheumatology and Physical Medicine, 11,* 334–348.

Burns, D. D. (1980). *Feeling good: The new mood therapy.* New York: W. W. Morrow.

Cohen, J. (1985). Vocational rehabilitation of the severely brain damaged patient: Stages and processes. *Journal of Applied Rehabilitation Counseling, 16,* 25–30.

Cowood, L. T. (Ed.). (1975). *Work oriented rehabilitation dictionary and synonyms.* Seattle, WA: Northwest Association of Rehabilitation Industries.

Cull, J. G. & Hardy, R. E. (1972). *Vocational rehabilitation: Profession and process.* Springfield: Charles C. Thomas.

Dikman, S. & Reitan, R. M. (1977). Emotional sequelae of head injury. *Annals of Neurology, 2,* 492–494.

Ellis, A. (1962). *Reason and emotion in psychotherapy.* New York: Lyle Stuart.

Feuerstein, R. (1980). *Instrumental enrichment: An intervention program for cognitive modifiability.* Baltimore: University Park Press.

Field, T. F. & Field, J. E. (Eds.). (1982). *Classification of jobs according to worker trait factors.* Athens, GA: VDARE Service Bureau.

Gajar, A., Schloss, P. J., Schloss, C. N. & Thompson, C. K. (1984). Effects of feedback and self-monitoring on head trauma youths' conversation skills. *Journal of Applied Behavior Analysis, 17,* 353–358.

Gardner, D. C. & Warren, S. A. (1978). *Careers and disabilities: A career education approach.* Stanford, CA: Greylock Publishers.

Gazzaniga, M. (1985). *The social brain.* New York: Basic Books.

Gilchrist, E. & Wilkinson, M. (1979). Some factors determining prognosis in young people with severe head injury. *Archives of Neurology, 36,* 355–359.

Ginzberg, E. (1972). Toward a theory of vocational choice: A restatement. *Vocational Guidance Quarterly, 20,* 169–176.

Glasser, W. (1965). *Reality therapy.* New York: Harper & Row.

Glenn, M. B. & Rosenthal, M. (1985). Rehabilitation following severe traumatic brain injury. *Seminars in Neurology, 5,* 233–246.

Goldstein, A. P., Heller, K. & Sechrest, L. B. (1966). *Psychotherapy and the psychology of behavior change.* New York: John Wiley & Sons.

Goldstein, G. & Ruthven, L. (1983). *Rehabilitation of the brain damaged adult.* New York: Plenum Press.

Gronwall, D. & Wrightson, P. (1974, Sept.). Delayed recovery on intellectual function after minor head injury. *The Lancet,* 605–609.

A guide to job analysis: A "how-to" publication for occupational analysts. (1982). Menomonie, WI: Materials Development Center, University of Wisconsin-Stout, Stout Vocational Rehabilitation Institute.

Hardy, R. E. & Cull, J. G. (Eds.). (1973). *Vocational evaluation for rehabilitation services.* Springfield, IL: Charles C. Thomas.

Helffenstein, D. & Wechsler, F. (1982). The use of interpersonal process recall in the remediation of interpersonal and communication skill deficits in the newly brain injured. *Clinical Neuropsychology, 4,* 139–143.

Holland, J. L. (1966). *The psychology of vocational choice.* Waltham: Blaisdell.

Humphrey, M. & Oddy, M. (1980). Return to work after head injury: A review of post-war studies. *Injury: The British Journal of Accident Surgery, 12,* 107–114.

Kagan, N. (1969). Interpersonal process recall. *Journal of Nervous and Mental Disease, 148,* 365–374.

Kelly, G. A. (1955). *The psychology of personal constructs.* New York: W. W. Norton.

Levin, H. S. (1979). Long term neuropyschological outcome of closed head injury. *Journal of Neurosurgery, 50,* 412–422.

Levin, H. S., Benton, A. L. & Grossman, R. G. (1982). *Neurobehavioral consequences of closed head injury.* New York: Oxford University Press.

Lezak, M. D. (1978a). Living with the characterologically altered brain injured patient. *Journal of Clinical Psychiatry, 39,* 592–598.

Lezak, M. D. (1978b). Subtle sequelae of brain damage. *American Journal of Physical Medicine, 57,* 9–15.

Lishman, W. A. (1973). The psychiatric sequelae of head injury: A review. *Psychological Medicine, 3,* 304.

Lynch, R. T. (1983). Traumatic head injury: Implications for rehabilitation counseling. *Journal of Applied Rehabilitation Counseling, 14,* 32–35, 46.

Lynch, W. J. & Mauss, W. K. (1981). Brain injury rehabilitation: Standard problems list. *Archives of Physical Medicine Rehabilitation, 62,* 223–227.

May, V. R. (1985). Physical capacity evaluation and work hardening programming: The Carle Clinic Association model. In C. Smith & R. Fry (Eds.), *National forum on issues in vocational assessment.* Menomonie, WI: Materials Development Center, University of Wisconsin-Stout, Stout Vocational Rehabilitation Institute.

McGowan, J. & Porter, T. (1967). *An introduction to the vocational rehabilitation process* (Rev. ed.). Washington, DC: U.S. Government Printing Office.

Meers, G. D. (1985). Certification for teachers and vocational evaluation specialists. In C. Smith & R. Fry (Eds.), *National forum on issues in vocational assessment.* Menomonie, WI: Materials Development Center, University of Wisconsin-Stout, Stout Vocational Rehabilitation Institute.

Meichenbaum, D. (1977). *Cognitive-behavior modification: An integrative approach.* New York: Plenum Press.

Mercer, C. D. & Snell, M. E. (1977). *Learning theory research in mental retardation: Implications for teaching.* Columbus: Charles E. Merrill.

Newmark, S. R., Sublett, D., Black, J. & Geller, R. (1981). Nutritional assessment in a rehabilitation unit. *Archives of Physical Medicine Rehabilitation, 62,* 279–282.

Okun, B. F. (1982). *Effective helping: Interviewing and counseling techniques* (2nd ed.). Monterey, CA: Brooks/Cole.

Osipow, S. H. (1968). *Theories of career development.* New York: Appleton-Century Crofts.

Patterson, C. H. (1980). *Theories of counseling and psychotherapy* (3rd ed.). New York: Harper & Row.

Prigatano, G. P., Fordyce, D. J., Zeiner, H. K., Roueche, J. R., Pepping, M. & Wood, B. C. (1986). The outcome of neuropsychological rehabilitation efforts. In G. P. Prigatano and others, *Neuropsychological rehabilitation after brain injury* (pp. 119–133). Baltimore: Johns Hopkins University Press.

Rimel, R. W., Giordani, M. A., Barth, J. T., Boll, T. J. & Jane, J. A. (1981). Disability caused by minor head injury. *Neurosurgery, 9,* 221–228.

Rusch, F. R. & Mithaug, D. E. (1980). *Vocational training for mentally retarded adults.* Champaign, IL: Research Press.

Rutherford, W. H., Merrett, J. D. & McDonald, J. R. (1977). Sequelae of concussion caused by minor head injuries. *Lancet,* 1–4.

Salamone, P. (1971, June). A client-centered approach to job placement. *Vocational Guidance Quarterly,* 266–270.

Sankovsky, R., Arthur, G. & Mann, J. (Eds.). (1971). *Vocational evaluation and work adjustment.* Auburn, AL: Materials Information Center, Auburn University.

Sax, A. (1981). New V.E.W.A.A./C.A.R.F. standards for work evaluation and adjustment. *Vocational Evaluation and Work Adjustment Bulletin, 14,* 141–143.

Shontz, F. C. (1975). *The psychological aspects of physical illness and disability.* New York: Macmillan.

Silver, S., Ben-Yishay, Y., Rattok, J., Ross, B., Lakin, P., Piasetsky, E., Ezrachi, O. & Diller, L. (1983). Occupational outcome in severe TBD's following intensive cognitive remediation: An interim report. In *Working approaches to remediation of cognitive deficits in brain damaged persons* (Rehabilitation Monograph No. 66, pp. 79–91). New York: New York University Medical Center, Institute of Rehabilitation Medicine.

Smith, P. C. & McFarlane, B. (1984). Work hardening model for the 80's. In C. Smith & R. Fry (Eds.), *National forum on issues in vocational assessment.* Menomonie, WI: Materials Development Center, University of Wisconsin-Stout, Stout Vocational Rehabilitation Institute.

Stokes, T. F. & Baer, D. M. (1977). An implicit technology of generalization. *Journal of Applied Behavior Analysis, 10,* 349–467.

Super, D. E. (1957). *The psychology of careers.* New York: Harper & Bros.

Super, D. E. (1980). The preliminary appraisal in vocational counseling. In B. Bolton & D. W. Cook (Eds.), *Rehabilitation client assessment* (pp. 6–18). Baltimore: University Park Press.

Thomsen, I. V. (1984). Late outcome of very severe blunt head trauma: A 10–15 year second follow-up. *Journal of Neurology, Neurosurgery, and Psychiatry, 47,* 260–268.

Wehman, P. (1981). *Competitive employment: New horizons for severely disabled individuals.* Baltimore: Paul H. Brookes.

Wehman, P. & McLaughlin, P. (1980). *Vocational curriculum for developmentally persons.* Baltimore: University Park Press.

Wilcox, B. & Bellamy, G. T. (1982). *Design of high school programs for severely handicapped students.* Baltimore: Paul H. Brookes.

Wolfensberger, W. (1972). *The principle of normalization in human services.* Toronto, Canada: National Institute on Mental Retardation.

Woodworth, R. S. & Schlosberg, H. (1954). *Experimental psychology.* New York: Holt.

Zahara, D. J. & Cuvo, A. J. (1984). Behavioral applications to the rehabilitation of traumatically head injured persons. *Clinical Psychology Review, 4,* 477–491.

CHAPTER 6

Treatment Aspects of Vocational Evaluation and Placement for Traumatically Brain Injured Adults

James F. Wachter
Heidi L. Fawber
Mason B. Scott

Because of the relatively young age of head injured individuals and the consequent economic impact in loss of productivity if they are unable to return to work, vocational rehabiliation must be seen as a keystone in the total rehabilitation process (Lynch, 1983). ccording to Lynch, the traditional vocational rehabilitation service delivery model — which focuses on vocational evaulation and work placement to the neglect of cognitive and psychosocial treatment — has not served this population well, due to the complex interaction of physical, cognitive, and psychosocial sequelae of closed head injuries. Tabaddor, Mattis, and Zazula (1984) emphasize that quality of life for head injured adults depends on cognitive recovery and successful handling of concomitant psychosocial problems. Effective vocational management of these problems requires specialized programs which include an interdisciplinary approach to treatment along with vocational evaluation.

Severe head injury can produce: (a) physical limitations such as quadriplegia or hemiplegia, slowness and incoordination, visual problems, or seizures; (b) cognitive limitations such as impaired memory, attentional deficits, concentration problems, slowed information processing skills, or shallow and disorganized thinking and problem solving; or (c) emotional and behavioral changes such as depression, disinhibition, lability, or irritability (Benton, 1979; Goethe & Levin, 1984). These and other deficits can exist in isolation, or, as is usually the case, in varied combinations. It is the manner in which the sequelae interact that complicates the vocational rehabilitation of this group. Although a commonality with respect to deficits exists (see Chapter 1), the specific brain injury that is sustained, in interaction with pre-traumatic characteristics and post-traumatic environment, makes each head injured adult unique. Further complicating their vocational rehabilitation is the fact that head injured young people often have no work history to draw upon. The formulation of tentative vocational objectives is, therefore, extremely challenging.

Case illustration: J.D. was a 21 year old male with a history of low academic achievement, low average intelligence, and a spotty work history which included lost jobs due to absenteeism and tardiness. As a result of a severe closed head injury, J.D. had residual balance problems, significantly impaired fine and gross motor skills, and mildly to moderately impaired information processing and memory skills. This combination of deficits precluded concrete, repetitive motor tasks working with small objects (e.g., assembly line work); moderate or heavy physical tasks (e.g., materials handling); and also training or educational programs that require reasonable new learning potential. J.D.'s pre-traumatic work behaviors further complicated vocational rehabilitation planning. His profile of skills is not, however, atypical within a population of head injured young adults and illustrates how the interaction of deficits can limit vocational choices. His memory and learning potential would at best allow him to perform repetitive manual tasks, but his physical deficits ruled out most jobs of this sort. Similarly, most sedentary or light jobs that his physical characteristics would allow him to perform were ruled out by memory and general information processing deficits.

Vocational rehabilitation services for head injured adults are too often added at the end of the rehabilitation process in a way that is not integrated with other types of intervention. Traditional vocational rehabilitation programs offer vocational counseling, vocational evaluation, work adjustment and personal adjustment services, sheltered employment, limited medical and psychological services, and job placement. In our opinion, vocational services for this group should be integrated in the context of a well-defined and focused head injury program and should include cognitive rehabilitation, psychosocial counseling, and specialized placement services. Furthermore, many patients continue to benefit from physical therapy, occupational therapy, and speech-language therapy months and even years following their injury. Joint programs or other networking arrangements among rehabilitation facilities may be the most efficient way to bring together appropriate services that are at the same time broad enough to meet the many needs of head injured individuals and also consistently directed to the unique characteristics of this population (see Chapter 10). In Pittsburgh, such a program has been created through a networking arrangement between The Vocational Rehabilitation Center and The Rehabilitation Institute of Pittsburgh. It has been our experience that this combination of services has promoted more efficient vocational rehabilitation and more successful community reentry for head injured adults.

In this chapter, we discuss the vocational rehabilitation of head injured individuals, including vocational evaluation, training, and job placement. Because vocational rehabilitation for these individuals cannot be viewed as a discrete step, independent of cognitive and psychosocial treatment, a model of vocational rehabilitation is presented that deliberately integrates cognitive and psychosocial intervention with vocational services. Early in the vocational rehabilitation process, vocational evaluation is used as a treatment vehicle to mitigate cognitive and psychosocial deficits.

COGNITIVE AND PSYCHOSOCIAL ISSUES

The literature on outcome following severe closed head injury has emphasized the significance and pervasiveness of cognitive and psychosocial sequelae (Ben-Yishay et al., 1982; Ben-Yishay & Diller, 1983; Diller & Gordon, 1981; Lezak, 1978a; Prigatano and others, 1986). Problems in these areas affect all aspects of life and certainly must be addressed directly by vocational rehabilitation professionals. Gogstad and Kjellman (1976) suggested that any return to normalcy for head injured individuals must address the complex issues stemming from cognitive and psychosocial deficits.

Impaired cortical functioning and weak coping mechanisms create problems that are easily misdiagnosed as psychiatric (Ben-Yishay et al., 1982; Long, Gouvier & Cole, 1984). "Insight therapies" are predictably ineffective in dealing with these problems, since many head injured clients lack the self-awareness, ego functions, and cognitive abilities presupposed by such therapies. Ben-Yishay and colleagues (1983) argue that "insight therapies" can be effective only if the head injured client (a) is aware that a problem exists; (b) is willing to admit that help is needed; (c) is able to change; and (d) possesses intact ego functions. More commonly, according to Ben-Yishay, the severely head injured client requires a much more directive approach to the amelioration of psychosocial and emotional problems.

Generally, head injured individuals are faced with the demands of returning to community life at a time when their abilities to cope are most diminished. During the initial stages of recovery, emphasis is placed on physical rehabilitation. Physical deficits are easier for the client and family to accept since they are observable, concrete, and more likely to be understood as a direct consequence of head injury. However, in the later stages of recovery, the client and family are often left to struggle, with little understanding or advance preparation, with the cognitive, emotional, and behavioral problems that are observable and may not be understood as a consequence of the injury to the brain. The family and the client can be overcome with guilt or shame for behaviors that have no observable origin. For many, it is hard to understand why the person who now can walk and talk as he did before the accident cannot think and behave as before.

Improved cognitive functioning may result in improved emotional adjustment to the injury. However, as the head injured client becomes more aware of cognitive, vocational, and psychosocial deficits, it is common for functioning to deteriorate (Fordyce, Roueche & Prigatano, 1983). Obviously, in such a state there would be little point in developing vocational plans without emphasizing supportive therapies that address cognitive and psychosocial issues. In many cases, the initial stages of the vocational evaluation process can be used as a treatment modality for cognitive rehabilitation and psychosocial therapies. In essence, planning therapies around vocationally oriented tasks provides the client and family with a sense of "face validity" in that such a program is oriented toward community re-entry.

In our experience, head injured clients and their families see greatest value in rehabilitation therapies and activities that are clearly related to community re-entry: employment, school, or community life in general. Thus, therapies utilizing situations that resemble these activities generally receive greater support from the client and family. For this reason, treatment for cognitive and psychosocial deficits is often more openly embraced when dealt with in the context of employment or school issues. This is not to suggest that cognitive therapy and psychosocial counseling are not effective in a nonvocational environment, but that the effect can be enhanced when the client is able to see a direct relation between these therapies and community re-entry.

A SERVICE DELIVERY MODEL FOR VOCATIONAL REHABILITATION

The need for cognitive and psychosocial treatment in head injury rehabilitation is well-established (Ben-Yishay et al., 1982; Diller & Gordon, 1981; Gogstad & Kjellman, 1976; Lezak, 1978a; Prigatano, et al., 1984). Unfortunately, in traditional vocational rehabilitation settings such treatment is not an integral component of the evaluation and placement process and often little attempt is made to integrate the treatment received at a medical rehabilitation facility with the subsequent vocational program.

In this section we briefly outline the program model that we use in Pittsburgh. It consists of three stages, each stage consisting of three elements: cognitive, psychosocial, and vocational (see Figure 6–1). This model assumes tight interdisciplinary coordination of the cognitive, psychosocial, and vocational elements. The interdisciplinary team consists of a psychologist, social worker, cognitive therapist, community re-entry specialist, and vocational counselor. The cognitive, psychosocial, and vocational elements are directed by specialists in the respective element. The program elements are not discrete, but rather work in concert to attain the overall program goals. Thus, the roles of the specialists overlap. If, for example, it is predicted that a client's "bossiness" will interfere significantly with successful work placement, this will be made a target of intervention in all three program elements. The vocational counselor can use a work context to illustrate and highlight for the client the negative effects of this behavior. Within the context of psychosocial counseling, the social worker can impress upon the client — perhaps using video feedback — how such behavior interferes with social goals as well as job placement. Finally, the cognitive therapist can use the "bossiness" issue as the content of exercises to improve problem-solving skills and self-monitoring. The model further assumes that clients will progress from one stage to the next in all three elements simultaneously. For example, Stage 2 vocational issues generally cannot be addressed if the client is still at Stage 1 in the cognitive and psychosocial elements.

As with any sound rehabilitation plan, goals must be established and clearly defined. Goals are established by the interdisciplinary team under the direction of a psychologist. A psychologist, broadly trained in brain functioning, in the effects of brain injury on behavior, and in the process of brain injury rehabilitation, is an appropriate professional to provide clinical supervision for services required by head injured individuals. The team reviews referral information,

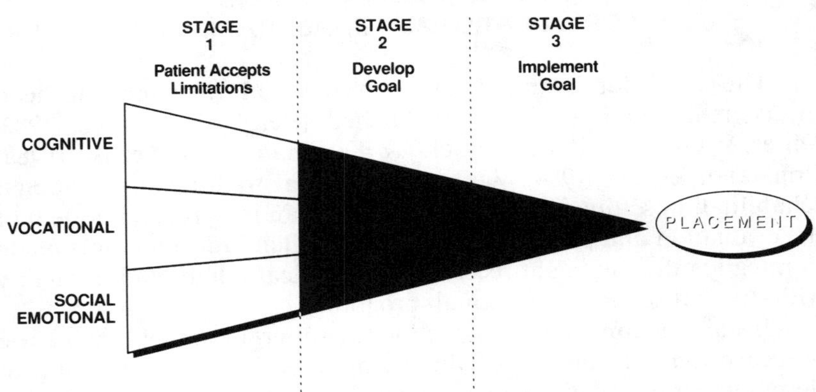

Figure 6–1. Three-stage model of a vocational rehabilitation program.

including medical records, previous psychological or neuropsychological testing, work history, initial interview notes, information from previous rehabilitation facilities, anecdotal information from the family, and referral requests, to establish initial objectives for each element (cognitive, psychosocial, and vocational).

Programming Stages

In this section we describe the three stages of programming leading to community re-entry. Each stage has cognitive, psychosocial, and vocational goals that are interrelated and addressed simultaneously. The program emphasis for a particular client will, of course, depend upon that client's needs and profile of strengths and weakness. Vocational evaluation takes place during Stages 1 and 2, concurrent with the development of strategies to lessen the impact of deficits; Stage 3 emphasizes specific preparation for community re-entry.

Stage 1

Stage 1 is defined by the following goals:

- *Vocational* — the client will realistically estimate the vocational implication of deficits and accept vocational program goals; staff will identify appropriate program goals
- *Cognitive* — the client will demonstrate the use of previously acquired strategies to compensate for cognitive deficits and

acquire new vocationally oriented strategies; and

- *Psychosocial* — the client will accept program goals based on a realistic estimate of vocational potential. Clearly, vocational and psychosocial goals at this stage are strongly interdependent and will therefore be discussed together.

In our model, Stage 1, which focuses on the client's awareness of deficits and estimation of the effects of these deficits, is the most critical stage since there can be no serious thought given to a job placement until the client has begun to demonstrate a realistic awareness of the implications of deficits, both cognitive and physical, on vocational planning. Musante (1983) asserted that awareness of deficits and ability to estimate their vocational implications is a critical element in the vocational rehabilitation of head injured clients. Awareness of deficits alone is not sufficient; a client might be able to verbalize the presence of a memory deficit, but continue to insist on returning to work as an on-the-road salesman, thus indicating a failure to understand the implication imposed by the deficit. The ability to evaluate one's performance with respect to established criteria is often extremely hard for head injured clients to achieve, but is essential to successful functioning in a work environment. For example, a client whose motor speed is impaired to the extent that it takes three times as long to assemble a component as required by an employer, demonstrates impaired self-evaluation if, after being made aware of the criteria, he continues to stress that he is able to return to work as an electronics assembler. Thus, the primary task of the head trauma team at this stage is to help clients to understand and accept the vocational implications of their individual physical, cognitive, or psychosocial deficits.

EVALUATING SELF-ESTIMATION OF DEFICITS. Evaluating a client's ability to estimate the implications of deficits begins in the initial interview. By relating the client's stated vocational goals to the relevant background information (medical and neuropsychological reports, pre-traumatic work and educational history), the vocational counselor can make a preliminary judgment about this crucial ability. Additional information about the client's goals and about the family's understanding of the client's vocational potential can be obtained by interviewing family members.

During the vocational assessment, the client is given tasks including job samples with specific instructions and real-world performance expectations. Upon completion of the task, the client is asked to evaluate that performance over a number of variables (e.g., speed, accuracy, efficiency of plan, correctness of direction following).

At the same time, the evaluator assesses performance over the same variables. Thus, clients are able to record their perceptions of their performance against established criteria. That record is compared with the counselor/evaluator's assessment. The degree of congruence indicates awareness of limitations in a functional setting. This awareness can in turn be used as the foundation for attaining an understanding of the implications of deficits. (Additional techniques are discussed in Chapter 5.)

The Functional Assessment Inventory (FAI) and Personal Capacities Questionnaire (PCQ) developed by Crewe and Athelstan (1981, 1984) provide the vocational counselor with a means of evaluating a client's self-perception over a broad range of variables. The PCQ is completed by the client and the FAI by the vocational counselor, with the degree of congruence again reflecting the accuracy of the client's self-perception with respect to community standards. These methods are not foolproof or fully objective assessment techniques, but they do provide the vocational counselor with insight into the head injured client's self-perception.

Case illustration: B.L. was a 35 year old head injured client whose cognitive deficits included impaired memory, impulsive problem solving, poor planning skills, and impaired concentration. Physically, his dominant right upper extremity was moderately involved due to peripheral nerve damage. Ours was the second facility he attended; he left the first facility stating that once his right arm and hand healed he would return to work repairing automatic transmissions. All medical reports clearly stated that his right arm would not recover to the degree needed to do this work. Not only was he physically unable to perform the work, but his cognitive deficits also precluded such employment. Thus, the first objective of our program for B.L. was to increase his awareness of the implications of his deficits with respect to his selected vocational objective. The team felt he would consider no vocational alternative until he accepted the idea that he was unable to repair automatic transmissions. During the 4 weeks that B.L. was in the program, the team was unable to bring about meaningful improvement in his ability to appreciate the implications of his deficits. He left the program continuing to believe that he would return to work repairing automatic transmissions.

Although successful vocational planning depends on the client's awareness of how deficits impact on vocational goals, the process of promoting more realistic self-awareness must occur within the context of support and encouragement from all staff members. In addition, the client's vocational strengths must be highlighted. An unrelenting focus on problems, deficits, and shortcomings is rarely successful in achieving the goal.

PROMOTING IMPROVED SELF-ESTIMATION OF DEFICITS. The same type of tasks or job samples that are used to evaluate a client's self-estimation of deficits can also be used to promote a more realistic self-perception. When each job sample is completed, the vocational counselor reviews in detail with the client how performance on that sample compares with real-world critieria (e.g., levels required for competitive or sheltered employment). For example, a woman 4 years post-injury who intended to return to work as a sales representative was asked to file 100 cards in numerical order. She took 40 minutes to complete the task, first looking through the entire set for card 1, then for card 2, and so on for each card. When she completed the task, she received the following feedback from the vocational counselor: (a) The time taken was not close to competitive standards; (b) her plan was very inefficient; (c) she did not evaluate the efficiency of her plan as she completed the task; and (d) the combination of these three aspects of her performance calls sharply into question her vocational goal.

Letting clients know that their performance has improved relative to their previous performance can provide needed encouragement and motivation. However, it is essential at the same time to measure progress against real-world criteria and to give the client feedback based on these standards. Failure to do so may simply prolong the resistance to realistic vocational goals.

COMPENSATORY STRATEGIES. The Stage 1 cognitive goal is to promote the acquisition and use of strategies to compensate for cognitive deficits that would likely interfere with vocational goals. The job samples in Stage 1 provide the client with the opportunity to implement such strategies and to observe their benefits. To help clients appreciate the value of strategies, they are assigned a task, first using a designated strategy and later performing the same task without the strategy. The client and counselor then compare the results and measure the effects of the compensatory strategy. A detailed account of compensatory strategies and appropriate teaching procedures is included in Chapter 4, along with a useful list of strategies, some of which are appropriate in work settings. In that chapter several cautions are issued. Our experience in a vocational setting underscores the importance of the client's comfort level with a strategy. If, for example, carrying a memory book is perceived as stigmatizing, it will not be used despite its potential benefits. To be useful in a work setting, strategies must be easy to use and their value must clearly outweigh the client's natural resistance to their use. Chapter 4 also lists some techniques for overcoming client's resistance to using compensatory strategies. In our own experience, strategic procedures that do not involve observable external aids — for example, a self-relaxation procedure to relieve anxiety — are more likely to be accepted.

Not all clients are capable of internalizing compensatory strategies to the point of functional, independent use in a work setting. In other cases, strategic procedures and external aids simply do not compensate adequately for the cognitive impairment. When this occurs, the team must be ready to provide the counseling needed to help the client begin the process of accepting an alternate vocational goal. This responsibility rests with the entire team in order to provide a consistent program theme. At the same time, the team must consider either modifying the work environment (e.g., create an isolated work area for a highly distractible person) or selecting jobs that are not compromised by the observed deficits. For example, clients with very significant memory problems may be restricted to jobs of a short, cyclical nature that do not require ongoing encoding and retrieval of information. Clients who are easily confused by new situations or who become disoriented with unexpected changes may require workplace modifications including firmly established routines, slow and gradual introduction of change, and adequate preparation for change. Just as personal strategies are accepted and used by clients only if their perceived value outweighs their difficulty of use and stigmatizing effects, so will employers accept job modifications only if they do not reduce productivity or create animosity or resentment among other employees.

Additional Stage 1 vocational objectives include: assessing the client's motor, perceptual, and vocational skills; assessing the extent to which a deficit impacts on vocational planning; and providing an opportunity for vocational exploration. Stage 1 is completed when the client's perception of vocational potential and acceptance of revised vocational goals are adequate to move programming into a more traditional vocational setting. This, of course, is a matter of degree, with no sharp line dividing Stage 1 and Stage 2.

Stage 2

Stage 2 is defined by the following goals:

- *Vocational* — the client will acquire specific vocational skills required by program goals; a vocational goal will be tentatively formulated;

- *Cognitive* — in specific vocational situations, the client will demonstrate the spontaneous use of strategies designed to compensate for cognitive deficits;
- *Psychosocial* — the client will demonstrate appropriate work-related behaviors.

GENERALIZATION OF COMPENSATORY STRATEGIES. The goal of strategy intervention is to have the client internalize the strategy and generalize its use to appropriate work situations. In Chapters 4 and 5, several methods for promoting generalization are presented. The vocational counselor can assist this process by gradually reducing the amount of cuing given the client to use the strategy. When the client reaches the point where the strategy is used independently in the training context, then systematic changes in task, materials, work area, and supervisor are made. Each change is made with the goal of maintaining independent use of the strategy.

Systematic observation of the client's success or failure in generalizing compensatory strategies allows the team to decide if a level of employment requiring such compensation is a reasonable goal, or if, on the other hand, efforts need to be directed to jobs not compromised by the deficit(s). Some clients are able to make functional use of strategies, while others — for various reasons including significantly impaired memory, self-monitoring, and self-direction — are not. For example, a client who has weak planning and organizational skills and who is unable to make functional use of organizing strategies would be unable to return to work as an office manager, but might be able to perform concrete, structured jobs such as a clerk typist or file clerk. For some clients, the team may decide to locate a particular job capable of being performed by the client, and "overtrain" the client on the skills for that specific job. This approach may require staff to train the client on the actual job. However, such a decision usually occurs toward the end of Stage 2 and the beginning of Stage 3.

FORMULATION OF A VOCATIONAL GOAL. The formulation of a tentative vocational goal assumes greater prominence in Stage 2 than Stage 1. Technically, the formulation of tentative vocational objectives begins before the client enters the vocational rehabilitation program, but the process becomes more formalized as the client progresses. The complex interaction of psychosocial, cognitive, and physical problems impacts greatly on the development of a vocational goal. Many head injured clients had a vocational identity before their accident which complicates the selection of vocational goals since those clients have an understandably strong desire to return to their former jobs and can become resistant to an evaluation program if they are confronted with having to select an alternate vocational objective too soon (before the issue of estimation of deficit has been addressed).

Chapters 5 and 9 include discussions of the type of counseling that may be necessary during this process of formulating a vocational goal. As Anderson (1981) has suggested, vocational potential is often restricted by cognitive impairments in the areas of memory, judgment, and rate of information processing. Thus, the vocational counselor needs to be cognizant of the cognitive demands of a variety of jobs in order to begin formulating tentative vocational choices based on the profile developed for the client. For the rehabilitation counselor working with head injured clients, the ability to perform a cognitive job analysis takes on a role as important as the traditional physical job analysis performed by the vocational counselor. Table 4-5 lists a large number of cognitive, perceptual, psychosocial, and academic variables that must be considered in a thorough analysis of the demands imposed by any job. Job analysis is discussed later in this chapter.

Stage 2 is completed when (a) maximum vocational skills and work-related behaviors have been developed; (b) either compensatory strategies have been generalized to work settings or a decision has been made to restrict work options to those not compromised by cognitive deficits, and (c) a tentative vocational goal has been formulated.

Stage 3

Stage 3 is essentially the transition from the vocational rehabilitation program to a community work placement (competitive, sheltered, or volunteer) and possibly an independent living arrangement. The ultimate direction Stage 3 takes is based on the client's performance in Stage 2. Once a decision has been reached with respect to community placement, Stage 3 emphasizes specific preparation for that placement.

The goals of Stage 3 are:

- *Vocational* — staff will identify specific jobs appropriate to the client's skills; the client will secure appropriate employment and demonstrate the skills required by that job;
- *Cognitive* — the client will demonstrate the use of strategies in the new work setting or the job requirements will be altered to fit the client's functioning;
- *Psychosocial* — the client will accept this level of employment and demonstrate appropriate behavior in the work place.

Consider a young male whom the head trauma team considered capable of returning to work as a machine operator. Stage 3 could emphasize improving physical stamina, work speed, punctuality, interpersonal skills, or job seeking skills. At this point, the team knows the client has the potential to work competitively; therefore, efforts are centerd on improving areas of weakness while placement efforts in the community are begun. Stage 3 goals are in this way a function of the specific community re-entry objectives considered appropriate for the client. Placement issues are discussed at length later in this chapter.

SELECTED ISSUES IN VOCATIONAL EVALUATION

The field of vocational evaluation and assessment is far too broad to be discussed in detail in this chapter. This section is limited to selected issues in the vocational evaluation of traumatically brain injured individuals. Textbooks such as Smith and Fry (1985) offer detailed information on vocational evaluation.

In the model that we have sketched, vocational objectives in all three stages should be addressed within the context of vocational evaluation. These objectives include treatment objectives which necessitate an extended evaluation period. The additional time allows for vocational exploration, for counseling in the notoriously stubborn area of self-estimation of deficits, and for attempts to compensate for cognitive weakness with strategic procedures or external aids.

This view is supported by Prigatano and colleagues (1984) who stated that only one-third of severely head injured clients are returned to competitive employment utilizing the traditional rehabilitation service delivery model (evaluation, work adjustment, and job placement). While there is little empirical evidence supporting any particular type of vocational evaluation for head injured clients, Musante (1983) suggested that the traditional, short, cost-effective evaluation models that focus on the transfer of skills and that are favored in today's economy are not effective for this population. These evaluation systems are designed to gather large amounts of data in relatively short periods of time. This shortened evaluation period does not allow for cognitive and psychosocial treatment needed by most head injured clients. In the proposed model, vocational evaluation includes treatment procedures in addition to the more standard vocational assessment.

Botterbusch (1982), in a review of commercially available evaluation systems, describes four basic assessment techniques used in the vocational evaluation process: (a) on-the-job evaluation; (b) sheltered employment; (c) work samples; and (d) psychological testing. Of these, work samples and their derivatives comprise the bulk of vocational evaluation systems used in the rehabilitation process. Work samples can be further broken down into four types, according to Botterbusch: (a) actual job samples; (b) simulated job samples; (c) cluster trait samples; and (d) single trait samples. We do not wish to recommend one method to the exclusion of the others. However, the vocational counselor must be flexible in using any assessment technique and, above all, must allow ample time for treatment and learning. Psychological testing as the sole method of vocational evaluation is, therefore, too restrictive, given the special needs of the head injured client.

The keys to vocational evaluation are the creativity of the counselor/evaluator and caution in making predictions about work potential based on the results of commercially available evaluation systems that are not of demonstrated validity with head injured individuals. For example, timed tasks penalize the head injured adult whose ability to process new information quickly is typically impaired. Such an individual may be able to perform the task at competitive levels given sufficient repetition or familiarity. Performance on one or two trials, however, may mistakenly predict an inability to perform work tasks of that sort. This is not to suggest that normed tasks — or, more specifically, timed tasks — are inappropriate. Many jobs (e.g., typist, stenographer, assembly worker) have specific production standards which must be met in the competitive job market. The point is rather that the true vocational potential of a head injured individual is often determined only after a period of diagnostic intervention that focuses on strategies to compenstate for cognitive and physical deficits as well as on the acquisition of specific vocational skills.

In addition to thorough assessment of the client's vocational strengths and deficits by means of work samples and diagnostic treatment, a comprehensive vocational evaluation requires a careful analysis of the demands of possible jobs. In addition to the standard analysis of the physical and environmental factors, job analysis for head injured individuals must include careful consideration of cognitive factors. The content of a job analysis is discussed later in this chapter. In general, the vocational evaluator attempts to outline the salient cognitive skills required to perform a job (see Table 6–2). Analyzing jobs from a cognitive point of view and relating those cognitive requirements to the client's profile of cognitive strengths and weaknesses are most effectively done by the head injury team, including vocational evaluator, psychologist, and cognitive rehabilitation therapist.

Given the heterogeneity of closed head injury sequelae and the frequently scattered pattern of cognitive skills, a hierarchial approach to vocational evaluation tends to unduly restrict the vocational possibilities for the head injured client. For example, a client may be unable, because of specific cognitive deficits, to perform certain jobs requiring a Reading, Math, or Language (R,M,L) Development level 2 as defined by the Dictionary of Occupational Titles (U.S. Department of Labor, 1977), yet be able to perform jobs at higher R,M,L levels if the cognitive demands are more consistent with the patient's strengths or if the work environment can be adequately modified. For example, a client with spatial orientation problems may not be able to perform the job duties of a janitor, yet be able to perform adequately as a bench mechanic.

During the course of a head injured client's evaluation, it is often essential to modify a job sample to accommodate for a physical or cognitive deficit, to assess a specific cognitive skill, to train a particular skill, or enhance the client's self-awareness. It is in these situations that the creativity of the counselor/evaluator is of paramount importance. Standardized evaluation techniques need to be compromised in these situations.

Case illustration: K.S. was a 29 year old head injured woman with moderate right hemiparesis and overall decreased motor coordination. Cognitively, she was unable to plan or organize complex tasks. Without step-by-step instructions her work was disorganized and ineffective. Her goal was to return to work as a sales person and she would not accept the team's judgment that her poor planning skills would preclude this type of work. To help demonstrate her poor planning skills, a job sample was selected that required her to reproduce a simple wooden article from a diagram and picture of the finished product. Given her physical involvement, the counselor performed the physical aspects of the job as dictated by K.S. The finished product bore little resemblance to the pictured model. Since the session was videotaped, K.S. was able to review her performance and not only see that she lacked a plan, but also see her errors along the way. To highlight her need for assistance in planning, her performance on this task was reviewed along with a similar task which she completed flawlessly because she had detailed written instructions.

A standardized evaluation would not have permitted such an intervention without invalidating the results. In this case, the counselor/evaluator used the evaluation procedure for a nonstandard, but very important purpose, namely, to assess and promote the client's ability to perceive cognitive deficits. Assessment and treatment goals of this sort are as important as the more customary evaluation of the transfer of vocational skills.

Selection of work samples to use during the evaluation process involves consideration of the client's pre-traumatic personality and work history, cognitive strengths and weaknesses, physical characteristics, and stated vocational goals. As in any sound rehabilitation plan, the client's interests and goals are part of the plan development. Initially, stated goals can provide insight into the client's awareness of how the residual effects of the head injury impact on vocational planning. Later, when selecting work samples, the counselor may choose tasks that have "face validity" in relation to the client's goals — that is, tasks that are clearly perceived by the client to relate directly to vocational goals. This is useful in helping the client to become actively engaged in the rehabilitation process. Selection of samples that are consistent with the client's goals but unrealistic relative to his or her abilities may also be useful in asesessing self-estimation of deficits and promoting a more realistic self-estimation. Alternatively, the vocational evaluator may choose work samples that do not relate directly to the client's goals, but are designed to guarantee success. These tasks are important for those client's whose fragile egos need to be boosted by successful performance. The decision to use samples for guided success or guided failure rests with the head trauma team's assessment of what would be most consistent with the client's needs and the program goals. With careful integration of the vocational and psychosocial program elements, a point should be reached in Stage 2 at which the vocational counselor/evaluator can simply explain to the client the objectives of a particular task without fear of the client becoming unduly upset.

DETERMINANTS FOR SELECTING VOCATIONAL OBJECTIVES

The development of an appropriate vocational objective depends on a number of factors. During the acute recovery stage, little serious vocational development can be undertaken except to gather data with respect to pre-traumatic work, education, and personality history. As Long et al. (1984) suggested, the acute stage centers on physical recovery. However, during the chronic stage, reality in the form of cognitive limitations begins to take shape. It is at this time, when physical recovery is relatively stabilized, that the client and family begin to give serious thought to community re-entry. For those head injured adults who worked or attended school before the accident, the goal is usually to return to pre-traumatic activities. Thus, the objective of a vocational program is to assess the appropriateness of such a goal and, if necessary, provide alternatives based on performance in the rehabilitation program.

A well-conceived neuropsychological evaluation can be an invaluable aid to the vocational counselor. The assistance of a psychologist with special expertise in the assessment of brain functioning can help the vocational counselor to understand what cortical functioning is intact and what cognitive abilities remain. Properly interpreted, this information can be used to suggest broad job families. Of course, owing to the complex interplay among various cortical areas, the issue is never as simple as an analysis of a neuropsychological evaluation. Neuropsychological assessment by itself does not accurately indicate how effectively a client may be able to compensate for a cognitive or perceptual deficit. For example, patients with strong visual perceptual skills and solid problem-solving ability but impaired language processing may be able to perform jobs that normally require intact verbal skills. This fact again supports the need for a comprehensive, longitudinal vocational assessment.

Case illustration. J.W. was a head injured young adult whose neuropsychological report indicated significantly impaired auditory memory. The vocational evaluator, therefore, assumed that the client would be unable to independently perform multistep tasks from verbal instructions alone. However, upon observing the client complete a fairly involved task from verbal instructions, it became obvious that he was able to determine how to complete the task by examining the finished product and by picking up cues from the material at hand. It is, therefore, incumbent upon the vocational counselor to avoid concluding prematurely that a client will be unable to perform a job that, on paper, requires a skill that the client, on paper, lacks.

With this qualification in mind, neuropsychological assessment results, together with medical data, academic achievement levels, and physical aptitudes, can be used to formulate tentative vocational objectives that may be different from those verbalized by the client. Using the Dictionary of Occupational Titles as a guide, a profile for the client can be developed using a computerized program such as JOBS by Train Ease (Zorn, 1984). Specific jobs and job families can be generated from such a profile. For the head injured client with no stated vocational objective, such a profile can be the springboard for vocational exploration. Similar profiles can be generated from the client's work history. Comparing the profile that is developed from the assessment data with a profile based on the client's work history enables the client to understand in very practical terms the results of the evaluation.

In addition to the difficult task of matching job characteristics with client abilities and interests, it is imperative that the vocational counselor consider community resources, the local economy and employment outlook, transportation, and other pertinent external determinants in selecting vocational goals. Placement issues are discussed in detail later in this chapter. However, their impact cannot be ignored when selecting tentative vocational objectives. A head injured client may be employable but not placeable because appropriate jobs do not exist in the community, or other external factors mitigate against placement. This problem exists not only in the competitive job market but also in the sheltered employment market, which in many cases is not prepared to handle the needs of head injured clients.

Case illustration: R.M. was a head injured young man whose residual deficits included mild memory impairment, mildly depressed motor speed, poor planning and organizational abilities, and a back injury that limited him to light or sedentary work. His work history included moderate and heavy work. He lived in a rural, economically depressed area. His evaluation suggested the ability to perform a variety of light or sedentary jobs competitively. However, such jobs did not exist where he lived, and the team felt that job modification was unlikely since very few jobs existed in the area and an employer with access to a large labor pool would be reluctant to modify a job. Thus, characteristics of the community dictated the direction that needed to be taken in developing a vocational plan for this client. Since the team was aware of these circumstances early in the program, appropriate steps could be taken. Since the client agreed to relocate, the team objectives focused on developing appropriate job skills and improving independent living skills.

Vocational evaluation, psychosocial counseling, work adjustment, cognitive rehabilitation, and job preparation mean little if the appropriate community work placement cannot be found. As with other rehabilitation services, vocational placement for head injured clients demands special attention. The remainder of this chapter is devoted to discussing those specialized services that have been found to be effective in placing head injured adults in the community.

VOCATIONAL PLACEMENT ISSUES

Traumatic brain injury can have a significant effect on return to gainful employment. In general, the more severe the injury, the greater the impact on the ability to return to work. However, even in mild and moderate cases, problems can be encountered. Table 6–1 summarizes several studies that specifically address vocational outcome.

In most of these studies, the severely injured subjects had received some type of rehabilitation, although the nature of the services was not specifically discussed. Variability in these outcome data is most likely a consequence of methodological differences among the studies, including varying criteria for classifying severity of injury and varying follow-up intervals, possibly combined with differences in rehabilitation services. One can safely conclude from this review, however, that vocational reintegration is often jeopardized by traumatic brain injury.

Table 6–1. Vocational Outcome Following Closed Head Injury

Study	N	Severity	Follow-Up	Employment Status*
Rimel, Giordani, Barth, Boll & Jane(1981)	424	mild	3 months	66%
Klonoff & Snow (in press)	47	mild	2–4 years	93%
Rimel, Giordani, Barth & Jane (1982)	170	moderate	3 months	31%
Klonoff & Snow (in press)	8	moderate	2–4 years	75%
Matheson (1982)	50	severe	6 months	32%
Gilchrist & Wilkinson (1979)	72	severe	9 months–15 years	39%
Klonoff & Snow (in press)	23	severe	2–4 years	52%
Bruckner & Randle (1972)	88	severe	3–14 years	64% (40% at same-level job)

*Percent of the subjects who had been employed pre-traumatically and had returned to work at the time of follow-up.

Mild: Glasgow Coma Scale: 11–15

Moderate: Glasgow Coma Scale: 8–12

Severe: Glasgow Coma Scale: 7, or 24 hour coma

Matheson study: post-traumatic amnesia: 5 days

These studies highlight the importance of appropriate vocational rehabilitation services and careful job placement for head injured individuals. Unfortuately, there is limited experience and research to date which specifically address the rehabilitation methods or processes necessary to facilitate their successful vocational placement. The two programs that are most thoroughly described in the literature on adult head injury rehabilitation are the Head Trauma Program at the Institute of Rehabilitation Medicine, New York University Medical Center (Ben-Yishay et al., 1982) and the Neuropsychological Rehabilitation Program at Presbyterian Hospital in Oklahoma City (Prigatano and others, 1986). Both programs have been successful in improving vocational outcome.

Outcome data from the first eighteen head injured patients to complete the Oklahoma City program indicated that the initial rate of successful work placement was an optimistic 60 to 65 percent, but dropped to 50 percent on subsequent follow-up. Of the control group that had not received intensive rehabilitation services, 36 percent were employed at the time of follow-up (Prigatano et al., 1984; Prigatano and others, 1986).

Prigatano's program included (a) a minimum of 6 months in program — 4 days per week, 6 hours per day; (b) individual and small group therapies dealing with increased awareness and acceptance of injuries and residual deficits, cognitive retraining and development of compensatory strategies, and increased understanding of the emotional issues resulting from the injury; (c) an emphasis on continuity and consistency in programming; and (d) family involvement on a weekly basis. In 1984, actual work samples were added to the program. This work trial program is composed of three stages: (a) staff supervised volunteer work, (b) staff supervised volunteer/pay work placements at a different site, and (c) gainful employment with staff supervision as needed (Prigatano and others, 1986). It should be noted that the modest gain in employment outcome relative to controls (50 percent versus 36 percent) is based on those head injured patients who completed the program *before* the work trials were added. It is reasonable to speculate that the effectiveness of the program will be enhanced by this direct focus on work, given the notorious difficulty that brain injured people have generalizing treatment gains to different and more functional settings (Fowler, 1981).

The New York University program, in many respects similar to that in Oklahoma City, includes a 20-week, 4 day per week program, intensive cognitive remediation, daily group sessions with a psychosocial emphasis, daily community meetings, and occupational trials (Ben-Yishay & Diller, 1981). Ben-Yishay and colleagues (1985) reported that, of the 90 head injured clients who had completed the program, 65 percent were competitively employed, 15 percent were placed in a sheltered workshop, and 20 percent were unemployed one year after completing the program.

These two studies suggest that employability can be enhanced with specialized rehabilitation services. The standard practice of treating job placement as a separate, discrete step which follows the completion of vocational evaluation and training (Revel, Wehman & Arnold, 1984) and neglecting targeted cognitive and psychosocial intervention during the vocational evaluation/training phase poorly serves the needs of head injured individuals. We have emphasized the understanding and acceptance of deficits and their implications, and the ability to generalize newly learned skills — including compensatory strategies — as central to successful vocational placement. Both considerations argue for a gradual and well-planned transition from evaluation/training to job placement.

For many head injured clients, it is useful to modify the traditional process by providing specific job training after a placement has been secured. In this way, difficulty generalizing skills and strategies has a reduced effect on successful placement.

Case illustration: C.N. was a head injured client with poor verbal memory, impaired planning and organizational skills, and weak problem-solving ability. His vocational evaluation indicated that he was capable of performing jobs of a very concrete nature in a structured setting, but that he could not independently generalize skills from one setting to another. Consequently, the team located an appropriate job for C.N. that involved filing material in an already organized filing system. This job was then replicated in the vocational rehabilitation setting, and C.N. was thoroughly trained in the task. He was then placed on the job and, with staff support and no variation in his job responsibilities, was able to function adequately.

C.N.'s vocational rehabilitation would probably not have been successful using the traditional approach of evaluation followed by training followed by placement. "Supportive employment," which refers generally to modifications of this approach in the direction of increased vocational services following job placement, is receiving growing recognition and is discussed later in this chapter.

Issues to Consider Prior to Vocational Placement

1. Selectivity: Job placement must be consistent with all that is known about a client's work history, work behaviors, aptitudes, and

interests as well as the client's ability to generalize compensatory skills and acquire new information.

Case illustration: P.N. was a 26 year old head injured male with poor memory, impulsive behavior, a short temper, and significant spatial disorientation. He was placed as a materials handler in a spatially complex warehouse without the job site being reviewed by a placement specialist. It was later learned that P.N. was fired after a short time on the job because he was unable to remember how to get from place to place in the warehouse. With prior knowledge of the demands of the job site, this placement could have been successful with either modifications in job responsibilities or adequate training on the actual job site.

2. *Job Analysis:* Job analysis is the process of collecting, organizing, and evaluating information about a job, which can be done with a variety of techniques. The purposes of job analysis include classifying jobs, establishing work standards, and developing employment medical standards (Lytel & Botterbusch, 1981). Effective job placement of head injured individuals requires careful analysis of the physical, environmental, cognitive, and behavioral/interpersonal factors of the job. *Physical factors* include walking, standing, sitting, stooping, crouching, kneeling, lifting (specific weights), handling (large objects with both hands versus small objects requiring refined dexterity), reaching, stretching, and bending in addition to endurance requirements and visual and auditory acuity demands. *Environmental factors* include noise levels, hazards, ventilation, temperature, lighting, elevated surfaces, type of flooring, and types of tools and/or equipment. *Cognitive factors* include the demands imposed on the worker in the following areas: rate at which information must be processed, amount of information to be processed, visual complexity, environmental distractions, temporal and spatial orientation, attention span, sequential organization, analyzing and planninng, language comprehension, language expression, memory and new learning, integration of information over time, content-specific knowledge, flexibility, goal setting, initiation, self-monitoring and evaluating, problem solving and decision making, safety judgment, strategy use, and academic levels (reading, writing, mathematics). *Behavioral/interpersonal factors* include demands in the following areas: independence/ability to work alone, self-control, interpersonal relations (cooperation, interaction, ability to accept supervision), frustration tolerance, and response to interpersonal stress.

These lists are not exhaustive. They do, however, underscore the complexity and importance of job analysis in making job placements for head injured clients. Table 6–2 sketches a job analysis in the often neglected area of cognitive factors. Job analysis serves several purposes:

1. It gives the treatment team information needed for a responsible decision about the appropriateness of placement for a client.
2. It serves to focus intervention on functional objectives that are known to make a difference on the job.
3. It helps to establish terminal behaviors for the training program.
4. It may yield information essential to job modification or employer counseling and education.

3. *Placement site education and training:* Proper training of potential employers and work site supervisors serves two broadly different purposes. First, with such training it is possible to avoid misinterpretations that are likely to occur in the absence of an understanding of head injury or of the client's deficits. In our experience, "head injury" as a diagnostic label is often confused with psychiatric disability, thus creating in the minds of employers groundless fears and suspicions. It is even more common for people unfamiliar with head injury to misinterpret specific behaviors of head injured clients. A flat affect and problems with initiation — both very likely cortical in origin — are easily mistaken for disinterest or lack of motivation. Behavior resulting from disinhibition or impaired concentration may be taken as disrespect or deliberate defiance. Specific information processing deficits can be confused with global intellectual retardation. With education and advance preparation, employers and supervisors can avoid such misinterpretations and place the workers behavior in proper context.

Second, problem solving between rehabilitation staff and placement site personnel can occur in advance of anticipated problems. The young man with significant spatial disorientation mentioned in an earlier case illustration may not have failed in his warehouse job if staff and employer had anticipated the problem and worked out an effective map-following strategy for the client. Another head injured client, who had been very successfully placed in a competitive job, experienced major problems when promoted to a position that was thoroughly incompatible with his profile of strengths and weaknesses. Again, this could have been avoided with a more complete exchange of information between rehabilitation staff and employer. Fortunately in this case ongoing communication with the placement counselor resulted in a resolution of the problem before it could lead to failure and termination.

Table 6–2. Illustration of a Cognitive Job Analysis

JOB: Accounts Receivable Assistant
JOB SITE: S&A Hardware Company
CLIENT: K.T.
DOT: Accounting Clerk 216.482–010

JOB SUMMARY: This position involves three main tasks:

1. collating invoices
2. extending and mailing invoices
3. receiving payment through the mail

The work area is in an office which is located in a separate part of the hardware warehouse. Supervision is provided by the company accountant who is the only other employee housed in this work area. The position is rated as sedentary as defined by the *Dictionary of Occupational Titles.*

COGNITIVE ANALYSIS BY JOB TASK:

1. Collating Invoices
   The employee alphabetizes the invoices by last name and places them in alphabetized bins. This involves the ability to:
   - read (7th grade level)
   - alphabetize
   - sort
   - organize a task
   - visually scan a complex invoice
   - remember and remain oriented to the task
   - maintain attention to repetitive work for extended periods
   - self-monitor for accuracy
2. Extending and Mailing Invoices (See sample invoice, Fig. 6–2)
   A. The employee takes each alphabetized invoice in turn and lists the total price in the "Terms" column. This involves the ability to:
   - attend to detail
   - maintain attention and remain oriented to repetitive work
   - visually process a complex invoice
   - sequentially organize a task
   - self-monitor for accuracy

   B. The employee adds the sales tax, then totals the amount at the bottom of the invoice (using an adding machine). This involves the ability to:
   - add (accurately use adding machine)
   - remember and remain oriented to the task
   - visually process a complex invoice
   - coordinate eye-hand movements (using the adding machine and writing on the invoice)
   - attend to detail
   - sequentially organize a task
   - self-monitor for accuracy

C. The employee separates and distributes the four copies of the invoice: the yellow copy is filed alphabetically; the white and pink copies are mailed to the customer for payment; the goldenrod copy (if not already given to the customer) is thrown away. This involves the ability to:
    - maintain attention and remain oriented to repetitive work
    - sequentially organize a complex task
    - spatially organize a complex task
    - discriminate colors
    - coordinate eye-hand movements
    - self-monitor for accuracy

D. The employee folds the invoice and places it in an envelope in such a way that the name and address appear in the window of the envelope. This involves the ability to:
    - sequentially organize a task
    - maintain attention and remain oriented to repetitive work
    - coordinate eye-hand movements
    - organize a spatially complex task

3. Receiving Payment Through the Mail:

A. The employee opens the envelope and retrieves the invoice from the file. This involves the ability to:
    - read
    - sequentially organize a task
    - remember the filing system
    - search the files in an organized manner

B. The employee checks the payment against the invoice and marks the invoice "paid" if correct. This involves the ability to:
    - read
    - attend to detail
    - scan invoice and payment for amounts
    - make decisions
    - compare numbers
    - organize a complex task
    - self-monitor for accuracy

C. The employee enters into the logbook: (a) the check number; (b) the check amount; and (c) the company invoice number which appears in the upper right hand corner of the invoice. This involves the ability to:
    - process complex visual information
    - coordinate eye-hand movements
    - attend to detail
    - organize a complex task
    - self-monitor for accuracy

D. The employee places the check in a designated envelope and sets the envelope in a bin on the accountant's desk. This involves the ability to:

continued

Table 6–2 *(continued)*

- orient effectively in space
- remain oriented to a job despite a change of location

E. The employee refiles the invoice. This involves the ability to:

- alphabetize
- orient effectively in space
- process complex visual information
- attend to detail

In certain cases, prior contact with the prospective work site supervisor is undesirable or impossible. Head injured clients who are well recovered and efficient at compensating for residual deficits may not want their supervisors to know about those deficits. Short of compelling reasons to the contrary, such wishes should be respected. In other cases, the work site supervisor may be unwilling to learn about head injury generally or about the worker's specific problems. In these cases, efforts must be directed toward making the client well prepared for the job and ensuring that the client will communicate with the rehabilitation staff if significant problems arise on the job.

4. *Staff supports:* In certain cases, employable head injured clients can succeed on the job only with the help of a community reentry specialist or job coach. The job coach is a key member of the treatment team whose role is to implement on the job those skills and compensatory behaviors that were developed by the vocational rehabilitation team. The job coach must know how to cue and reinforce target behavior, to shape behavior to fit different settings, to withdraw cues and reinforcement on an appropriate schedule, to modify job tasks if necessary, and to solve problems on the spot — in general, to serve as an extension of the treatment team on the job. Perhaps most importantly, the job coach must be able to develop an effective working relationship with the work supervisor. Depending on client needs, the job coach is essential for a longer or shorter period of time.

5. *Family support:* The family in most instances assumes as important a role in head injury rehabilitation as the client. Family expectations and support are critical, and need to be addressed along with the client's own expectations. Stages of denial, anger, frustration, and acceptance are as much a natural process for the family as for the client (see Chapter 9). Since family support is critical, education programs for families should address not only the effects of brain injury on the injured family member, but also the dynamics of the

SOLD TO

R+R Electric
Route 910
Gibsonia, PA

Date

Customer Order No.

MDSE RET'D	TERMS:

QTY. ORDERED	QTY. SHIPPED	DESCRIPTION	PRICE	TERMS	
12		4" White Globes	5.50		
1		Case brown - single hole switch plates	15.24		
1		Case 50' Rolls black friction tape	22.74		
5		Multi-outlet strips #E7452	5.70		
1		Case 12 oz cans Gum Turpentine	25.74		
		TAX			
		TOTAL			

ALL CLAIMS AND RETURNED GOODS MUST BE ACCOMPANIED BY THIS BILL.

Figure 6–2. Sample Invoice.

family's response. Families need to know that the emotions they experience — including anger, frustration, and guilt — are natural reactions when living with a brain injured adult (Lezak, 1978b). In a vocational setting, indifference or resistance from family members can adversely affect vocational outcome.

Rosenbaum, Lipsitz, Abraham, and Najenson (1978) emphasize the importance of the family's involvement in and support for the vocational rehabilitation program. Early in the process, family understanding and support are keys to the client's acquiring an adequately realistic perception of vocational potential. Later, families can facilitate the placement process by distinguishing their hopes and dreams for their loved one from what they know to be realistic vocational options, by supporting the decisions of the treatment team, and by placing realistic demands on the client in vocationally relevant areas such as punctuality, reliability, self-responsibility, and productivity. Counseling may be necessary to help family members and also the client understand the reasons for a particular work placement. The likelihood of successful placement is substantially increased if all parties are in agreement with the recommendation. (Family counseling is further discussed in Chapter 9.)

Case illustration: R.B. was a 23 year old male who suffered a severe closed head injury and underwent extensive rehabilitation, including inpatient medical rehabilitation, followed by vocational rehabilitation as a dormitory resident. As his vocational program was nearing its end, staff members complimented themselves on the progress R.B. had made, particularly with respect to independence. Staff members were aware of the family's tendency toward overprotectiveness, but because the family verbally supported the goal of competitive employment this issue was not addressed directly. As part of his program, R.B. was placed in a transitional job near the rehabilitation facility so that staff could closely monitor his progress. Having successfully completed the transitional job, R.B. returned home while attempts were made to secure a job for him near his home. After several weeks of having their son at home, R.B.'s parents told staff that the uncertainties of holding a job were outweighed by the securities of SSDI and long-term disability benefits. In effect, the family was saying that financial security and their own need to protect their son were of greater concern than R. B.'s obtaining a job and becoming independent, despite having verbally supported the team's and client's objective of competitive employment. In this case, failing to include the family as active members of the rehabilitation team was the single factor that blocked an otherwise very successful rehabilitation program.

Vocational Placement Options

In this section we present an overview of vocational placement options in the following order: sheltered employment, volunteer placement, supported work, transitional employment, and competitive employment. This order represents a graduated increase in the complexity of demands and level of expected productivity. In each case, characteristics of the placement that are important to consider for head injured clients are highlighted.

Sheltered Employment

Sheltered employment is most often available within sheltered workshops, although sheltered employment can occur in other settings as well. In our experience, great caution must be exercised in selecting a sheltered workshop as the most appropriate work setting for a head injured client. The type of work associated with workshops — repetitive and physically oriented — is inappropriate for those clients with significant motoric involvement. Second, the limited type of work available does not allow for increasingly complex or demanding tasks as a head injured client recovers cognitive or motor skills. Because the recovery period following head injury is long (Thomsen, 1984), it is essential not to place clients in a situation that may actually limit their vocational potential over time.

More importantly, sheltered workshops are very often inappropriate from a social and emotional standpoint. Traditionally, sheltered workshops have served mentally retarded individuals or those with a psychiatric diagnosis. Cognitive profiles and social functioning of these groups typically differ in important ways from those of head injured people. Social interaction for the head injured client is, therefore, limited. Furthermore, clients often react in a strongly negative way when such placement is proposed, even if for just a short period of time. Hackler and Tobis (1983) reported that a number of head injured patients in a program designed to secure placement in a sheltered workshop failed because they felt that the "work assignments were insulting and menial and their co-workers were unacceptable" (p. 423). Aves (1985) noted that sheltered workshops are perceived as primarily serving mentally retarded and mentally ill individuals whose behavior and work characteristics differ significantly from those of head injured adults.

Our experience at the Vocational Rehabilitation Center (VRC) of Allegheny County generally supports these observations. Many head injured clients whose degree of impairment would suggest a sheltered level of employment have strongly refused to be placed in our sheltered workshop. B.C. was a 27 year old male, 10 years post-injury, with severe expressive and receptive aphasia, significant right hemiparesis, and poor temporal sequencing ability. The results of his evaluation indicated that very few job placements could realistically be considered, and that therefore securing work for B.C. would take a long time. He was not economically secure and lived in an area that resulted in social isolation for him. For these reasons, it was recommended that he work temporarily in our workshop. This work would provide him with some income and daily activity until a more appropriate placement could be secured. Despite these reasons — which B.C. recognized to be good reasons — he flatly rejected the suggestion because it would mean working with people who were "crazy" or "retarded." He chose rather to return home despite the limited opportunity for social contact.

The general population's perception of a sheltered workshop as an environment appropriate solely for mentally retarded individuals — together with the generally negative and ill-informed understanding of mental retardation — also exercises a powerful influence on the acceptance of family and friends of such a placement. That these perceptions are inaccurate may be immaterial; it is very difficult to change attitudes that are deeply rooted in societal thinking.

Nevertheless, for some head injured clients, a sheltered workshop is the most appropriate work placement. As a general rule, the best candidates for workshop placement are years post-injury, no longer improving spontaneously or in response to rehabilitation efforts, and frustrated by the inability to find meaningful work. The following characteristics further define this group: generally depressed cognitive functioning requiring a highly structured work environment, severely impaired learning potential (possibly learning impaired pre-traumatically), relatively improved performance on repetitive tasks, adequate fine motor skills, and weak social cognition. Indeed, not all head injured clients resist this type of placement. The desire to "work," to earn money, and to have some type of regular productive activity may outweigh negative associations with workshops. Skilled adjustment counseling for both the client and the family may be necessary to promote acceptance of workshop placement. Some sheltered workshops offer work adjustment services and independent living training which may add to the appropriateness for selected head injured clients. Follow-up should occur at regular intervals to identify those clients whose improvement may indicate a need for re-evaluation and to guarantee that the services offered are as complete and appropriate as possible.

The future may offer a wider variety of options to head injured clients. At least one workshop — Genesis Manufacturing in Michigan — was created specifically for head injured adults (Zivanovic, 1984).

Other efforts, short of creating separate facilities, should also be undertaken to make sheltered workshops more appropriate for those head injured clients with severe disabilities. For example, special jigs can be designed to compensate for motor problems; job routines can be defined in such a way that profound memory impairments do not interfere with performance; areas within sheltered workshops could be designated as work areas for head injured individuals; and finally, counseling and information campaigns may begin to break down stereotypes based on diagnostic labels and allow individuals to feel comfortable with other individuals regardless of their label.

Volunteer Placement

Volunteer placements — also called work trials, therapeutic work placements, or internships — are often an essential component of the vocational rehabilitation process for head injured adults. Competitive employment, even with staff support, job coaching, and the like, may initially be too demanding for the client. For this reason VRC uses volunteer placements as part of its "vocational residency" program. Clients can be prepared for competitive employment in small, carefully graded increments. Since no wages are involved, volunteer placements can be more flexible and less demanding than a similar competitive placement. Furthermore, our experience suggests that treatment objectives are often more efficiently met within the context of a volunteer placement than in a treatment environment. Because clients can see a clear relation between this activity and their long-term goals, motivation is enhanced. In addition, invaluable feedback is available as clients measure their progress against real-world criteria. As with any placement, a job analysis is necessary to create an adequate match of the job with the client's profile of skills and interests. In addition, the volunteer placement supervisor should be aware of the client's strengths and weaknesses, objectives, strategies, and other relevant treatment issues.

Rehabilitation professionals have successfully used community-based and/or hospital-based therapeutic work placements for traumatically brain injured adults. Smith (1983) noted that a hospital or community placement can be an invaluable resource for providing valid and demanding yet protected work experiences for the emerging vocational candidate who has completed prevocational programming. Weiss (1980) described an individualized vocational evaluation program for a head injured young man who had a nursing background. Assuming that head injured individuals function at their highest level in a familiar setting, Weiss chose a rehabilitation medicine ward as the vocational evaluation site. She found that this procedure was a valid method of determining vocational potential for the young nurse.

The New York University Head Trauma Program, described earlier in this chapter, uses "systematic occupational trials," specifically designed for each client within the program (Ben-Yishay et al., 1982; Ben-Yishay & Diller, 1981). These volunteer placements are used as an intervention method following completion of the 20-week intensive remedial program which consists of cognitive remediation, group therapy, individual counseling, and community activities. Their occupational trials have included work as an assistant librarian and accounts payable clerk.

The Neuropsychological Rehabilitation Program (NRP) in Oklahoma City (Prigatano and others, 1986) added work trials to the already intensive program because "brain injured patients need a guided and at times protected work trial if the ultimate goal is for them to return to the community as productive individuals" (p. 134). Clients are placed in volunteer work stations in the hospital as part of their daily programming. These work trials are graded from volunteer work sites in the hospital to limited pay work placements in the community outside the hospital to competitive placements. Throughout this process, staff support is gradually reduced.

Our own Vocational Residency Program has used such volunteer placements in the Pittsburgh community as recreation aide at a boys' club, data entry clerk at a hospital, mail room assistant at a planetarium, and hospital escort. Each of these placements was used as a step between an in-house rehabilitation program and competitive employment. For clients who lack potential for competitive employment, volunteer placements of this sort could become long-term placements and be thought of as alternative to sheltered workshops.

Supported Work Placement

The evaluate-place-and-then-train model of vocational rehabilitation, which reverses the traditional order of training and placement, has in recent years received well-deserved recognition in the form of supported work projects. Although most of the literature on supported work deals with mentally retarded individuals (Kraus & MacEacheron, 1982; Sowers, Connis & Thompson, 1979; Williams & Vogelsburg, 1980), the approach appears to have value for all severely disabled persons (Wehman, in press). Supported employment is characterized by: (a) a paid job; (b) work in an integrated setting; (c) publicly subsidized, ongoing support throughout the client's life of employment; and (d) a severe disability which necessitates this form of support in order for employment to occur. A supported work approach to competitive job placement requires specialized assistance locating an appropriate job, intensive job site training, and permanent ongoing follow along services (Wehman, in press).

The supported work model also provides preplacement planning and intervention to address transportation arrangements, family adjustment counseling, employer education, and related problems. The client is then placed on the job and a rehabilitation professional provides initial and ongoing training for that client. The professional normally has daily contact with the client and the work supervisor during the initial phase of the client's work experience. Contact is then reduced as warranted by the client's performance, but is maintained in some form indefinitely.

Supported employment can include a variety of approaches to improving a severely disabled person's opportunities for achieving paid work. The 1984 U.S. Department of Education, Office of Special Education and Rehabilitation Services Initiative characterizes supported employment as paid work which usually occurs in regular competitive work settings, but may involve sheltered enclaves, mobile work crews, sheltered industries, or other creative approaches to improving employment opportunities (Wehman & Kregel, 1983).

The concept of supported employment is ideally suited for many severely head injured individuals. It provides for selective placement, for intensive on-the-job training to accommodate weak learning and generalization skills, and for indefinite follow along services. However, only a small number of supported work programs exist. The more successful programs have operated with shared funding from state vocational rehabilitation departments and mental health/mental retardation services. Since head injury is not commonly included under the MH/MR umbrella, creating a program of this sort for head injured adults may require a different funding source.

Transitional Employment

Supported employment is ideally suited to the needs of many severely brain injured clients, but, unfortunately, is not widely available. Transitional employment (TE) is similar in concept and more generally available. The primary difference between TE and supported competitive employment is that TE is time limited in staff involvement. TE can be used as a vocational assessment technique, as a treatment phase in the vocational rehabilitation process (like volunteer placement) or as a temporary job placement. For the client who is beginning to "burn out" with the rehabilitation process or who needs to improve job skills, the use of compensatory strategies, vocational behaviors, or interpersonal skills, a transitional employment placement may be appropriate.

As with supported employment, job site training and support services are essential to success. During the first several weeks of the placement, the job site trainer (job coach, re-entry specialist) is involved with the client on a one-to-one basis much of the time. As the client progresses, staff involvement is reduced, depending on the specific situation and the client's specific needs. It is important that staff support not be terminated completely. Periodic visits will at least remind the client that support is always available. To observe a more "natural" work performance, unscheduled spot checks are also recommended.

The Sister Kenny Institute in Minneapolis developed a Transitional Employment Program for head injured adults in 1984 (Aves, 1985). The program begins with a 2-week vocational assessment to establish appropriateness and eligibility for the TE program. This is followed by situational assessments to establish baselines for work behaviors and skills. A work site is then selected on the basis of job interests, tested work skills, work history, training, and education along with the client's ability to learn new information, follow instructions, interact with others, and monitor work quality and speed. The TE placement can extend from 3 to 12 months. The client is hired by the company and paid minimum wage; the program staff determine the number of work hours per day. A Transitional Employment Program counselor provides daily training for both the client and the work supervisor. In addition, work supervisors are enrolled in a program of training and orientation as part of the TE program. Following successful completion of this temporary placement, clients are assisted with job placement. Data on the long-term effectiveness of this project will be useful for future vocational rehabilitation planning for head injured adults.

Competitive Employment

Competitive employment is an attainable goal for many head injured clients. Depending on the severity of injury, this may be possible following the initial hospitalization or following a period of rehabilitation or, finally, only as a result of a series of increasingly demanding work placements. Our experience suggests that competitive placement is successful for clients with significant residual deficits only if certain conditions are met: (a) They accept realistic vocational goals, which frequently include jobs at a lower level than those held pretraumatically; (b) they have a reasonable awareness of their deficits and the vocational implications of those deficits, and have made adequate emotional adjustment to their disability; and (c) they either demonstrate functional use of compensatory techniques or accept work that is not compromised by their deficits.

In most cases, obtaining competitive employment requires active participation by the client. Even with the help of an experienced and successful job placement counselor, a competitive job is still obtained by individuals "selling" themselves. It remains a hard fact of life that employers hire people who have the skills necessary to perform a particular job. Indeed, if a client lacks the necessary skills, it would be a disservice to support that vocational goal.

There are many resources that can and should be used in the attempt to secure competitive employment for head injured clients. As a rule, the more resources used, the greater the chances of obtaining employment.

1. *Projects with Industry (PWI):* PWI programs were initially funded by the vocational rehabilitation amendments of 1968 (U.S. P.L. 90-391) and were later expanded under the Rehabilitation Act of 1973 (U.S. P.L. 93-112). Over 50 PWI programs exist in the United States which work together with over 2500 private companies (National Association of Rehabilitation Facilities, 1980). The Vocational Rehabiliation Center's PWI Program has enjoyed considerable success. The 1985-86 Project Progress Report indicated that 74 of the 104 clients accepted into the project during the first half of the project year have been competitively placed and have completed at least 60 days of work (Vocational Rehabilitation Center, 1986). The PWI Program at VRC also reported a 93.7 percent job retention rate (VRC, 1986).
2. *Placement Services:* Clients who previously attended a college, university, or training program can frequently use the placement services of that facility. The rehabilitation counselor should work closely with this placement office to ensure that appropriate positions are sought.
3. *Friends and Relatives:* Since jobs are often acquired through personal contacts, clients and their families should be encouraged to use friends and relatives as contact persons.
4. *National Head Injury Foundation:* The local chapter of the National Head Injury Foundation (NHIF) can be used in the job placement effort. NHIF may be able to improve local employer awareness of head injury and, thereby, encourage the hiring of head injured persons. Local NHIF chapters, working together with vocational rehabilitation professionals, can encourage the development of business advisory councils to promote the placement of head injured persons.
5. *Vocational Rehabilitation Programs:* Most vocational rehabilitation programs have trained job placement counselors who can assist with placement, primarily by establishing ongoing working relationships with local employers. In this way, job openings are posted through the vocational rehabilitation facility. The job place-

ment counselor can also be of benefit to the employer by intervening and assisting with problems which may arise with the disabled employee. Having this resource available generally makes prospective employers more comfortable with the hire.

6. *State Vocational Rehabilitation Agencies:* Placement counselors are also part of the state vocational rehabilitation system and can provide these services to active clients of the state system. State vocational rehabilitation clients are also eligible for certain employer incentives, such as on-the-job training monies, which can offer the employer some financial support while training the disabled worker for the new position.
7. *Employer Incentives:* Affirmative action requirements of the Rehabilitation Act of 1973 (U.S. P.L. 93–112) have greatly aided disabled citizens in securing employment in cases where they may have been discriminated against due to their disability. There are also income tax credits available to employers who hire state vocational rehabilitation clients. The Federal Targeted Job Tax Credit, established by the Federal Revenue Act in 1978, provides a tax credit of up to $3000 for the first year's wages and up to $1500 for the second year's wages for disabled citizens.

Despite these resources, securing competitive employment can be a very complex and demanding task. Many employers are reluctant to hire a disabled worker. The reasons given, which are mostly unfounded, include: (a) handicapped persons are more likely to have accidents; (b) worker's compensation insurance rates will increase; (c) necessary modifications of the work area will be expensive; and (d) other workers will not accept the disabled worker (Corthell & Boone, 1982).

These commonly given reasons for not hiring disabled workers are, in fact, inconsistent with available evidence. Research done by E.I. du Pont de Nemours and Company, which employs 110,000 people of whom 1452 are disabled, yielded the following conclusions: (a) There were no increases in workers' compensation costs; (b) most disabled workers required no special work arrangements; (c) 96 percent of the disabled workers were rated average or better both on and off the job with respect to safety; (d) the disabled workers wanted to be treated like regular employees, without special privileges; (e) 91 percent of the disabled workers were rated average or better in job performance; (f) 79 percent were rated average or better in attendance; and (g) there were no differences between disabled and nondisabled workers in their ability to get along with co-workers (Corthell & Boone, 1982). Although this information does not pertain specifically to head injured workers, it is nevertheless useful to placement counselors. Data which similarly support the hiring of head injured persons needs to be gathered and disseminated.

Follow-Up Services

Follow-up services, designed to ensure retention of successful vocational placements, are critical for traumatically brain injured individuals who often require support and job intervention indefinitely (Aves, 1985). Since large amounts of time, money, and energy are invested in bringing the client to the point of successful placement, it would be unwise not to provide the services needed to maintain that placement. Follow-up services should include work site visits by a rehabilitation professional familiar with the worker and the employer. Visits should initially be frequent (e.g., two to three times per week), and later gradually reduced to occasional "spot checks," depending upon need. Most programs do offer some form of follow-up services for 3 to 6 months following discharge. In our experience, a much longer period of follow-up is required by many head injured clients.

FUTURE DIRECTIONS

1. *Programs:* As the number of head injured adults returning to the community grows, the need for vocational rehabilitation services — particularly in the area of community placement — will correspondingly grow. Due to the heterogeneity of this group, a wide variety of vocational placement options must be available. There currently exists in the United States a very uneven distribution of quality vocational rehabilitation programs. Some parts of the country lack even the most rudimentary vocational rehabilitation services for this group, while other areas have several high quality programs available. Condeluci, Fawber, and Gretz-Lasky (1986) reported the results of a national survey designed to gather information from rehabilitation professionals regarding perceived needs of head injured clients. The survey revealed a wide-spread desire for more long-term rehabilitation programs specifically for head injured clients. These professionals ranked the following needs as most pressing: (a) supervised apartment programs for persons without insurance funding; (b) programs that accept clients with severe behavioral disorders; and (c) transitional employment programs. Many of the respondents indicated a desire to create such programs in their area; of these, 65 percent cited lack of funding as their reason for not implementing needed programs.

2. *Funding:* Program development within the field of vocational rehabilitation for head injured adults continues to be at the mercy of state and federal funding. As a disability group, this population does not receive consistent funding from a consistent source. Support from private insurance carriers, state vocational rehabilitation programs,

and mental health/mental retardation services is rarely sufficient to implement the programming that is needed. This is particularly true in the field of vocational rehabilitation which frequently requires long-term, costly, and individualized services not funded by these sources. All too often services are terminated at the point when the client is entering the most critical phase of community placement. This resistance to protecting the enormous investment of resources in previous rehabilitation is economically short-sighted and particularly frustrating when funding is terminated at the point of vocational placement. It makes little sense to fund expensive medical rehabilitation and an expensive vocational evaluation, but not fund services needed to secure a supported work placement or provide the follow-up services necessary to maintain the client in the community placement.

3. *Research:* Longitudinal studies are needed to measure the relative effectiveness of different approaches to vocational rehabilitation , with a special focus on long-term vocational outcome. Data from such research is needed to plan the most cost-effective programming for head injured clients, and also to support the need for funds to pay for specialized programming.

Effective vocational rehabilitation for head injured clients requires flexibility, creative problem solving, and keen observational skills (Musante, 1983). Given the broad spectrum of deficits and occupational outcomes, no one program or intervention method will work with every head injured client. In this chapter, we have emphasized the need for individualized programs that exist within a framework that emphasizes cognitive and psychosocial intervention and systematically graded community placement.

REFERENCES

Anderson, T. (1981). Stroke and cerebral trauma: Medical aspects. In W. Stolov & M. Clovers (Eds.), *Handbook of severe disability* (pp. 119–126). Washington, DC: U.S. Government Printing Office.

Aves, D. K. (1985). Transitional employment model for adults with brain injuries. *Proceedings of the 1985 Annual National Association of Rehabilitation Facilities Conference.* Washington, DC: NARF.

Benton, A. (1979). Behavioral consequences of closed head injury. In G. Odom (Ed.), *Central nervous system trauma reserach status report* (pp. 220–231). Washington, DC: National Institute of Neurological and Communicative Disorders and Stroke.

Ben-Yishay, Y. (Ed.) (1980). *Working approaches to remediation of cognitive deficits in brain damaged persons.* (Rehabilitation Monograph No. 62). New York: New York University Medical Center, Institute of Rehabilitation Medicine.

Ben-Yishay, Y. & Diller, L. (1981). Rehabilitation of cognitive and perceptual defects in people with traumatic brain damage. (Brief Research Report) *International Journal of Rehabilitation Research, 4*(2), 208–210.

Ben-Yishay, Y. & Diller, L. (1983). Cognitive deficits. In M. Rosenthal, E. Griffith, M. Bond, and J. Miller (Eds.), *Rehabilitation of the head injured adult* (pp. 167–183). Philadelphia: F. A. Davis.

Ben-Yishay, Y., Lakin, P., Ross, B., Rattok, J., Piasetsky, E. & Diller, L. (1983). *Psychotherapy following severe brain injury.* (Rehabilitation Monograph No. 64. New York: New York University Medical Center, Institute of Rehabilitation Medicine.

Ben-Yishay, Y., Rattok, J., Lakin, P., Piasetsky, E. B., Ross, B., Silver, S., Zide, E. & Ezrachi, O. (1985). Neuropsychological rehabilitation: Quest for a holistic approach. *Seminars in Neurology,* 5, 252–259.

Ben-Yishay, Y., Rattok, J., Ross, B., Lakin, P., Ezrachi, O., Silver, S. & Diller, L. (1982). *Rehabilitation of cognitive and perceptual deficits in people with traumatic brain damage: A five year clinical research study.* (Rehabilitation Monograph No. 63). New York: New York University Medical Center, Institute of Rehabilitation Medicine.

Botterbusch, K. (1982). *A comparison of commercial vocational evaluation systems.* Menomonie, WI: Materials Development Center, Stout Vocational Rehabilitation Institute.

Bruckner, F. E. & Randle, A. P. H. (1972). Return to work after severe head injuries. *Rheumatology and Physical Medicine, 2,* 344–348.

Condeluci, A., Fawber, H. L. & Gretz-Lasky, S. (1986). A national survey: The need for long term independent living/vocational rehabilitation services. *NHIF, Inc. Newsletter, 5,*(4), 5, 8.

Corthell, D. W. & Boone, L. (1982). Marketing: An approach to placement. *Ninth Institute on Rehabilitation Issues,* St. Louis.

Crewe, N. & Athelstan, G. (1981). Functional assessment in vocational rehabilitation: A systematic approach to diagnosis and goal setting. *Archives of Physical Medicine and Rehabilitation* , *62*(7), 299–305.

Crewe, N. & Athelstan, G. (1984). *Functional assessment inventory manual.* Menomonie, WI: Materials Development Center, Stout Vocational Rehabilitation Institute.

Diller, L. & Gordon, W. (1981). Intervention for cognitive deficits in brain injured adults. *Journal of Consulting and Clinical Psychology, 49,* 822–834.

Fordyce, D., Roueche, J. & Prigatano, G. (1983). Enhanced emotional reactions in chronic head trauma patients. *Journal of Neurology, Neurosurgery and Psychiatry, 46,* 620–624.

Fowler, R. (1981). Stroke and cerebral trauma: Psychosocial and vocational aspects. In W. Stolov & M. Clowers (Eds.), *Handbook of severe disabilility* (pp. 127–135). Washington, DC: U.S. Government Printing Office.

Gilchrist, E. & Wilkinson, M. (1979). Some factors determining prognosis in young people with severe head injuries. *Archives of Neurology, 36,* 355–359.

Goethe, K. & Levin, H. (1984). Behavioral manifestations during the early and long term stages of recovery after closed head injury. *Psychiatric Annals, 14,* 540–546.

Gogstad, A. & Kjellman, A. (1976). Rehabilitation prognosis related to clinical and social factors in brain injured of different etiology. *Social Science and Medicine, 10,* 283–288.

Hackler, E. & Tobis, J. S. (1983). Reintegration into the community. In M. Rosenthal, E. Griffith, M. Bond, and J. D. Miller (Eds.), *Rehabilitation of the head injured adult* (pp. 421–434). Philadelphia: F. A. Davis.

Klonoff, P. S. & Snow, W. G. (in press). Employment outcome in a sample of Canadian closed head injury patients. *NATCON.*

Kraus, M. & MacEacheron, A. (1982). A competitive employment training for mentally retarded adults: The supported work model. *American Journal of Mental Deficiency, 86,* 650–653.

Lezak, M. (1978a). Living with the characterologically altered brain injured patient. *The Journal of Clinical Psychiatry, 39,* 592–598.

Lezak, M. (1978b). Subtle sequelae of brain damage. *American Journal of Physical Medicine, 57,* 9–15.

Long, C., Gouvier, W. & Cole, J. (1984). A model of recovery for the total rehabilitation of individuals with head trauma. *Journal of Rehabilitation, 70,* 39–45.

Lynch, R. (1983). Traumatic head injury: Implications for rehabilitation counseling. *Journal of Applied Rehabilitation Counseling, 14,* 32–35.

Lytel, R. B. & Botterbusch, K. F. (1981). *Physical demands job analysis: A new approach.* Menomonie, WI: Materials Development Center, Stout Vocational Rehabilitation Institute.

Matheson, J. M. (1982). The vocational outcome of rehabilitation in fifty consecutive patients with severe head injuries. In J. F. Garrett (Ed.), *Australian approaches to rehabilitation in neurotrauma and spinal cord injury* (pp. 32–35). New York: World Rehabilitation Fund.

Musante, S. (1983). Issues relevant to the vocational evaluation of the traumatically head injured client. *Vocational Evaluation and Work Adjustment Bulletin,* Spring, 45–49.

National Association of Rehabilitation Facilities. (1980). *Projects with industry training manual.* Washington, DC: National Association of Rehabilitation Facilities.

Prigatano, G., Fordyce, D., Zeiner, H., Roueche, J., Pepping, M. & Wood, B. (1984). Neuropsychological rehabilitation after closed head injury in young adults. *Journal of Neurology, Neurosurgery and Psychiatry, 47,* 505–513.

Prigatano, G. P., Fordyce, D. J., Zeiner, H. K., Roueche, J. R., Pepping, M. & Wood, B. (1986). *Neuropsychological rehabilitatition after brain injury.* Baltimore, MD: The Johns Hopkins University Press.

Revel, G., Wehman, P. & Arnold, S. (1984). Supported work model of employment for mentally retarded persons: Implications for rehabilitative services. *Journal of Rehabilitation, 50,* 33–38.

Rimel, R. W., Giordani, B., Barth, J. T., Boll, T. J. & Jane, J. A. (1981). Disability caused by minor head injury. *Neurosurgery, 9*(3), 221–228.

Rimel, R. W., Giordani, B., Barth, J. T. & Jane, J. A. (1982). Moderate head injury: Completing the clinical spectrum of brain trauma. *Neurosurgery, 11,* 344–351.

Rosenbaum, M., Lipsitz, N., Abraham, J. & Najenson, T. (1978). A description of an intensive treatment project for the rehabilitation of severely brain-injured soldiers. *Scandinavian Journal of Rehabilitation Medicine, 10,* 1–6.

Smith, C. & Fry, R. (Eds.). (1985). *National forum on issues in vocational assessment.* Menomonie, WI: Materials Development Center.

Smith, R. K. (1983). Prevocational programming in the rehabilitation of the head injured patient. *Physical Therapy, 63*(12), 2026–2029.

Sowers, J., Connis, R. & Thompson, L. (1979). The food service vocational training program: A model for training and placement of the mentally retarded. In G. T. Bellamy, G. O'Connor & O. C. Karan (Eds.), *Vocational rehabilitation of severely handicapped persons.* Baltimore: University Park Press.

Tabaddor, K., Mattis, S. & Zazula, T. (1984). Cognitive sequelae and recovery course after moderate and severe head injury. *Neurosurgery, 14,* 701–708.

Thomsen, I. V. (1984). Late outcome of very severe blunt head trauma: A 10-15 year second follow-up. *Journal of Neurology, Neurosurgery, and Psychiatry, 47,* 260–268.

U.S. Department of Labor. (1977). *Dictionary of occupational titles.* Washington, DC: U.S. Government Printing Office.

Vocational Rehabilitation Center. (1986). *Projects with industry interim report* (PWI Grant Number G0083C0100). Pittsburgh, PA.

Wehman, P. (in press). Supported competitive employment. *Journal of Applied Rehabilitation Counseling.*

Wehman, P. & Kregel, J. (1983). *A supported work approach to competitive employment of individuals with moderate and severe handicaps* (Contact No. 82-37-300-0357). Washington, DC: Innovative Programs for the Severely Handicapped, U. S. Department of Education.

Weiss, L. (1980). Vocational evaluation: An individualized program. *Archives of Physical Medicine Rehabilitation, 61,* 453–454.

Williams, W. & Vogelsburg, T. (1980). *Comprehensive vocational service model for severely handicapped adults.* (Center for Developmental Disabilities Monograph Series). Burlington, VT: University of Vermont.

Zivanovic, C. (1984, December 3). Barrier-free businesses. Corporations are starting to retain, promote the disabled. *The Detroit News,* pp. 1, 14.

Zorn, G. (1984). *The J.O.B.S. Program* [Computer Program]. Pleasantville, NY: Train-Ease Corp.

CHAPTER 7

Independent Living: Settings and Supports

Al Condeluci
Sue Cooperman
*Barbara A. Seif**

Perhaps the most challenging phase of rehabilitation following severe head injury is community re-entry and long-term care. The medical system invests massive resources in saving lives and providing early rehabilitation for those who have been injured. This effort may lose its impact if the individual is discharged into a setting that cannot meet long-term care needs. Strong gains can be made in the rehabilitation process, but if appropriate discharge settings are not available, the effects of rehabilitation are diminished.

Ducker (1983) reported that most of the adults with head injury who were discharged to home or a long-term care institution regressed in skills. Yet these are exactly the settings in which many severely head injured adults find themselves. Because of limited program options and financial support, all too many persons with head injury, who are still in need of rehabilitation supports, are inappropriately placed in a long-term care facility or are forced into a condition of unwanted dependence on family members.

For families who do take their injured family member back into the home, there are often no services available to meet long-term needs, which include all of the supportive services necessary to main tain an injured individual after discharge from an acute-care or community re-entry program; e.g., attendant care, home management, home health services, respite services, and general supervision in addition

* Authorship listed alphabetically at author's request.

to physical, occupational, speech, and cognitive therapy, and psychological counseling as indicated. Jacobs (1985) found that there are few services available to meet the long-term needs of families.

Although the complexities of head injury sequelae contribute to the need for long-term supportive services, the concerns are similar to those associated with other disabling conditions. Indeed, the long-term needs of severely disabled persons were acknowledged in 1978 when the Rehabilitation Act of 1973 was amended to initiate independent living services. These services developed from two main sources: the prompting of disabled individuals seeking a more meaningful life and the efforts of rehabilitation professionals to provide services for those people who lacked potential for gainful employment (DeJong, 1979). It was projected that if individuals with severe disabilities could become more self-directed through independent living, then they would have a greater chance to become gainfully employed should job opportunities become available.

It is essential for rehabilitation professionals to appreciate fully the strength of the term "independence" in the context of independent living services. Within traditional medical rehabilitation, independence is usually defined as maximization of physical functioning. In the vocational rehabilitation setting, independence is often measured by level of employment. Independent living is defined as control over one's life based on choice of acceptable options that minimize reliance on others in making decisions and in performing everyday activities (Pfluger, 1979). It is this emphasis on consumer control that often sets independent living services apart from traditional rehabilitation. In most rehabilitation settings, a counselor, social worker, program manager, or rehabilitation specialist either sets or helps to set goals and directions for clients. The concept of independent living in its strict sense requires that the disabled individuals (the consumers) choose their goals and lifestyle and then, as necessary, organize and manage the appropriate physical supports (Cole, 1979). For example, in a traditional rehabilitation program all individuals might be expected to learn to dress themselves. In an independent living arrangement, an individual would be expected to make a choice about self-dressing and then manage the choice. Thus a lawyer with a physical disability could choose to pay a personal care attendent to dress him so that he might spend more time working at the practice of law.

This focus on consumer choice can complicate independent living rehabilitation for individuals with head injury. Unlike many other disabling conditions, head injury typically affects cognitive functioning.

These cognitive deficits may significantly reduce an individual's potential for independent living, including making choices about goals and lifestyle, organizing and managing the necessary supports, and making safe decisions in emergency situations.

HEAD INJURY SEQUELAE AND INDEPENDENT LIVING

Chapters 1 through 4 explore in some detail the deficits commonly associated with severe closed head injury. In this chapter, we highlight those deficits that have the greatest impact on independent living. Disability following moderate and severe head trauma usually includes a unique combination of physical, cognitive, perceptual, and emotional problems. Cognitive deficits create an especially stubborn challenge for independent living.

Of the many head injuries sustained in the United States each year, approximately 14 percent are classified as severe or very severe while the remaining 86 percent are classified as mild or moderately severe. Many of those who survive severe head injuries are left with permanent physical, mental, or emotional deficits. Of those who sustain less severe injuries, many recover physically but may have difficulty resuming their previous lifestyle (Long, Gouvier & Cole, 1984).

Physical, cognitive, and perceptual functioning tends to improve over time, with the greatest recovery occurring during the first year. Emotional and social recovery may parallel improvement in cognitive functioning or it may actually deteriorate with the passage of time, as the client becomes more aware of residual deficits and must adjust to long-term changes in lifestyle (Fordyce, Roueche & Prigatano, 1983). Follow-up studies support the conclusion that cognitive and behavioral disorders are more common than physical impairments and, in turn, constitute the chief cause of long-term disability for individuals with head injury. In addition, head injury can reduce the essential means for coping with disability, including reserves of emotional drive, stability of personality, and intellectual resources (Jennett, 1984).

Physical Deficits

Most of the physical deficits associated with head injury are functionally similar to those that result from other disorders. Although these deficits are significant and challenging, rehabilitation specialists have learned many ways to remediate or compensate for them. Therefore, they generally do not present the greatest obstacle to independent living after head injury. Chapter 2 includes a discussion of physical sequelae and their treatment, emphasizing those compensations often critical to independent living.

Traumatic epilepsy is a deficit that is especially significant because of its social implications and its unpredictability. It may develop months or even years after the injury and can lead to significant problems for a person who has made a fairly good recovery (Jennett, 1983). Epilepsy not only prevents individuals from driving, it can also prevent them from obtaining automobile, health, and life insurance. Although the public attitude toward epilepsy has improved over the years (Sands & Minters, 1979), many people are still reluctant to associate with those who have this disorder, while others may regard them as needing to be closely watched and cared for — in other words, unable to be left completely alone.

Behavioral Deficits

After a head injury, subtle personality changes may only be noticed by relatives or close associates. These changes frequently take the form of exaggeration of pre-traumatic personality traits, but occasionally they may be a reversal of them. According to Long and colleagues (1984), post-traumatic behavior may be viewed as the combined effect of the client's premorbid personality adjustment, response to cognitive impairment, and level of perceived stress. In their view, inadequate coping skills resulting from impaired cognitive functioning combined with sustained stress during the chronic phase of recovery are the primary factors contributing to psychological complications following head trauma. Prigatano et al. (1984) similarly state that anxiety, anger, and depression are often in response to not knowing how to handle the cognitive, perceptual, and motor limitations imposed by the brain injury. Other behavioral problems commonly evidenced by head injured adults include: emotional lability, irritability, lack of initiation, impulsivity, loss of inhibition, and withdrawal from social interaction.

Cognitive and Perceptual Deficits

Spontaneous neurologic recovery, including recovery of cognitive and perceptual deficits, continues at a decelerating rate for months and often years following severe closed head injury. It is, however, common for some combination of cognitive and perceptual deficits to remain. The most commonly reported persisting sequelae (according to both clients and their families) are difficulties in remembering and concentrating (Oddy, Coughlan, Tyerman & Jenkins, 1985). Memory impairment may range from a general state of confusion and disorientation, in which the client remembers very little from day to day, to more subtle problems such as failure to keep appointments, take medication, or pay bills. Problems with concentration are also common. Individuals may be easily distracted and have difficulty screening out irrelevant visual and/or auditory environmental stimulation. They may also have problems dividing their attention, limiting their ability to perform two tasks simultaneously such as talking on the telephone and tending something on the stove.

Of particular importance to independent living specialists is the frequently reported inability of head injured clients to plan, organize, and execute a task efficiently. Getting oneself up and out to work in the morning involves planning what to wear and what to eat for breakfast, and leaving on time to catch a bus. Many head injured clients demonstrate the ability to perform such tasks during formal assessment or in a structured therapeutic environment, but when on their own either lack the processing abilities to deal with the increased demands of a natural environment or lack the initiative to follow through with the activities. Assessment must, therefore, include observation of these and other daily living activities in a natural setting. A reduced ability to initiate activities leads to an increase in dependence and, therefore, affects a person's ability to live independently.

Impaired safety and social judgment has a similarly powerful effect on independent living, and is also commonly reported following severe head injury. How safe is the client around the stove and in the kitchen in general? Does he or she relate appropriately to strangers? Due to impaired judgment and deficient problem-solving abilities, many head injured clients are limited in their ability to make well thought out decisions, especially under stress. Therefore, they have the potential to be hazardous to themselves or others, and they easily may be taken advantage of by unscrupulous individuals.

In addition to cognitive deficits, head injured clients often demonstrate a variety of visual-perceptual-motor deficits. Assessment of perceptual functioning is frequently neglected in routine follow-up examinations, and therefore its full effect cannot be determined (Bond, 1983). Although perceptual deficits may be subtle, they can significantly affect an individual's ability to perform activities of daily living successfully (Wahlstrom, 1983). Impaired form and space perception interferes with many daily activities. Form and space perception includes the ability to perceive similarities and differences in the shape, color, and size of objects as well as the position and orientation of an object and its relationship to other objects. As a result of a severe deficit in this area, an individual who knows the sequence and steps for dressing might put a shirt on inside out or backwards or with an arm through the neck hole. Spatial disorientation can also result in difficulty learning routes and frequently becoming lost in the community or in a complex building. The case of S.J. illustrates the effects of the combination of residual deficits following head injury as they relate to independent living.

Case illustration — Background: S.J. was admitted to the Rehabilitation Institute of Pittsburgh in 1982 with a diagnosis of organic brain syndrome secondary to head injury. At the time of her admission she was 28 years of age, 7 years post-injury, and expecting a child. Deficits from the head injury included right hemiplegia as well as significant cognitive and behavioral deficits. Following the accident, S.J. was not involved in a formal rehabilitation program, but she did receive occupational therapy, physical therapy, and speech-language therapy in her home for a brief period of time. She was not able to return to her former job as a secretary. Although she was able to secure several jobs as a receptionist, she was unable to hold a job for any length of time. Since the accident, she had also been hopitalized several times for psychiatric problems and at the time of admission was taking Lithium, Ativan, and Mellaril. Until her marriage in September 1981, S.J. lived at home with her parents.

The family eventually became involved with the National Head Injury Foundation. Their concern about their daughter's ability to manage a household and care for a young child prompted them to seek professional help for her. When S.J. was initially evaluated at the Institute, she denied the existence of cognitive deficits other than mild memory problems, which she dismissed as an occasional need "to write things down." She was concerned with her fine motor functioning — expecially her handwriting which was slow, but legible. Her overall physical status had improved dramatically since the accident. A mild right-sided weakness was the only persisting deficit. S.J. also stated that her psychiatric hospitalizations were precipitated by her failure to take her medications.

S.J.'s husband presented a totally different picture of his wife's capabilities. He stated that prior to the marriage, he had no idea of the extent of his wife's cognitive and emotional problems. He reported that, although she was physically able to perform most homemaking tasks, she lacked the ability to initiate or complete these activities and usually she just sat and watched TV all day long. He felt that she was lazy and resented that he had to assume responsibility for washing the clothes, shopping, and managing the family finances. He was hurt when she forgot things that were important to both of them, such as plans to go out to dinner. He was also embarrassed by her almost constant, and often inappropriate, talking and lack of social judgment. He was especially upset because S.J. had stopped taking birth control pills without his knowledge. He questioned his wife's ability to cope with the stress of caring for a child, but interpreted her family's concern as meddling.

Implications for independent living: S.J. typifies several of the common difficulties in developing independent living options for individuals with head injuries. During her brief home therapy program she may have functioned adequately because of the structure created by the therapy. Although S.J. had made an almost complete physical recovery and, on the surface, appeared to have only minor and insignificant cognitive deficits, she was still not able to function independently. Her inability to self-initiate activities caused her to be unable to use her skills without assistance. Only with the assistance of her parents, sisters, and husband was S.J. able to carry out her homemaking responsibilities. Her lack of awareness of cognitive deficits made her reluctant to use compensatory strategies and significantly increased her dependence on others. It is important to recognize that because S.J. was physically able to perform homemaking tasks, she would not be a candidate for most independent living programs. The professional community has yet to apply the entire spectrum of independent living services to head injury rehabilitation due to the challenge of the cognitive and emotional deficits which often accompany head injury.

HISTORY OF THE INDEPENDENT LIVING MOVEMENT

In the fall of 1985, a consumer-related newsletter, the *Disability Rag,* devoted an entire edition to a review of independent living as a concept, a movement, and a service system. In a summary statement, the editors captured the spirit of this movement with these words:

> The desire to live independently is in the best tradition of the American dream. Dependency has always been the lot of the disabled people, and it is only natural that the cornerstone in

'disability rights' should be the right to live independently, which in more explicit terms, means the right to be in charge of our lives. (p. 11)

Indeed, independent living is at the same time a philosophy, a movement, and a service system. Although this chapter is devoted to the application of independent living services in head injury rehabilitation, these services must be understood in relation to the independent living philosophy and history. Initially, most rehabilitation services were understood within a medical model; disabled individuals were perceived to be "sick" and in need of treatment. Following medical stabilization, services tended to be justified in economic terms — that is, in terms of what a disabled individual could return to society. A more appropriate justification for rehabilitation services, and one that is consistent with the spirit of independent living as a sociopolitical movement, is that services are provided because it is morally and politically right to do so.

In order to fully appreciate the importance of independent living, it is essential to understand Wolfensberger's (1972) principle of normalization. Wolfensberger outlined how, historically, groups of people, including those with physical disabilities, have been devalued by the society in which they live. The principle of normalization emphasizes the need to reverse this process of devaluation to enable people to lead normal lives. In more recent writings, Wolfensberger has used the phrase "social role valorization" in place of the term "normalization" which, in his opinion, had become overused and confusing (Wolfensberger & Thomas, 1983). According to Wolfensberger, the new phrase, which means giving value to the social role, is more consistent with his views.

The process of devaluation begins with a group of people who are perceived as "different" and are thought to be less valuable than everyone else. Society then ascribes specific roles to these people; these roles, in turn, lead to expected behaviors and therefore to stereotypes. Once a group is stereotyped, it is easy to lose sight of the individuality of the members of the group and therefore to devalue the entire group.

According to Wolfensberger, the process of devaluation has, historically, been managed by societies in three major stages. Initially, people who were "different" were simply destroyed or deported. A sobering example of this approach can be found in Nazi Germany where Jews and other non-aryan groups were eliminated or deported.

The second stage in the management of devalued people is segregation. In this approach, devalued people are set apart from society and at best tolerated from afar. In many cases, the needs of the devalued group are served entirely within the segregated setting. Isolated state schools and hospitals for retarded individuals are clear examples of this approach.

In the third management stage, reversal, a more enlightened society attempts to reinstate the devalued group into the mainstream. The ultimate goal is to eliminate the stereotypes that created the devalued state in the first place. It is at this point that Wolfensberger's concept of social role valorization becomes especially important. He proposed that the way to "valorize" individuals is, as much as possible, to bring them back into the mainstream. He advocates treating the devalued people as equals and avoiding situations that isolate or single out these individuals.

An important facet of the principle of social role valorization is the dignity of risk. Often devalued individuals are protected from risky situations because they are judged to be unable to handle the consequences. Although there are legitimate concerns for retarded individuals or persons who are head injured and have residual judgment impairments, we must recognize the impact of overprotection. It is natural in life to take risks, and all of us have taken some chances in decisions we have made. This is reflected in popular expressions such as "the school of hard knocks" and "no pain, no gain." Yet we are quick to protect and buffer disabled people from situations that involve risk. The implication is that the disabled person is not capable of deciding, even in the most basic sense. Professionals who work with head injured clients must be cautious that their protective instincts do not overshadow the individual's right to choose and to risk.

A number of movements, including the civil rights movement, have paved the way for the emancipation of the physically disabled and for development of independent living. DeJong (1979) identified the self-help movement of the 60s, the consumer movement of the 70s, and the deinstitutionalization movement of the mid-70s as powerful contributing forces. Through all of these efforts, disabled individuals have gained greater control over their lives and we have begun to recognize that they are entitled to basic rights and are viable consumers of many things, including human services. In this spirit, the independent living movement took hold.

Throughout the 1970s, there was recognition of disabled individuals as consumers and an acknowledgement of their rights. During this period, several important laws were enacted that identified needs and mandated services for disabled individuals. These include the Architectural Barriers Act of 1968, the Urban Mass Transit Act of

1970, the Rehabilitation Act of 1973, the Housing and Urban Development Act of 1973, the Federal Highway Aid Act of 1973, The Education for All Children Act of 1976, the Developmental Disabilities Act of 1976, State and Local Fiscal Assistance Amendments of 1976, Domestic Volunteer Service Act Amendments of 1978, Constitutional Protection for Handicapped Persons, the Civil Service Reform Act of 1978, the Foreign Service Act of 1980, the Omnibus Budget Reconciliation Act of 1981, the Job Training Partnership Act of 1982, the Community Development Act of 1974, and the Full Employment and Balanced Growth Act of 1978. All of these measures identified needs of disabled people and promoted the concept of control over one's life based on a choice of acceptable options.

Traditional independent living services have primarily been available to physically disabled individuals. More recently, however, leaders in the movement have become aware of the growing number of disabled people whose cognitive and perceptual impairments significantly limit their options for independent living. This shift is best seen in the newer independent living programs that have developed specifically for head injured individuals. The National Head Injury Foundation's (NHIF) Directory of Head Injury Rehabilitation Services (1983) identifies such programs.

Although housing concerns are central to independent living, the concept of independent living includes many other components which must be viewed as an integrated whole. Where one lives, how one lives, how one recreates, who one recreates with, and what one does to give meaning to life are all critical components of independent living (DeLoach, Wilkins & Walker, 1983).

In 1978 the Amendments to the Rehabilitation Act of 1973 were signed officially introducing and defining independent living as a service system and authorizing the development of centers for independent living throughout the United States. This initiative launched a formal advocacy and created a structure for the independent living movement.

ASSESSMENT

As with any area of rehabilitation, the application of independent living services requires an effective assessment to identify strengths and deficits of the individual. In addition to life skills functioning, a thorough assessment for head injured individuals should include physical, cognitive, perceptual, behavioral, social, educational, and vocational areas. Because a discussion of each of these areas of assessment is far beyond the scope of this chapter, we will focus our brief discussion on the process of assessment for independent living.

Over the past decade, a number of independent living assessment instruments have been developed. Most of these assessments focus on basic life skills and are in a checklist format. Commonly used checklists include: Camelot Behavioral Checklist (Foster, 1976); Independent Living Behavioral Checklist (Walls, Zane & Thuedt, 1979); Inventory of Essential Skills (Brigance, 1981); and National Independent Living Skills Assessment Instruments and Curriculum Guide (Woosley, Harden & Murphy, 1984). Life skills typically assessed are:

- health/hygiene
- parenting/child care
- home maintenance
- money management
- activities of daily living
- community awareness and mobility
- legal awareness
- social/interpersonal skills
- family involvement

Of particular importance in the assessment of head injured individuals is the validation of responses. Most assessment instruments are paper and pencil tests. In this type of format the evaluator asks questions of the individual and/or the family. Sometimes the individual or family does not answer the questions accurately. Memory or processing ability may be impaired to the point that individuals are confused or mistaken with their answers. Furthermore, impaired self-awareness of deficits is a frequent consequence of severe head injury (see Chapter 1). In other cases the family might be embarrassed by the individual's inability to perform the task or deny the severity of the deficits and therefore imply that their loved one has capabilities beyond his or her actual scope.

It is important, therefore, that the evaluator directly assess any life skills that are questionable on the basis of client or family interviews or the client's history. This may require that the client actually perform an activity. However, care must be taken in this effort to avoid humiliating the client by the results of the assessment.

The rehabilitation professional must realize the limitations of independent living assessments. As a dynamic concept, independent living needs to be considered as an integrated totality. Assessments by their very nature isolate areas and explore them without this isolation. They often do not account for the logical or natural "tie-in" of concepts. For example, a client may have difficulty doing mathematical computations as part of an assessment, but may be able to do the computations necessary for basic cooking. Alternatively, a client may demonstrate adequate computational skills under the conditions of formal assessment, but be unable to apply those skills in a more natural or stressful setting.

Assessments can be conducted by one or several of the professionals on the rehabilitation team. The results of the assessment should be reviewed by the entire team, including the client and family, and a comprehensive independent living plan developed. This plan should identify that least restrictive environment for the client, necessary support services, areas of deficit which need to be remediated, and a plan for treatment.

When developing and implementing the independent living plan for head injured clients, it is important that demands and expectations be consistent and that all members of the support services team, including the family, be aware of the comprehensive plan (Schwab, 1981). It may be necessary to repeat all or part of the assessment as the individual progresses in life skills and revise the independent living plan accordingly.

INDEPENDENT LIVING SETTINGS

"Setting" refers to the place in which independent living support is provided. At times, the setting alone constitutes a type of support; but more often than not, the setting is just that — the structure in which services are offered.

Settings can best be understood as a continuum of options ranging from large instititutional situations to individual, autonomous environments. Within each of the settings a variety of supports can be offered to maintain and/or enhance the basic life skills necessary for success. Figure 7–1, developed for a national independent living training program (Condeluci, 1979), illustrates the continuum of settings which will be discussed in turn.

Institutions

Under most state regulations, an institution is a treatment facility with twelve or more residential beds (Laurie, 1977). Often institutions are large multi-bed facilities that by their very size create a dependent

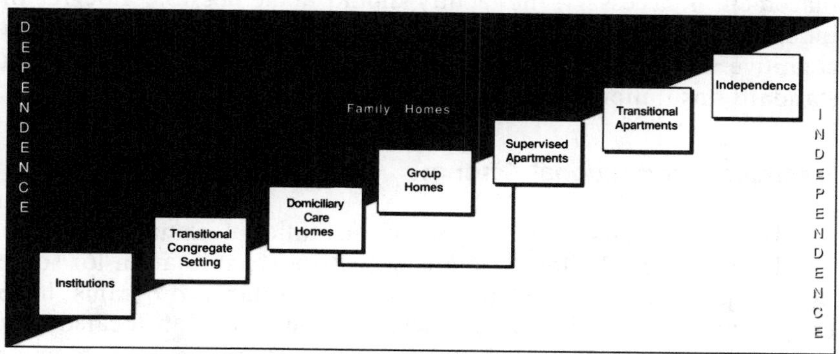

Figure 7–1. Continuum of residential settings.

environment. Size dictates that structure and routine be imposed, and at times this structure can limit residents' independence (Wolfensberger, 1972). Often residents have limited privacy and are usually treated as patients within the medical service structure.

Institutions can be private or public, and are usually focused on a particular population. Institutional settings for head injured individuals include acute-care facilities, rehabilitation facilities, community re-entry facilities, and, for those with life-time needs, intermediate-care or skilled nursing facilities. Each of these types of facility has a different focus, but all fit the definition of an institution.

The advantage of institutions is that they offer a comprehensive environment that can meet the medical needs, many of the rehabilitative needs, and some of the social needs of the residents. Because of their size and comprehensive service system, however, institutions can create negative images with the lay public and perpetuate stereotypes about certain populations. More importantly, institutional living can unwittingly reduce a resident's autonomy and independent functioning, thus interfering with the possibility of future independent living — particularly when the institutional admission is inappropriate or is continued longer than is necessary. This possible effect of institutional living must be considered when placing head injured young adults in nursing homes. In addition to reducing autonomy, large institutions can be impersonal and dehumanizing.

Institutional placement is, of course, appropriate during the period of acute care and early medical rehabilitation. Institutions can provide specialized treatment modalities and can support those patients with no functional skills. Later in recovery, if institutional placement is necessary, the facility should make possible a degree of independence and self-determination consistent with the client's cognitive and physical abilities, even if this requires deviation from standard institutional routines.

Transitional/Institutional Settings

In recent years, a new type of institutional setting has been developed. Given the long, tedious aspects of rehabilitation for some head injured individuals, transitional ranch/farm programs have been developed (NHIF, 1983). These facilities are often located in a rural setting and are communal in nature. Many have garden or ranch-type employment opportunities available on the grounds which help to sustain the facility.

On the positive side, transitional settings provide a comprehensive therapeutic milieu and a consistent program. Any aberrant behavior occurs within a supportive setting and residents are free to progress in the rehabilitation process at their own pace.

On the other hand, these settings can communicate a negative message to the community at large. To the lay person, they represent an isolated environment that can generate fear, misunderstanding, or stereotyping of the residents. Inaccurate inferences about the disabling condition are easily drawn by the public and may make actual community re-entry more difficult.

For entry into these facilities, individuals should have some basic skills in grooming, dressing, light housekeeping, simple laundry, and facility mobility. Usually these programs are best suited for head injured clients with mild physical disabilities and moderate cognitive or behavioral deficits.

Domiciliary Care Facilities

Domiciliary care is a recently developed independent living setting best described as a foster home. In this arrangement, families are contracted, usually by a state run agency, to host a disabled individual in their home. The family provides care and supervision, and in return is paid a monthly stipend from the state or local government. Although clients have more privacy and control than in an institution, they are still a guest in someone else's home. Choice is often limited to family wishes and independent opportunities are minimized.

Usually the required skills for "dom care" placement include basic independence in grooming, dressing, feeding, light housekeeping, toileting, bathing, simple money management, and community mobility. Appropriate referrals include those individuals with mild physical disabilities (or moderate if there are no architectural barriers) and moderate cognitive deficits.

For the appropriate population, domiciliary care homes can serve a useful purpose in the independent living continuum. They offer the security of a supportive family, enhance social interaction in the home and community, and help guide and improve personal care habits (Thompson, 1979).

For the individual who has moved beyond these areas of need, however, domiciliary care home can be too protective. It is important that the rehabilitation specialist or advocate recognize the point at which the individual needs a more challenging setting to develop independent living skills and abilities.

Group Homes

In this setting, most often eight disabled individuals share a home that is staffed and supervised by a support agency. Live-in house parents are on site 24 hours per day and the overall emphasis is on teaching and/or maintaining maximum life skills. In group homes, residents participate in decisions and are given opportunities to be independent, but the house parents and staff oversee or are aware of all activities.

Group homes have become popular as a result of the attempt in most states to reduce the number of people in residential institutions. They offer a secure setting and give the residents the opportunity to develop social and domestic life skills at their own pace. They offer much more privacy than institutions and make possible careful monitoring of the individual's re-entry into the community.

Again, as with all of the settings on the continuum, professionals must identify those individuals who have grown beyond the supports of group homes and give them the choice of more independent settings. Group homes are protective settings and have certain stereotypes in the community. In recent years, many communities have reacted negatively to the group home concept and have opposed their development through zoning laws (Thompson, 1979). Rehabilitation specialists must be aware of the undesirable image that group homes can project and should develop them in close cooperation with community leaders.

Individuals considered for group home placement should have basic skills in the following areas: cooking, toileting, bathing, grooming, cleaning, simple money management, laundry, community mobility, dressing, and feeding. Group homes can usually accommodate individuals with mild physical disabilities (or moderate if there are no architectural barriers) and moderate to severe cognitive deficits. In group homes, clients are supervised by staff who have had training and experience in dealing with head injured individuals with severe cognitive deficits. However, in domiciliary care facilities the family does not usually have the expertise to work with individuals who are severely cognitively impaired.

Supervised Apartments

With supervised apartments, typically a support agency leases a number of apartments in a housing development and places a live-in, full-time staff member in one of the apartments. This individual oversees the program and supervises a staff of scheduled employees who provide support services to the residents. Support services can be as intensive as needed, from case management to attendant care. Generally two or three residents live in each apartment which are scattered around the complex (Laurie, 1977). Although the residents have regular staff support, they can be on their own during the sleeping hours. In these cases, however, either an emergency beeper or call system is installed or an overnight awake staff member is available.

As the first setting on the independent living continuum that integrates and disperses the disabled individual into the residential community, supervised apartments offer a large step toward community perception of independence. Since staff do not live with the residents, it is possible for other community members to see them as independent. In a supportive way, the residents are given direct exposure to the community.

The supervised apartment approach also has drawbacks. There is often considerable risk involved in allowing residents to be alone at all times. Residents with impaired judgment or other cognitive deficits may make poor decisions and inappropriate behavior may jeopardize neighborhood relations and may be dangerous to the resident.

Individual skills usually associated with supervised apartments include familiarity with money management and the basic ability to manage supports, including attendant care, homemaker/chore support, and transportation. For individuals who lack some of these skills, an agency-sponsored independent living counselor can assist in the basic management of needed supports.

Appropriate referrals to supervised apartments would include head injured individuals with mild, moderate, or severe physical disabilities and mild to moderate cognitive deficits. Again, for individuals with severe cognitive limitations, an independent living counselor would be necessary.

Transitional Apartments

This setting also uses apartments, but in this case staff do not live on the premises. Rather, an agency-supported independent living counselor oversees services and supports on a scheduled basis to a number of residents who live essentially on their own in an apartment complex. As in the supervised apartment format, services can be as intensive as needed. In both the supervised and transitional settings, the agency can hold the apartment lease. However, it is much more normal to have the lease in the name of the resident.

A primary benefit of the transitional setting is that it allows the residents to demonstrate that they can live independently, with the support of the independent living counselor's scheduled visits. As residents demonstrate to their families, support agency, and themselves that they can be independent, confidence and honest acceptance can follow.

Transitional living is the first setting on the independent living continuum in which residents are truly on their own. Although there is an independent living counselor who makes scheduled visits to assist and evaluate progress, residents have extended periods during which they are in full control of their lives. From a rehabilitation point of view and in light of residual judgment problems, this step in the progression should be approached with caution. One only needs to think back to the first "on my own" experience to appreciate the potential dilemmas that can arise. Residents may feel that they can handle a situation — and under supervision may have demonstrated the necessary abilities — but when confronted on their own with the challenge, they may panic or take the situation too lightly.

As stated earlier, central to the concept of independent living is the right to take risks and to fail. It is at the level of transitional living where this right may be put to the test. This level naturally causes great concern to rehabilitation professionals and families alike. They want the client to move forward and recognize that this entails risk, but at the same time they do not want him or her to fail or get hurt.

Occasionally, clients at the transitional living stage attempt to exert their independence beyond the support staff or families. They feel that they can accomplish everything independently and need no help. They may want to be left alone and feel that their lifestyle is their own business. This push to be independent before one is ready can lead to poor choices.

Because of these potential difficulties, it is important that clients selected for transitional living programs have the ability and judgment to manage their supports, including attendant care, homemaker/chore support, money management, and transportation, and to utilize the services of an independent living counselor. As with supervised apartments, individuals with mild, moderate, or severe physical disabilities could be appropriate for transitional apartments. However, a thorough cognitive assessment must assure that the individual has the judgment and problem-solving abilities to make sound decisions.

Independent Living

As the most independent of situations, this setting has no generic definition. Rather, each setting is defined by the disabled person based on individual needs. Here the individual is in total control of the setting, and all necessary supports are self-managed. Again, as in the transitional phase, a good assessment and a firm sense of readiness for the independent life are essential. At this level individuals are truly on their own. Head injured clients who have progressed to this level must be ready not only to make basic life decisions, but they must also take responsibility for any compensatory needs dictated by their condition, e.g., using compensatory strategies and supervising personal care attendants and/or homemaker support. Along with apartments, options for independent living include a condominium, mobile home, return to the individual's private home, or any type of dwelling that may be appropriate or available.

Family Homes

Returning to one's family home is often the goal of independent living rehabilitation. For many clients, the family offers the most natural of settings and can have a positive influence on recovery.

Prior to discharge, however, the rehabilitation specialist must ensure that the client is ready to return home and that the appropriate support systems are available to the family. Often it is simply assumed that the family will readily adapt to changes in the client's behavior and new demands on their time and energy. In a recent study, however, Jacobs (1985) found that most of the returning head injured individuals could not resume work or school and were dependent upon others for many aspects of care, for financial support, and for securing resources outside the home. These demands seriously taxed the families capabilities and in some cases caused a severe family breakdown. During the months that a severely head injured person is away from home, it is likely that the family has adopted a new pattern in dealing with day-in, day-out demands, including new coping procedures and redefined roles within the family. When the injured family member returns to this revised and still fragile system needing care and behaving in ways that may be embarrassing and incomprehensible to the family, the effects on the family may be profound.

If the family is to be a viable stage in the continuum of independent living settings, the rehabilitation specialist must clearly identify needs and ensure that the necessary supports are available. The supports discussed later in this chapter can be understood as supports for families as well as for clients. It must not be assumed that families can handle or arrange for the needs of their returning loved one without assistance. Although families are a tremendous resource, they are often so emotionally involved that they have difficulty perceiving their situation objectively and making the best decisions.

INDEPENDENT LIVING SUPPORTS

Independent living supports are those services that are essential to successful community re-entry. Even though the settings may differ, supports can provide the necessary stabilization.

Two fundamental questions face the provider of independent living supports: (a) Should the supports be self-managed or managed by a case worker? and (b) should the orientation of the supports be medical or social? The definition of independent living as control over one's life based on choice of acceptable options implies that disabled individuals should, if possible, choose which supports are necessary and manage those supports. Autonomy and self-control are central to the concept of independent living.

Many head injured individuals, however, have significant cognitive deficits that impair their ability to make decisions. In these cases, someone else must manage the necessary supports. The decision between self-management and case management is complex and involves many factors. It must, however, be based on the principle of consumer control over decisions, combined with a caution against setting an unprepared client up for failure.

At the present time, the majority of community re-entry and independent living services for head injured clients emanate from medically oriented support systems. In a recent national survey (Condeluci, Fawber & Gretz-Lasky, 1986) it was found that 61 percent of the independent living programs surveyed have a physician on their team and 56 percent have nurses as active members of the team. These data suggest that the majority of respondents to this survey feel that they need to provide medically oriented case management. It could be, on the other hand, that these respondents simply feel that an element of security and safety is added when medical supports are directly attached to the program.

A pure definition of independent living, consistent with Wolfensberger's normalization principle, supports a more socially oriented management model in the independent living stage of the rehabilitation process (DeLoach et al., 1983). The medical orientation is treatment oriented and is based on a physician's prescription of treatment services (Hahn, 1985); consequently, the injured individual may have little control over the services. Conversely, the social orientation is consumer driven and all program activity is driven by the client. Although the identified needs of the head injured individual should determine the program orientation, the independent living approach is to strive for the most socially oriented program consistent with these needs.

After decisions are made regarding the orientation of the services (medical and social) and the responsibility for managing the services (self-management or case management), the spectrum of available services or supports must be reviewed. Regardless of who makes the decision or where the client is on the independent living continuum, there are standard supports that need to be considered. The following supports are designed to maximize independence and minimize reliance on others:

- training
- independent living counseling
- attendant services
- homemaker/chore support
- medical support
- transportation
- advocacy
- respite services

Training

This type of support can be offered in any independent living setting or in a separate facility. Clients receive training in areas that include both the "hard" life skills (e.g., domestic skills, money management, meal preparation) and "soft" life skills (e.g., self-care skills, sexuality, and communication skills). Typically, head injured clients will already have received activities of daily living (ADL) training during their rehabilitation stay. However, because the home environment may be quite different from the earlier training environment and because head injured clients have difficulty transferring skills from one setting to another, ADL training may need to be repeated.

When training is provided in the living environment — which is often the most appropriate place for the acquisition and practice of life skills — care must be taken to ensure that clients are not thereby unwittingly confined to their living setting. Being in the same place day and night is not conducive to social growth and is certainly not normal. The principle of normalization requires that disabled people have varied experiences in many community settings. All of us need change and movement to maintain a healthy perspective (Wolfensberger, 1972).

Independent Living Counseling

Sometimes referred to as case management, this support offers basic independent living supervision, monitoring, or management. For head injured individuals who lack the cognitive skills to make appropriate life decisions, the independent living counselor is essential. Depending upon need, this support can range from assistance with money management, meal planning, or other life skills, to assistance with accessing needed community resources. Independing living counseling can be offered within any setting.

Since the overall goal of independent living programs is to maximize participation of the consumer, the independent living counselor must be as consumer-oriented as possible. For many head injured individuals, supports need to be managed or at least monitored by someone else. From a theoretical point of view, this can pose a sizable challenge. Professionals have a natural inclination to make decisions for the client based on their own values and attitudes. This practice, however, can interfere with clients' growth in autonomy and self-responsibility and is clearly inconsistent with the consumer orientation of independent living services. Programs that use independent living counselors must, therefore, ensure that individuals who hold these positions represent the consumer to the best of their abilities.

Attendant Services

For the head injured client with residual physical deficits, personal attending is a key support. This service can be retained privately by the injured individuals or dispatched through a variety of home health agencies. Attendant services are direct "hands on" assistance in the personal areas (e.g., bathing, dressing, feeding, toileting) essential to independent living (DeJong & Wenker, 1979). In some cases the independent living counselor must help to manage the personal attendant.

It is interesting to note that in the national survey mentioned earlier (Condeluci, et al., 1986), only 6 percent of the independent living programs described attendant services as a gap or need for their head injured clientele despite the fact that only 39 percent of these programs reported offering classes to teach attendant service management in their life skills training program. Apparently, those who administer independent living programs for head-injured individuals need to better understand attendant care services and how they can enhance independent living options.

Homemaker/Chore Support

This refers to those household tasks that are not personal in nature but are nevertheless essential to independent living (e.g., cooking, shopping, cleaning, and other household chores). In some settings, the independent living counselor or the attendant can perform some of these tasks. However, for purposes of clarity in supports, we list homemaker/chore services separately. In many cases, the head injured person may be able to perform the chore or household tasks but only with cuing or management.

Medical Supports

For some head injured adults, the need for medical support continues throughout life. When these needs are identified, home health support can be scheduled. Like personal care and homemaker/chore supports, medical supports can be retained privately or through home health agencies. By medical supports, we mean any specialized medical or nursing services required as a result of the injury and needed on an ongoing basis. These include skilled or semi-skilled nursing tasks that are essential to health, such as respirator care, catheter irrigation, and ulcer dressings. Routine health care is not included in this category. Standard medical and dental care needs should be met by disabled individuals as anyone else would, through clinics, emergency rooms, and other community-based medical support systems.

Transportation

When clients move into any of the settings, they or rehabilitation specialists must seriously plan for transportation supports. Some settings offer transportation routinely, whereas in others it needs to be scheduled. Options include an adapted van or station wagon, or an accessible public transportation system.

Respite Services

Respite services are short-term intervention programs designed to offer residential support. Usually respite services are offered in one of two ways. One type of respite care is provided in a facility where an individual can stay for a short period of time to receive needed services. These facilities can be used if the injured individual has a medical or physical relapse that requires special attention or if the primary caretaker is not available. Usually these facilities offer all of the needed supports and are available on a per diem fee basis.

The second type of respite care is provided by staff dispatch services. A support person is sent to the injured individual's home on an hourly basis or on a short-term live-in basis. Respite services offer relief or specialized care on a temporary basis.

Advocacy

Although not directly necessary for independent living, advocacy is a service that is always associated with the independent living concept. Because disabled individuals are often subject to discrimination, there can be systemic difficulties when they attempt to re-instate themselves within the community. Architectural and attitudinal barriers can be overwhelming. In such cases, advocacy becomes essential.

Two tiers of advocacy must be distinguished. The first is advocacy for the individual in the case of discriminatory acts directed against the person. In these situations, the advocate works directly with individuals to uphold their rights through the courts or other governmental agencies such as the Human Relations Commission.

The second tier of advocacy relates to the system as a whole and targets general problems such as attitudinal and architectural barriers. Here, the advocate works through public or private sectors to change regulations, laws, or corporate practices that are discriminatory.

Both types of advocacy should be available to head injured individuals and their families. In some cases, the independent living counselor can serve as an advocate while other cases may call for a more sophisticated approach.

The Centers for Independent Living (CILs) offer a viable outlet for advocacy services. Most CILs include professionals knowledgeable about the law and rights of the disabled. They can be a valuable resource to ensure a head injured individual due process in the legal system.

PREPARATION FOR INDEPENDENT LIVING

The skills necessary to live independently are not an automatic consequence of standard physical rehabilitation programs. Rather, these skills must often be retaught to severely head injured clients. In normal development, children gradually learn independence skills from their parents — e.g., budgeting their allowance, making sure that their homework is finished, and being in by curfew. This is a gradual learning process that occurs primarily in the context in which the skills will be used and according to the individual's needs. This classic developmental process continues throughout life as new circumstances arise that require new or revised skills. For many individuals with head injury, memory deficits coupled with reduced speed of information processing make the learning and generalization of skills to new situations especially difficult. Physical deficits may further complicate this process by requiring the individual to learn new techniques for accomplishing previously learned activities of daily living.

Since learning or relearning to be independent is a lengthy and complex process for head injured clients, it is important to begin this process early in the rehabilitation program. Throughout the process, consideration must be given to the individual client's physical and cognitive skills and needs, and the treatment program should be adjusted and revised as the patient progresses. The type of intervention undertaken must also be compatible with the patient's stage of recovery (Ben-Yishay, 1980), with goals progressing from basic survival skills to more complex tasks (Panikoff, 1983). Decisions regarding treatment priorities and realistic expectations should be made by the entire treatment team including the patient and the family.

There are a variety of rehabilitation programs in which an individual with a head injury can obtain training in independent living skills. The initial skills should be taught in the early phase of rehabilitation in acute care hospitals and rehabilitation centers. Additional training is often available at independent living centers. Even more specific training may occur in actual living settings (e.g., community living arrangement [CLA] or supervised apartment). Regardless of the site, it is essential that the treatment staff include professionals with expertise in physical, behavioral, and cognitive functioning.

Ideally, the client's day is filled with nonfatiguing physical and cognitive activities interspersed with rest breaks (Long, et al., 1984). Activities should be challenging, interesting, and realistic, but at the same time designed to guarantee the client success. Initially, they should be selected from those already in the client's repertoire, that is, activities that were performed routinely prior to the injury. Whenever possible, the client should select and direct treatment activities. This not only enhances motivation, but also is part of training in self-management. If the client cannot perform an activity because of physical limitations, he or she should be encouraged to direct a caregiver in completing the task.

Brain injured individuals characteristically have difficulty generalizing skills to new situations. Therefore, it is particularly useful to determine, as soon as possible, where the individual will be living after discharge from the rehabilitation facility. Then the skills taught can be directly applicable to the discharge situation which can be simulated in the treatment setting. Even small details, such as the arrangement of clothes in the dresser, are factors to be considered in teaching skills for independent living. However, such simulation does not eliminate the need for additional assistance in transferring learned skills to the new situation.

The following are examples of skills necessary for independent living and suggestions for promoting these skills during the rehabilitation phase.

Making Choices: Throughout the day, encourage the client to make choices. Do you want apple juice or orange juice to drink? Do you want to write with a pen or pencil? Which shirt would you like to wear today? What would you like to do after supper? What could you do in therapy today to make your walking better?

Organizing and Sequencing Activities: Make use of daily activities to facilitate improved organizing. What clothes do you want to wear today? What are you going to put on first? What will you need in order to write a letter home?

Assuming Self-responsibility: Encourage the client to take responsibility for activities. What time are you going to set your alarm for?

You have therapy at 9:00 a.m. and need to wash up, get dressed, and eat breakfast, if you wish, first. What can you do to make sure that you get to your therapies on time?

As clients develop the skills necessary to be independent, they must be allowed to make decisions and to experience the outcomes of those decisions. When the outcome is not successful, staff must use the occasion to guide and teach the client rather than react punitively. For example, if clients choose to sleep late and consequently miss breakfast and are hungry by mid-morning, staff should help them to understand that if they choose to sleep late, then they will miss breakfast and may be hungry; the choice is theirs. This approach is more demanding of staff than highly regimented approaches that leave little room for client autonomy and therefore requires a conscious effort and commitment from the entire treatment team.

Cognitive deficits, if severe, significantly interfere with the learning or relearning of life skills. Consequently, special attention must be given to the methods used in teaching these skills. We will outline four useful techniques: task analysis, backward chaining, overlearning, and the use of compensatory strategies. Behavioral techniques such as reinforcement, encouragement, and immediate feedback have been used effectively in conjunction with these methods. Teaching should occur in individual or small group settings.

Task analysis is the process of breaking tasks down into small, manageable units, which helps to make the learning of a new or complex task easier (see Figure 7–2). For example, it is difficult to learn to make a complex meal. However, it is easier to learn to make one simple dish; it is easier yet to learn to make a simple dish by breaking it into individual steps. This process can also be applied to other activities. (Chapter 8 includes a more detailed discussion of task analysis.)

In *backward chaining,* the client completes the last step and receives the satisfaction of successfully completing the activity. After mastering the last step, the client is expected to complete the last two steps, and so on. The advantage of this technique is that each time an activity is presented, the client is able to complete it successfully and is therefore motivated to continue working.

It has been shown (Miller, 1980) that with extensive training and continued practice, many severely head injured clients are able to learn new tasks, although often at a slow rate. *Overlearning* involves repeating a task a sufficient number of times for it to become habitual. For example, overlearning safety procedures for crossing a street until they are habitual would enable a client to safely cross the street while at the same time carrying on a conversation. Unfortunately, there is no guarantee that a task once learned will be remembered

Structured Thinking

Task Prepare Jello

Time Constraints 1/2 hour

Materials Needed:

	✔
measuring cup (1 cup size)	☐
water	☐
1 3 ounce package of Jello	☐
1 mixing bowl	☐
1 large spoon	☐
4 individual serving dishes	☐
1 pot holder	☐

Steps Involved:

a. boil water	☐
b. turn off stove	☐
c. pour Jello into mixing bowl	☐
d. add 1 cup boiling water	☐
e. stir until Jello is dissolved	☐
f. add 1 cup cold water	☐
g. stir	☐
h. pour into serving dishes	☐
i. place Jello in refrigerator	☐
j. clean up	☐

Self-Evaluation: ______________________

____

Figure 7–2. Illustration of a structured thinking form for analyzing complex tasks into components and monitoring the completion of each component.

from day-to-day, initiated without prompting, or generalized to other settings.

Compensatory strategy development and implementation (discussed at length in Chapter 4) are crucial elements of most programs designed to teach independent living skills to head injured clients. A compensatory strategy is a deliberate, self-initiated application of a procedure in order to accomplish a desired goal otherwise difficult to accomplish because of impaired functioning (Szekeres, Ylvisaker & Holland, 1985). Not all clients, however, are suitable for strategy training. Certain prerequisites such as the ability to attend for a specified amount of time and to learn, retain, and generalize new information are assumed. In addition, for clients to become actively engaged in strategy training, they must recognize the need for using a particular strategy and be able to see the potential benefits to be derived from using it. The training and integration of strategies to facilitate independent living should begin as early as possible in the rehabilitative process. Several strategies for independent living that have been developed at our facilities and that we have used effectively with head injured clients are listed by deficit area in Table 7-1. Figures 7-2, 7-3, and 7-4 are examples of how the strategies may be implemented.

Regardless of the quality and length of the training and the motivation of the client, it may not be possible to remediate cognitive deficits or to equip the client with effective compensatory strategies. Due to the severity of their cognitive deficits, lack of judgment, and poor impulse control, some clients may require ongoing supervision for many independent living tasks.

MATCHING INDIVIDUALS TO SETTINGS AND SUPPORTS

The process of matching an individual client's physical and cognitive skills and choices, on the one hand, with the ideal setting and supports, on the other hand, is complex and difficult. This process requires the rehabilitation team, including the head injured client to be creative in putting all of the pieces together into a successful independent living arrangement. Decisions regarding living arrangements should result from discussion that includes all of the rehabilitation team members, including the client and family. Availability of services in a community may limit the options, forcing those involved to be especially creative and enterprising.

Table 7–1. Strategies for Independent Living

Deficit	**Strategy**
Memory/Orientation	Memo book for note taking; timer; alarm wrist watch; tape recorder; large wall calendar; schedule (for cleaning, medication, etc.); photographs of persons not readily identified; task-specific direction sheet; checklists; labels on closets, drawers, etc.; log book/diary; appointment book; maps with landmarks; designated places for personal items.
Attention/Concentration	Eliminate distractions (turn off TV or radio, unplug phone); cue cards in strategic locations; self-talk, e.g., "What am I supposed to be doing?"
Planning/Organizing	Pre-planning sheets (can be used to pre-plan the day's activities and reviewed with spouse, staff, etc.); structured thinking sheets detailing the materials needed and various steps required to perform a specific task (see Figure 7–2); master lists for grocery shopping, cleaning, bill paying (see Figure 7–3); time lines for accomplishing tasks.
Initiation	Written or tape-recorded messages to oneself to cue activities; pre-planned telephone call from significant other; self-talk, e.g., "At 4 o'clock I must start dinner"; environmental cues, e.g., getting ready to retire after the 11 o'clock news.
Judgment/Problem Solving	Problem-solving guide sheet (see Figure 7–4); self-questioning for alternatives and consequences; self-talk, e.g., "Slow down and think."

The case of J.N. illustrates the comprehensiveness of this process and also some of the problems commonly encountered by severely head injured clients in their attempt to succeed in living independently.

Case illustration: J.N. is a 24 year old male who was struck by a hit and run driver in April 1982. He was taken to a local

Month *May*

Monthly Bill	Date Received	Date Due	Date Paid	Check No.	Mailed
Mortgage		5/10	5/7	952	✓
Car		5/12	5/9	955	✓
Orthodontist		5/4	5/1	942	✓
Cable TV	4/28	5/10	5/7	951	✓
Credit Union		5/15	5/10	964	✓
Department Store	5/1	5/25	5/19	973	✓
Electric	5/1	5/30	5/26	975	
Telephone	5/10	5/30	5/26	976	
Water	4/20	5/15	5/10	963	✓
Insurance (Car)	4/28	5/20	5/15	970	✓
School Loan		5/10	5/7	950	✓
Dr. Smith	5/3	5/15	5/10	962	✓
Gasoline	4/20	5/14	5/10	961	✓
Misc. Bills					
Air Cond. Repair					
Book Club	5/6	5/30	5/26	977	
Mag. Sub.					
Taxes					
Car Repair	5/17	5/17	5/17		NA

Figure 7–3. Illustration of a form used as a strategy to organize and monitor bill paying.

emergency room where he was found to be responsive only to deep pain, to have multiple abrasions, a subdural hematoma, and an alcohol level of 0.275. J.N. remained comatose for 20 days. J.N. was a high school graduate and had been employed as a construction worker for 3½ years.

Six weeks after the injury, J.N. was transferred from acute care to The Rehabilitation Institute of Pittsburgh. The admission diagnosis

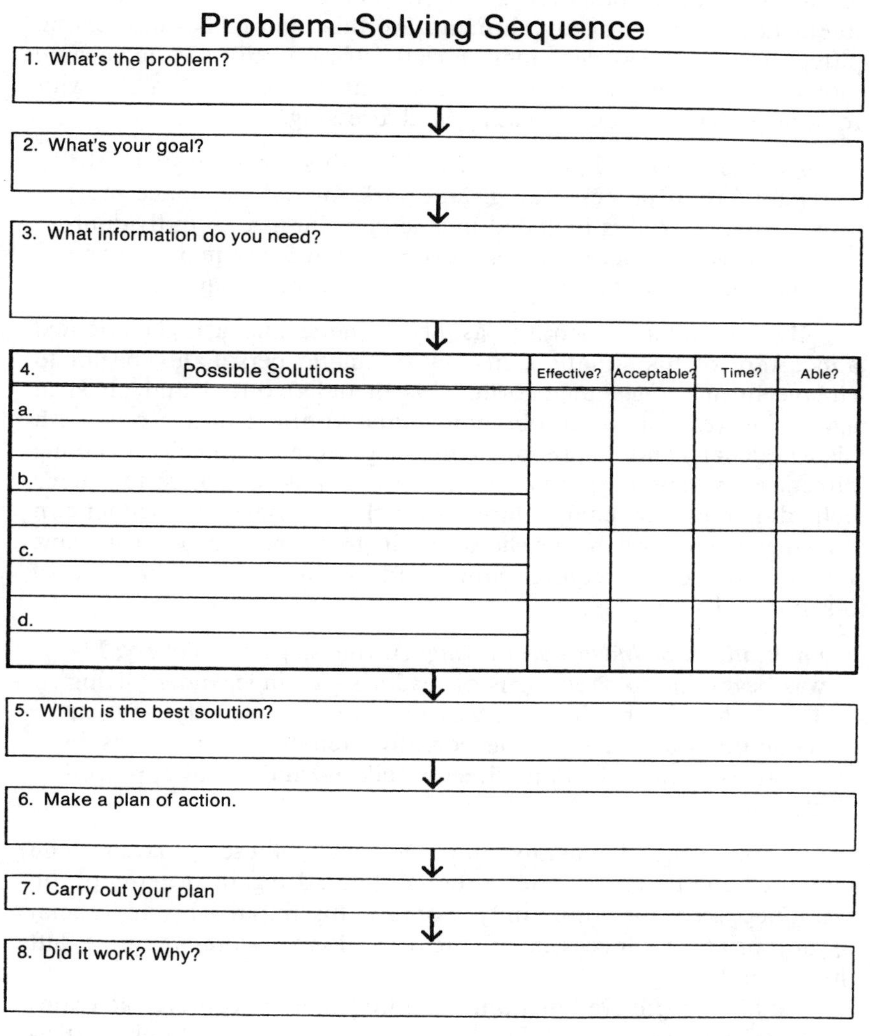

Problem–Solving Sequence

1. What's the problem?

2. What's your goal?

3. What information do you need?

4. Possible Solutions	Effective?	Acceptable?	Time?	Able?
a.				
b.				
c.				
d.				

5. Which is the best solution?

6. Make a plan of action.

7. Carry out your plan

8. Did it work? Why?

Figure 7–4. Illustration of a form used to facilitate organized problem solving.

was post-traumatic encephalopathy with severe motor and cognitive dysfunction. He appeared to be functioning at level II on the Ranchos Los Amigos Scale of Cognitive Recovery (Hagen, 1981). J.N.'s initial program emphasized physical rehabilitation and sensory stimulation to improve his responsiveness to stimulation and to increase his interactions with the environment. At this time, J.N. was eating pureed food and was dependent for all self-care skills. As he became more alert and aware of his environment, he began to assist with routine activities such as eating and dressing.

> *Implications for Independent Living:* At this early stage in the rehabilitation process, the groundwork for independence must be set. For J.N. this included independent eating, an individualized dressing program, a cognitive program for sequencing and organizing, and an individualized grooming program.

By 5 months post-injury, as J.N. became increasingly oriented and aware of his situation, his pre-traumatic personality began to emerge in an exaggerated form. This included verbal and physical aggression (e.g., shouting obscenities and running into people with his wheelchair) and inappropriate dressing. He had difficulty accepting direction or limitations imposed by others. His resistance to other's help did, however, enable him to quickly become independent in dressing, except for tying his shoes, and in grooming, except for shaving. J.N. continued to require cuing and assistance for the rest of his life skills.

> *Implications for Independent Living:* At this stage of recovery, J.N. was beginning to show signs of readiness for independent living. The focus of rehabilitation was therefore to intensify physical rehabilitation and continue cognitive rehabilitation efforts in the areas of organization, direction taking, and social appropriateness.

While J.N.'s behaviors improved with these programs, he remained emotionally labile. Although he had regained many of the skills necessary for community mobility, his impulsivity and social inappropriateness necessitated the use of an escort when he left the grounds.

As J.N.'s cognitive functioning improved, more complex activities were gradually introduced. J.N. loved to eat and thus willingly participated in the planning and preparation of simple meals. He became more appropriate in the community when he recognized that this was the key to his leaving the grounds unescorted. Since J.N.'s expectation was eventually to return to his mother's home, he did not see the need for, and was unwilling to participate in, other less interesting activities necessary for independent living. Such activities included: setting his alarm clock, monitoring his medication, managing money, writing checks, doing laundry, and general housecleaning. While J.N. had the potential to live independently, his impulsivity and lack of motivation interfered with his relearning of the necessary skills.

As the time for discharge approached, J.N.'s family indicated that it would not be possible for him to return home; an alternative setting had to be found. J.N. was functioning between levels VII and VIII of the Ranchos Los Amigos Scale of Cognitive Recovery (Hagen, 1981). He was able to walk with a cane and was independent in dressing and hygiene, except for shaving. Cognitively, he was well oriented, but continued to demonstrate poor judgment, impulsivity, and social inappropriateness. The combination of these deficits resulted in frequent shouting matches with his mother and other clients, and in temper tantrums which included overturning furniture and throwing objects.

> *Implications for Independent Living:* At this point, the process of determining settings and supports was crucial to J.N.'s continued progress. Given his physical functioning, no specific modifications to an apartment were necessary. The critical factors, however, were J.N.'s behavior and his need for additional training in independent living. Because United Cerebral Palsy's (UCP) independent living program addressed these two issues, it was selected as the most appropriate setting in which to advance J.N.'s rehabilitation.

In January 1983 (9 months post-injury), J.N. was enrolled in United Cerebral Palsy's Independent Living Rehabilitation Program for day program and in the Shaler Highlands Head Injured Community Living Arrangements (CLA) residential program. He reported that all of the classes that he attended within the Independent Living Rehabilitation Program were meaningless for him except his individual counseling. J.N.'s general attitude was one of disinterest and lack of concern for others. He made fun of instructors and clients, and was generally unsympathetic to others with disabilities. He wore excessive jewelry, head bands, and arm bands. In the CLA, he displayed similar behavior. His roomate was physically disabled and had minimal cognitive deficits. J.N. again made negative comments (supposedly jokes) about the disabilities of his roommate and other clients in that program. He often made racial comments towards staff members. He frequently screamed and swore at the woman who worked directly with him and occasionally threw things at her. These behaviors generally occurred when he was confronted with issues that were problems for him, such as budgeting, housekeeping chores, or his negative comments towards others.

Implications for Independent Living: Given the change in his environment from the Rehabilitation Institute of Pittsburgh to United Cerebral Palsy, some disruption was expected. The important independent living focus was to lessen the disruption through courses and counseling sessions at UCP where he could vent his concerns. The appearance issues were addressed to help J.N. understand how his attire could affect the way people treated him. Also at this point, plans were initiated to assess J.N.'s vocational potential. Self-esteem is often tied to one's vocational identity, and with J.N., the return to work was a very important goal.

By mid-term J.N. was learnng to control his behavior. He looked forward to his individual counseling sessions in which he was able to express himself openly. This was also an opportunity to deal with issues such as his disruptive behaviors in class and in the CLA, his appearance, and his general attitude toward placement at United Cerebral Palsy. J.N. was living in the CLA and taking classes oriented toward increasing his independence. His behaviors and appearance had improved, but his lack of motivation continued to interfere with his ability to live independently.

In September 1983, J.N. was scheduled for the same courses because of his previous lack of participation. He was also referred to the Vocational Rehabilitation Center's (VRC) Head Trauma Program for a vocational evaluation. As he became involved in vocational rehabilitation, J.N.'s attitude improved in all areas and he began making progress in his classes at UCP. In the CLA, he had moved in with another roommate who was less physically involved than his first roommate but had more cognitive deficits. Initially, the two young men got along well. However, after 3 months, very serious problems arose between the two, eventually resulting in another move for J.N. Again, the behaviors exhibited were excessive use of profanity, loud screaming, insults directed toward the roommate because of his disability, and, on occasion, physical confrontation.

Implications for Independent Living: This new setback necessitated a change in environment as J.N. was not ready for a roommate relationship. After agreement with all parties including J.N., he moved into a two-bedroom apartment alone. A plan was devised to attempt to lessen the effects of this renewed disruptive behavior. In addition, his day program staff and staff providing residential support continued efforts to assist J.N. in social appropriateness and appearance.

After 3 months of training at VRC, J.N. was placed in the extended employment workshop in that program. He is presently waiting for a job placement at the Easter Seals Society. Until such time, he will continue in the extended employment program at the Vocational Rehabilitation Center and will continue to take classes at United Cerebral Palsy. As J.N. has become more confident of himself and his future, he has made additional social gains. He made a good friend at UCP and invited this fellow to move in with him. He has joined a spa and works out 2 days per week. His disposition is much more even tempered and he is developing more refined social skills.

In the 2½ years since his accident, J.N.'s rehabilitation program has been complex and intensive. The program began in the acute care hospital and continued through his stay in a rehabilitation center, a CLA with classes at UCP, and now a supervised apartment with involvement with VRC. His rehabilitation program is not yet complete — the goal is for J.N. to some day live independently. Throughout his program, the health care professionals working with J.N. strived to help him to be as independent as possible. This necessitated periodic reassessment of J.N.'s status and, when appropriate, revision of his program. At each juncture, the team, which included J.N., reviewed the reassessment findings and determined the most appropriate setting and supports.

When determining the setting for an independent living arrangement, more than the specific house or apartment should be considered. As much as possible, the individual should be able to integrate into and have access to the surrounding community. Factors including curb cuts for wheelchairs, specialized public transportation, assistance in grocery stores, neighbors who are understanding, and community recreation programs are important in allowing the individual to participate fully in community life.

In establishing an independent living arrangement, it must be remembered that this will probably not be a life-long arrangement. Most adults live in several apartments and/or houses during their lifetime. So, too, individuals with head injury may choose to live in several settings. In addition, the skills and needs of the individuals may change over time, necessitating changes in the supports and setting so as to allow them to be as independent as possible.

Table 7–2 provides guidelines and suggestions for matching individuals to appropriate independent living settings and supports. The categories are broad and, in addition, an individual might fit into two or more categories, for example, mild physical disability, mild-to-moderate visual impairment, and moderate cognitive deficits. In all cases, therefore, the suggested settings and supports should be used only as guidelines which must be customized to meet individual needs and desires.

FUTURE DIRECTIONS

Independent living as a component of rehabilitation for head injured individuals is at an interesting juncture. After years of focus on the development of quality trauma centers and medical rehabilitation services, professionals are now confronted with questions associated with long-term supports. Families who have advocated specialty services within the medical and rehabilitation systems often find their head injured family member back at home (Jacobs, 1985). Their loved one may have regained many physical abilities but, because of residual cognitive and psychosocial deficits, must now shape a new life. These families need new options and independent living may offer a solution.

The national survey mentioned earlier in this chapter (Condeluci et al., 1986) polled the 265 programs listed in the National Head Injury Foundation (1983) Directory to determine what independent living and vocational rehabilitation programs for head injured individuals exist at the present time and to expose gaps in the service delivery system as perceived by rehabilitation professionals. This survey offers some interesting perspectives on future directions for independent living for head injured individuals. Of the 265 programs, 36 percent responded. To ascertain future needs, the survey asked the following questions:

- What services would you like to offer in addition to your current head injury programs?
- What is preventing your facility from offering the head injury services previously mentioned?
- Please identify and rank order the gaps you perceive?

Forty-six percent of the independent living respondents indicated that they would like to offer supervised apartments; 44 percent would like to conduct group homes; and 39 percent stated that

Table 7–2. Guidelines for Matching Individuals to Settings and Supports.

Disability	Functional Implications	Adaptations/Support	Setting Alternatives
Physical Disability: Mild	Ambulatory with or without brace, cane, etc. May be slightly unsteady in walking. Can ascend/descend steps. Mild difficulty/incoordination of hands/arms. Some difficulty with fine motor activities.	Adaptations: • Railing on stairs, grab bars in shower. • Push button appliances. Enlarged phone dial. Modified knobs and handles. Support: • Little or no support services other than initial training with and maintenance of brace, cane, etc.	Full range of alternatives. Close Proximity to transportation in order to limit distance of ambulation. May prefer: building with elevator or single level building, undercover parking.
Physical Disability: Moderate	Ambulatory with devices (walker, cane, braces). Unable to ascend/descend steps. Moderate difficulty with hands/arms. May have use of only one arm. Decreased coordination.	Adaptations: • Ramps, elevators, hand railings. • Possibly: automobile with hand controls. • Bathroom with grab bars, possibly: shower chair, raised commode seat. • Adaptive equipment and/or minor kitchen adaptations.	Any setting without steps or with appropriate modifications, e.g., ramps, elevators (including independent setting, transitional apartment, supervised apartment, group home, or domiciliary care). Undercover parking.

(continued)

Table 7-2 *(continued)*

Disability	Functional Implications	Adaptations/Supports	Setting Alternatives
Physical disability Moderate *(continued)*		• Adaptations to clothing and shoes. Support: • Training for mobility, safety in transfers, use of adaptive techniques for activities of daily living. • Possibly: homemaker/chore support attendant care.	Additional requirements of setting: • Close proximity to public transportation in order to limit distance of ambulation. • Availability of homemaker/chore support and attendants • Availability of emergency medical assistance.
Physical Disability: Severe	Non-ambulatory, uses manual or electric wheelchair. Significant deficits in function of arms/hands; minimal function.	Adaptations: • Wheelchair accessible housing including ramps, elevators, wide doorways, electric doors, accessible bathrooms. • Wheelchair with customized seat insert and possibly headrest. • Customized switch to control wheelchair. • Customized environmental control unit to access: lights,	Any setting which is wheelchair accessible and has access to appropriate public transportation (including independent setting, transitional apartment, supervised apartment, group home). Additional requirements of setting: • Availability of homemaker/chore support and attendant care.

		appliances, telephone, typewriter or computer, call button. Support: • Training in mobility and transfers of adaptive equipment and adaptive techniques. • Homemaker/chore support. • Attendant care. • Accessible public transportation. • Ongoing physical/occupational therapy or program to be carried out by attendant.	• Availablility of accessible adapted recreational opportunities. • Availability of emergency medical care.
Visual Impairment: Mild to Moderate	Perceptual deficits. Decreased visual field. Decreased visual acuity.	Adaptations: • Large dial telephone, enlarged print books, recipes, etc. Support: • Training in mobility and activities of daily living. • Development of compensatory strategies. • Independent living counselor.	Full range of settings. Additional requirements of setting: • Accessible public transportation.
Visual Impairment: Severe	Cortical blindness and/or severe visual perceptual deficits.	Adaptations: • Appliances with braille dials, reading machine, reader or talking books.	Full range of settings. Additional requirement of setting: • Availability of homemaker/ chore support and attendants.

continued

Table 7–2 *(continued*

Disability	Functional Implications	Adaptations/Supports	Setting Alternatives
Visual Impairment Severe *(continued)*		Support: • Attendant care. • Homemaker/chore support. • Training in mobility, activities of daily living. • Community resources for the blind.	Additional requirements *(cont.)* • Accessible public transportation. • Access to adapted recreation.
Auditory Impairment:	Decreased ability to process auditory information. Deaf.	Adaptations: • Adapted telephone and television. Support: • Training for mobility, lip reading, sign language.	Full range of settings with appropriate adaptations.
Cognitive Deficits: Mild	Difficulty with abstract reasoning. Mild memory deficits. Slow planning and organizing of tasks. Decreased rate of learning new information. Functional attention span. Adequate judgment in routine situations.	Adaptations: • Strategies such as appointment book and self-organizing system. Support: • Training and/or independent living counseling.	Full range of settings.

Cognitive Deficits: Moderate	Assistance and/or external cues needed for remembering appointments, chores, etc. Distractable from task by nonroutine events. Cues and external structure required to organize and initiate a multi-step activity. Judgment not reliable in any nonroutine situations, inconsistent for routine situations. Occasionally impulsive. Problem solving only with the help of someone else for supervision or cuing.	Adaptations: • Strategies such as appointment book, pre-planning sheets, and labels on closets and cupboards. • Prepared meals which only require heating. Support: • Training. • Independent living counselor. • Homemaker/chore support. • Transportation.	Transitional institutional settings, domiciliary care, group home, possibly a supervised apartment.
Cognitive Deficits: Severe	Poor orientation. Significant memory deficits. Difficulty with using strategies effectively. Cuing and supervision required for all activities. Severe limitation in ability to learn new information. Impulsive and distractible.	Adaptations: • Structured daily schedule. • Overlearning for simple tasks. • Additional time scheduled to perform tasks. • Memory and orientation cues such as: logbook, calendar, pictures of significant people. Supports: • Training. • Independent living counselor. • Homemaker/chore support. • Transportation.	Group home, possibly a transitional institutional setting.

transitional living programs are needed. Twenty-eight percent of the vocational rehabilitation professionals responded that they would like to provide supported work services, and 26 percent indicated that they wanted to add a day program to their existing head injury services. Funding was identified by 61 percent of the independent living respondents and 50 percent of the vocational rehabilitation respondents as the primary factor preventing these services from being offered.

To better understand the depth of the gaps perceived, the respondents were asked to rank program areas in order of importance (given a choice of seventeen areas). Results suggest that the types of programs most critically needed are:

1. supervised apartment programs for persons without insurance funding;
2. programs that accept clients with severe behavioral disorders; and
3. transitional (supported) employment programs.

Despite gains over the past decade, current programs and services are not adequate to meet existing needs. Professionals and planners must learn more about the specialty described in this chapter. Careful analysis of the services offered to other disability groups yields information and guidelines that can then be adapted and tailored for head injured clients.

So, where does one go? How are programs developed for people who often lack adequate financial support? Finding an answer to these questions is not easy, but answers must be consistent with the independent living philosophy outlined earlier in this chapter. Services for head injured individuals must become a sociopolitical issue. In order to accomplish this, individuals with head injury and their advocates must function as a viable political group and appropriate services must be seen as both politically prudent and socially correct (see Hahn, 1985).

In many cases long-term independent living programs need not be medical; the key supports for long-term independent living programs are independent living counseling and attendant services. Many states are presently looking to develop publicly funded community based programs and services. In 1984 the Commonwealth of Pennsylvania established a $4 million attendant services program. Although it does not address all the needs that can be associated with head injury, it does offer a start. Other states have developed programs in conjunction with their aging or welfare departments that offer community-based case management, homemaker/chore support, and attendant services. Since 1978, California has offered attendant services funded under Title XX of the Social Security Act. In 1985 the State of New Jersey expanded its Office of Mental Retardation to an Office of Developmental Disabilities and redefined developmental disability as any injury or illness acquired from birth to age 55 that affects life functions.

On the federal level, Senator John Chafee (RI) introduced in 1984 a bill that, for the first time, proposed the use of federal funds to create community-based services for disabled and elderly persons in need. Presently, billions of federal dollars (Title XIX of the Social Security Act) go to provide support services to disabled and elderly persons, but only if they reside in intermediate care or skilled nursing facilities. Senator Chafee's proposal would, in effect, eliminate the bias toward institutional settings and place community-based settings on an equal footing. The bill was not passed by Congress in 1984, but Senator Chafee has continued the fight for community-based services. Although this effort does not offer all of the supports needed by head injured individuals for community living, it does provide a strong core.

In addition to these small but positive steps toward developing less costly community-based programs, there is some reason to be optimistic about the availability of housing for independent living programs. To develop supervised living, transitional living, or independent living programs, one needs suitable housing. In many cases, using existing apartments is a reasonable and cost-effective alternative to building new housing. In Pittsburgh, United Cerebral Palsy has initiated a variety of independent living programs using preexisting apartments. By using apartments, this agency has avoided community objections and zoning problems often associated with institutions or group homes. Indeed, landlords who own or manage large unit projects often prefer to lease a block of apartments to agencies that then assist in the management of these apartments. Among other programs, UCP offers a cluster living arrangement in which four two-bedroom apartments are rented for head injured individuals. A live-in staff supervisor also resides at the apartment site. Therefore, necessary staff support is close enough to provide immediate assistance, yet the residents have their own apartments and privacy. UCP of Pittsburgh has also found that apartments lend themselves to easy architectural renovations to remove physical barriers. In 12 years of experience with this independent living program, the agency has had no major problems with communities or landlords.

Innovative programs, improvements in government funding, and pending legislation all point to a better future. It is the responsibility of rehabilitation specialists to demonstrate that community-based living arrangements and long-term supports can be successful and cost effective for head injured clients. We need to learn from experiences with other disability groups. Over the past 15 years, community-based programs serving the developmentally disabled have been found to be cost effective.

In 1985 a study was conducted by the Pennsylvania Association of Residential Facilities to ascertain the cost comparison between institutional programs and community living arrangements for mentally retarded individuals in Pennsylvania. This study found, on a basic comparison of residents' needs, that Community Living Arrangements cost, on an average, $25.50 per day per resident less than institutional care cost (Theodore Poister Associates, 1985).

Although these data are specific to the Commonwealth of Pennsylvania and are focused on programs that serve mentally retarded people, they offer some understanding of the cost differential between these two types of settings (supervised apartments/group homes versus institutions). This report shows that the most severely involved individuals are institutionalized, and the more severe the population the greater the cost. It also demonstrates vividly that in all direct comparison areas, the community-based settings are less costly than institutions. Although not all head injured individuals are appropriate for community-based settings, certainly there are individuals who have been placed in long-term institutions when it would be more cost effective (in addition to enhancing the quality of life) to have them live in less restrictive settings.

The development of independent living programs for head injured clients is challenging. It takes persistence, imagination, a knowledge of their needs, and an understanding of the community; but it can happen. There is a new awareness today of head injury and of the concept of independent living. As community-based services develop and more is learned about head injury recovery, it will be found that long-term independent living programs can work. No longer will severely brain injured persons have to be relegated to nursing homes. Nor will already burdened families have to be overburdened.

Independent living programs for head injured individuals offer viable solutions to complex problems. They provide humane alternatives to the injured persons and their families. They offer a new, less costly direction for third party vendors and state governments that are struggling with the mounting costs of health care. Most of all, however, independent living programs offer dignity to the person with a head injury. To live in a setting where one has choices among acceptable options and can exercise these choices to the best of one's ability is a fundamental right.

REFERENCES

Ben-Yishay, Y. (1980). Rehabilitating the severely head injured individual: Plain answers to complicated questions. In *Working approaches to remediation of cognitive deficits in brain damanged persons* (Rehabilitation Monograph No. 61, pp. 1–55). New York: New York University Medical Center, Institute of Rehabilitation Medicine.

Bond, M. R. (1983). Standardized methods of assessing and predicting outcome. In M. Rosenthal, E. Griffith, M. Bond & J. D. Miller (Eds.), *Rehabilitation of the head injured adult* (pp. 97–113). Philadelphia: F. A. Davis.

Brigance, A. (1981). *Inventory of essential skills.* North Billerica, MA: Curriculum Assoc.

Cole, J. (1979). What's new about independent living? *Archives of Physical Medicine Rehabilitation, 60,* 458–462.

Condeluci, A. (1979, March). *Continuum of independent living options.* Paper presented at the meeting of Handicapped Technical Assistance Project, Milwaukee, WI.

Condeluci, A., Fawber, H. & Gretz-Lasky, S. (1986, Winter). A national survey: The need for long term independent living/vocational rehabilitation services. *National Head Injury Foundation Newsletter.*

DeJong, G. (1979). Independent living: From social movement to analytic paradigm. *Archives of Physical Medicine Rehabilitation, 60,* 435–456.

DeJong, G. & Wenker, T. (1979). Attendant care as a protype independent living service. *Archives of Physical Medicine Rehabilitation, 60,* 468–475.

DeLoach, C., Wilkins, R. & Walker, G. (1983). *Independent living: Philosophy, process and services.* Baltimore, MD: University Park Press.

Ducker, C. (1983). *A comprehensive approach to the long term rehabilitation center.* Unpublished manuscript.

Fordyce, D. J., Roueche, J. R. & Prigatano, G. (1983). Enhanced emotional reactions in chronic head trauma patients. *Journal of Neurology, Neurosurgery and Psychiatry, 46,* 620–624.

Foster, R. (1976). *Camelot behavioral checklist.* Lawrence, KS: Foster Assoc.

Hagen, C. (1981). Language disorders secondary to closed head injury: Diagnosis and treatment. *Topics in Language Disorders, 1,* 73–78.

Hahn, H. (1985). Toward a politics of disability definitions, disciplines, and policies. *The Social Science Journal, 22,* 89–103.

Jacobs, H. (1985). *The family as a therapeutic agent: Long term rehabilitation for traumatic head injury patients.* Manuscript submitted to publication.

Jennett, B. (1983). Post-traumatic epilepsy. In M. Rosenthal, E. Griffith, M. Bond & J. D. Miller (Eds.), *Rehabilitation of the head injured adult* (pp. 119–124). Philadelphia: F. A. Davis.

Jennett, G. (1984). The measurement of outcome. In N. Brooks (Ed.), *Closed head injury: Psychological, social and family consequences* (pp. 37–43). Oxford: Oxford University Press.

Laurie, G. (1977). *Housing and home services for the disabled.* New York: Harper & Row.

Long, C. H., Gouvier, W. D. & Cole, J. C. (1984). A model of recovery for the total rehabilitation of individuals with head trauma. *Journal of Rehabilitation, 50*(1), 39–45.

Miller, E. (1980). The training characteristics of severely head-injured patients: A preliminary study. *Journal of Neurology, Neurosurgery, and Psychiatry, 43,* 525–528.

National Head Injury Foundation. (1983). *National directory of head injury rehabilitation services.* Framingham, MA.

Oddy, M., Coughlan, T., Tyerman, A. & Jenkins, D. (1985). Social adjustment after closed head injury: A further follow-up seven years after injury. *Journal of Neurology, Neurosurgery, and Psychiatry, 48,* 564–568.

Panikoff, L. (1983). Recovery trends of functional skills in the head-injured adult. *The American Journal of Occupational Therapy, 37*(11), 735–743.

Pfluger, S. (1979). *Independent living.* Washington, DC: Institute of Research Utilization.

Prigatano, G. P., Fordyce, D. J., Zeiner, H. K., Roueche, J. R., Pepping, M. & Wood, B. C. (1984). Neuropsychological rehabilitation after closed head injury in young adults. *Journal of Neurology, Neurosurgery, and Psychiatry, 47,* 505–513.

Sands, H. & Minters, F. C. (1979). *The epilepsy fact book.* Philadelphia: F. A. Davis.

Schwab, L. (1981). *Independent living assessments for persons with disabilities.* Lincoln, NE: Department of Human Development & the Family Nebraska Agricultural Experiment Station.

Staff. (1985, Sept.). Independent living issue. *Disability Rag,* p. 11. Louisville, KY: Advocado Press.

Szekeres, S., Ylvisaker, M. & Holland, A. L. (1985). Cognitive rehabilitation therapy: A framework for intervention. In M. Ylvisaker (Ed.), *Head injury rehabilitation: Children and adolescents* (pp. 219–246). San Diego: College-Hill Press.

Theodore Poister Associates. (1985). *A cost function analysis of private residential services for mentally retarded persons in the Commonwealth of PA.* Bellefonte, PA.

Thompson, M. M. (1979). *Housing for the handicapped and disabled.* Washington, DC: National Association of Housing and Redevelopment Officials.

Wahlstrom, P. E. (1983). Occupational therapy evaluation. In M. Rosenthal, E. Griffith, M. Bond & J. D. Miller (Eds.). *Rehabilitation of the head injured adult* (pp. 271–278). Philadelphia: F. A. Davis.

Walls, R., Zane, T. & Thuedt, J. (1979). *Independent living behavioral checklist.* Morgantown, WV: West Virginia Rehabilitation Research & Training Center.

Wolfensberger, W. (1972). *The principle of normalization in human services.* Toronto, Canada: National Institute of Mental Retardation.

Wolfensberger, W. & Thomas, S. (1983). *Passing.* Toronto, Canada: National Institute of Mental Retardation.

Woosley, T., Harden, R. & Murphy, P. (1984). *National independent living skills project.* Talladega, AL: Alabama Institute for Deaf and Blind.

CHAPTER 8

Avocational Programming for the Severely Impaired Head Injured Individual

Eva Marie R. Gobble
Lucille Dunson
Shirley F. Szekeres
Jacquelin Cornwall

Individuals who have severe and multiple handicaps as a result of traumatic brain injury may have no meaningful vocational options, even with the comprehensive vocational services described in Chapters 5 and 6. Following diffuse brain damage, characteristic of severe closed head injury, a combination of physical, cognitive, and behavioral factors often interfere not only with employment but also with recreational possibilities and even self-care and other activities of daily living (Bond, 1975; Bruckner & Randle, 1972; Gilchrist & Wilkinson, 1979; Lezak, 1978; Thomsen, 1984). In this chapter we discuss treatment for these significantly impaired individuals who need and deserve rehabilitative services to advance their pursuit of meaningful and satisfying career alternatives that can be a viable substitute for vocational activity. In this context, we use the term "career" broadly to include academic, vocational, avocational, familial, and civic roles (Super, 1976).

Severely injured patients may be impaired in any or all of the aspects of cognition outlined in Chapter 3. Particularly noteworthy are deficits in the areas of attention, memory and learning, organization, reasoning, problem solving, judgment, and "executive functioning" (goal setting, planning, self-directing, self-initiating and inhibiting, self-monitoring, and self-evaluating) (Gloag, 1985). Individuals with very severe cognitive deficits may remain indefinitely in a state of post-traumatic amnesia, that is, disoriented to some degree to person, place, and time, and unable to recall events effectively from day to day. Others may be adequately oriented in a highly structured and familiar environment, but may easily lose that orientation and become confused and inappropriate in a novel or stressful environment.

Physical impairments (e.g., neuromuscular problems such as hemiplegia, tremors, and incoordination; sensory deficits; seizures; and other physical complications described in Chapter 2), if present, further restrict the patient's range of activities by limiting mobility, endurance, dexterity, and sensory functions. Furthermore, physical and cognitive problems do not combine in a simple additive manner but rather interact to exaggerate their effects. For example, individuals with limited attentional "space" (impaired working memory) have further reduced cognitive capacity if some of that "space" in working memory is occupied by an effort to maintain balance or control a tremor. Conversely, sensory deficits are exaggerated in their functional effects if the client lacks the cognitive skill to capitalize on intact sensory modalities or to compensate for the sensory weakness by deliberately doing whatever is possible to maximize the residual sensory function.

These disabilities create obstacles to finding meaning in life — obstacles that are not easily overcome by time or by rehabilitative efforts (Panting & Merry, 1972). Too often the tragic outcome is a life of inactivity and consequent anger and depression (Lezak, 1978). Family members may attempt to create meaningful activity and entertainment for their loved one, but then frequently suffer the stress and frustration that results from their predictable failure to make possible those kinds of activity that the injured person would find truly satisfying (Brooks, 1984; Oddy, Humphrey & Uttley, 1978; Romano, 1974; Rosenbaum & Najenson, 1976). Many families state on follow-up that their primary need is for help in finding or developing constructive and satisfying leisure-time activities for their disabled family member (Karpman, Wolfe & Vargo, 1986).

Interactive problems, disinhibition, and impulsive and inappropriate behavior contribute to social isolation and feelings of hopelessness and depression (Bond, 1975; Lezak, 1978). Egocentricity and depressed interpersonal skills are a natural result of severe injury or illness (Shontz, 1975). Neuropathological changes may result in socially awkward or unusual behavior. Severely brain injured individuals may seem to be unaware of social rules, to act impulsively, and to communicate ineffectively.

Rehabilitation programs that purport to promote community re-entry for head injured adults must include adequate training and planning for avocational activity for these severely injured individuals. In this chapter, the word "avocational" is used to refer to those activities that promote constructive and enjoyable use of time in order to satisfy individual patient's needs (Overs, Taylor & Adkins, 1977). Recreational therapists, occupational therapists, rehabilitation counselors, cognitive rehabilitation therapists, and teachers may separately or as a team be responsible for planning avocational services. The term "avocational therapist" will be used to refer to the professional who delivers avocational programming, regardless of professional background. Ideally, the group of therapists with skills related to avocational planning will work together as a team to facilitate the most effective and efficient delivery of services.

There is a growing literature on avocational programming and leisure for various disability groups (Adams, Daniel & Rullman, 1975; Amary, 1975; Gedde, 1978; Wehman, Abramson & Norman, 1977; Wehman & Schleien, 1979). However, little has been published that addresses the specific problems and needs of severely head injured individuals. This chapter discusses some of these issues and focuses on developing avocational activity for severely impaired individuals as a career substitute for paid work. We do not address the avocational needs of those individuals whose impairments are less severe, but who may, nevertheless, require professional help in developing satisfying avocational options to complement their vocational career. By omitting less severely impaired patients from discussion, the authors do not wish to suggest that their need for a rewarding avocational life is less deserving of attention.

This discussion focuses on the following areas:

1. basic principles of avocational programming
2. avocational assessment
3. treatment planning
4. treatment techniques to facilitate development of skills
5. basic self-care and communication skills to enhance potential for integration into community-based programs and recreational facilities
6. counseling to facilitate acceptance of avocational goals and participation in avocational programming
7. community resources

BASIC PRINCIPLES OF AVOCATIONAL PROGRAMMING

Many problems encountered in other areas of rehabilitation for head injured individuals also pose obstacles to avocational programming. These include inadequate motivation on the patient's part, problems adapting equipment to meet unique needs, and funding problems. In addition, a new set of possible problems emerges with avocational rehabilitation, including (a) the patient's and family's failure to recognize the implication of deficits, which results in resistance to avocational programming; (b) the patient's lack of avocational interests; (c) lack of knowledge of community resources; or (d) lack of community resources, transportation, and accessibility.

The following general principles of treatment are derived from the avocational and rehabilitation literature (Kraus, 1973; Overs et al., 1977; Wehman et al., 1977; Wehman & Schleien, 1981; Wolfensberger, 1972) together with the authors' experience in working with head injured adults:

1. Comprehensive assessment is the key to the development and maintenance of avocational activity.
1. Modification of avocational activities reduces barriers to performance and enhances satisfaction and enjoyment.
3. Normalization and integration into a peer group should guide the modification of activities.
4. Skills needed to perform an avocational activity should be trained to proficiency to promote generalization and facilitate ease of performance.
5. Appropriate intrinsic or extrinsic reinforcement should be established to maintain the client's motivation.
6. Task analysis and skill analysis should both be used to develop a plan of therapeutic intervention.
7. Counseling services for the client and family should be provided, as needed, to promote acceptance of avocational programming and implementation of the avocational plan.

Table 8-1 presents a framework within which the basic principles of avocational programming can be successfully implemented. The framework supports a systematic approach to assessment, identification of specific avocational activities, thorough training, and generalization of activities into the community setting. This avocational programming guide can be a tool for establishing a plan of action which will provide meaningful, enjoyable activity for an individual in a setting that is as close to normal as possible.

EVALUATION

To provide a foundation for effective avocational intervention, the evaluation should include an exploration of the patient's leisure

TABLE 8–1. Avocational Programming Guide

Phase 1	Phase 2	Phase 3
Evaluation		
• Identify pre- and post-trauma leisure history • Determine family avocational interests • Determine community resources • Assess the client's interests and motivational, cognitive, physical & psychosocial status	• Establish a diagnostic profile • Generate an avocational hypothesis and tentative activities	• Provide therapy • Determine feasible avocational options
Therapeutic Intervention		
• Establish a treatment plan - specify goals and objectives - implement appropriate training procedures	• Generate a community re-entry action plan • Implement appropriate training procedures to facilitate generalization	• Follow-up in community settings • Provide necessary therapeutic intervention

history and community resources in addition to an assessment of physical, cognitive, and behavioral skills and current interests. Information from these sources allows the avocational therapist to generate a diagnostic profile which, in turn, suggests an avocational hypothesis — that is, a tentative avocational plan that is "tested" during a period of diagnostic therapy. Evaluation of the individual's skills, behavior, and interests continues throughout the treatment program so that the resulting avocational action plan best fits the needs, interests, and abilities of the individual and the resources of the family and community.

Leisure History

Because past preferences are often a good predictor of future interests (Overs et al., 1977), it is useful to explore the individual's leisure and recreational history. In most cases, interviews with the patient, family members, and close friends yield reliable information.

Families often have insight into the types of activities that are intrinsically motivating for the patient, even if he or she did not engage in the activity before the accident. Activities that were preferred pretraumatically may, with appropriate adaptation, be reasonable avocational goals.

It is equally useful to explore the family's leisure interests, the amount of time the family can devote to the patient's activities, and present social networks that may play a role in supporting his or her avocational pursuits. Overs and colleagues (1977) found that there is a strong correlation between the leisure interests of individuals and their families.

Community Resources

Because community resources have a major impact on avocational options, it is essential to determine likely discharge destinations for the patient before proceeding with avocational intervention. Community resources include organizations (e.g., YMCA, Garden Clubs, Community College, Red Cross), financial resources, and support services (e.g., National Head Injury Foundation, Center for Independent Living, self-help groups). In addition, it is important to determine if the family or significant others are available as resources to the client. Family attitudes toward disability and toward the importance of avocational pursuits strongly influence their availability as a resource, as do financial constraints. Avocational programming will have no meaningful effects if the activities that are planned cannot be afforded or are not available in the individual's community.

Practical considerations including architectural barriers, transportation, hours of operation of community facilities, supervision available, attitudes toward disabled people, and costs also need to be investigated. Everyone is familiar with leisure programs that look good when described in a brochure, but on closer examination are found to be inappropriate. Staff members in community facilities may be unable to meet the physical or behavioral needs of head injured individuals.

Patient Assessment

Careful assessment of the patient's physical, cognitive, and psychosocial strengths and weaknesses must be added to a detailed interest inventory to ground an effective treatment program. This assessment is best accomplished by a combination of consultation with other professionals (physical therapist, occupational therapist, speech-language pathologist, social worker, and psychologist) and informal activity probes. Informal probes are essential because a patient's performance in complex avocational activities may be lower than that reported during individual therapy sessions or on formal tests. Alternatively, the individual may perform at a cognitively or motorically higher level given the motivation provided by interesting activities. Consequently a variety of tasks should be used, varying in difficulty level and level of skill integration required, and performed in a variety of environments (Knapczyk, 1975).

Cognitive Functioning:

In Chapter 4, Table 4–5 lists a set of cognitive variables that influence performance of tasks and that can be graded to facilitate more successful performance. In assessing an individual's cognitive skills for avocational programming, it is useful to first determine skill levels in a natural environment without special cuing or structuring of the task. Systematically decreasing difficulty levels or processing demands by manipulating the variables listed in Table 4–5 until activities can be accomplished successfully and with relative ease suggest the type of structure and help that the individual will require in order to enjoy avocational activities. Answers to the following questions are particularly important in making decisions about appropriate activities in relation to their cognitive demands:

1. How long can the patient attend to a task and under what conditions? What are the effects of increasing environmental distractions?
2. How functional are the patient's perceptual abilities? How effectively can he or she scan the environment to locate objects and make sound safety judgements?
3. How much information can the patient hold in working memory? Can he or she use strategies like "rehearsal" to hold information longer when it serves some purpose to do so (e.g., repeat numbers while scanning a bingo card)?
4. How much of long-term memory (previously acquired knowledge and procedures) can be retrieved by the patient?
5. How efficiently can the patient learn new information and procedures (simple/complex; concrete/abstract; verbal/nonverbal)?
6. How does the patient interact with others (verbal/nonverbal; spoken/written; gesture)?

7. Can the patient understand basic language and follow instructions (simple/complex; spoken/written; gestural)?
8. How much external structure does the patient need to adequately organize behavior or materials?
9. What kind of reasoning and problem solving is the patient able to do independently (including safety judgment)?
10. To what extent can the patient independently monitor task performance or products?

Physical Functioning

Avocational planning requires accurate information about mobility, coordination, fine motor skills (handling of materials), visual skills, endurance, and ability to accomplish activities of daily living. Key questions include:

1 1. Does the patient walk? use a wheelchair independently? transfer independently?
2. Does the patient sit upright? require support?
3. Can the patient reach? lift? bend? stoop?
4. If upper extremity functioning is limited, can the patient use adaptive equipment functionally (see Chapter 2)?
5. Does the patient have a functional pincer grasp? How effectively are small/large objects manipulated?
6. Can the patient identify and track objects visually?
7. How effective is eye-hand coordination?
8. Is hearing functional?
9. What is the patient's endurance level for sedentary/moderate/strenuous activity?
10. Does the patient manage functional needs (feeding, toileting, dressing) independently?

Psychosocial Functioning

Behavioral and social characteristics are often the chief determinants of successful reintegration of head injured individuals into community social and recreational life (Oddy, 1984). In addition to current psychosocial functioning, information regarding pre-traumatic social behavior is helpful; having previously been comfortable in a particular social context increases the likelihood of adapting to that environment following the injury. Conversely, those who were uncomfortable in particular social contexts are likely to remain so. The assessment should provide answers to the following questions:

1. Does the patient initiate and maintain social/communicative interaction? with whom? appropriately or inappropriately?

2. Does the patient display positive affect during activities that are enjoyed?
3. Does the patient display unusual mannerisms? Is he or she aware of this behavior?
4. How does the patient respond to success? failure? stress? What is the threshold of tolerance for frustration? Does the client evidence catastrophic reactions? Under what circumstances?
6. To what degree has the patient accepted or adjusted to the disability?
7. What is the patient's attitude toward other disabled people?

Interest/Motivation

The goal of this essential phase of the evaluation is to identify activities or situations that are preferred by the patient or appear to be motivating. Again, both formal and informal means of assessment are useful. Informal assessment of interests includes observation of the individuals' responses when given choices among activities, observation of relative amounts of time engaged in various activities, informal interviews with the patient and family members, and a review of leisure interest patterns in the family.

Observation of the patient's choices of leisure activities should take place over a period of at least several days and occur in natural settings (e.g., the nursing unit or home) and in therapy. Presentation of choices in therapy can be systematically varied so that an ordering of preferences is established. A latency measure — the time elapsed between presentation and selection of an activity — may also be useful in establishing preferences (Wehman & Schleien, 1981). Finally, the frequency with which an activity is selected and the amount of time spent engaged in the activity are both strong indicators of preference. Attentional impairments rather than disinterest may dictate the length of time a patient remains engaged in an activity. However, even individuals with apparently fleeting attention for most tasks may remain on task for extended periods of time if the task is sufficiently engaging. This important phenomenon is illustrated by a head injured young man who had evidenced great difficulty maintaining orientation to any task for more than a few minutes, but who surprised the entire treatment team by remaining engrossed in computer games for more than an hour.

Formal assessment of leisure-time preferences is accomplished using one of the many inventories that have been developed for this purpose, including the Leisure Activities Blank, the Leisure Interest

Inventory, and the Mirenda Leisure Interest Finder. Wehman and Schleien (1980) reviewed these and other leisure assessment instruments. Individuals with significant cognitive or communicative deficits may be unable to participate in a formal assessment of their interests. In many cases, creative modifications of the inventory procedures will allow the therapist to sample the patient's interests. Communicatively impaired patients, for example, can be asked to sort pictures of activities into two stacks — activities that are desirable and those that are not.

Throughout the avocational program, ongoing assessment is needed to monitor the patient's response to treatment and also to revise the program if certain activities that were thought to be preferences are, in fact, now too difficult, time consuming, or cumbersome. The patient may also revise preferences as a result of trying new activities or acquiring new skills. Flexibility, imagination, and creativity are hallmarks of effective avocational programming.

Diagnostic Profile

Results of all components of the evaluation — leisure history, specific skills and deficits, family and patient interests, and community resources — can be organized into a diagnostic profile that enables the therapist and patient to select realistic and potentially satisfying avocational activities and to plan treatment objectives. Table 8–2 represents a diagnostic profile of A.S., a 32 year old head injured male with severe cognitive and motor impairments. This diagnostic profile suggested the following guidelines for selecting avocational activities for A.S.: (a) The activities must be of high interest due to his attentional impairment; (b) the activities should allow A.S. to be a positive role model for his children and encourage active communication in the family; (c) it must be possible for the activities to be performed independently, with adaptive equipment if necessary; (d) the activities should be based on previous experience and knowledge (because of significant new learning problems); (e) the activities should incorporate themes related to sports and oceanography; and (f) it should be possible for the activities to become increasingly complex and varied as skills improve and interests expand.

Avocational Hypothesis

Based on the summary of evaluation information in the diagnostic profile, a tentative avocational plan is developed for the client. Selection of appropriate activities is facilitated by the use of Overs and

TABLE 8–2. Diagnostic Profile

Name: A. S.

Age: 32

Diagnosis: Severe cognitive dysfunction of component systems and processes; moderate bilateral hemiparesis, with greater involvement on the left; perceptual difficulties

Tentative Discharge Destination: Home environment; will live with wife and 2 children (ages 6 & 9 years)

Summary of Past Vocational History: Oceanographer for university; Retail salesperson for home improvement supplies

Pre/Post-Trauma Leisure History	Interest Survey	Cognitive Status
• Pre-trauma: - outdoor activity: biking, fishing, hunting, swimming - people-oriented activities; contact sports • Post-trauma: - watching TV; playing card games • Family leisure activities: - wife: sewing, reading - children: have interests in animals	• deep-sea diving • reading: wildlife & sport magazines • cooking • playing table games	• severe memory & organization deficits for new information: requires repetition & structure to learn • moderate attention & concentration difficulties; can remain on task for 1 hour with direct cuing and prompting • intact language & conversation skills • good memory for pre-traumatic experiences • impulsivity & poor judgment • impaired problem solving • difficulty attending to detail

continued

Table 8–2 *(continued)*

Physical Status	Psychosocial Status	Community Resources
• uses electric wheelchair independently • has intact hearing • has limited hand function for fine motor activities • has visual perceptual limitations: impaired tracking • is unable to reach above head • transfers & ambulates for short distances with assistance • feeds self independently • needs minimal assistance with dressing	• has a need to have children interact with him and respect him • is self-centered & demanding of family time • has a need to engage in productive activity • is often depressed	• extended family members available • wife available & willing to help with leisure activity, but has time constraints • family car available for transportation • supportive church group in which family is involved is possible source of volunteers & leisure activity • YMCA in community: accessible, volunteers sometimes available • limited to $50.00/month for leisure activity

Possible Avocational Activities	Modifications
• aquarium hobbyist	• accessible aquarium equipment; • needs cognitive modification to compensate for deficits in memory, judgment, organization
• swimming	• needs assistance in dressing, getting into pool • will need supervision in pool

and colleagues' (1977) comprehensive listing of activities grouped by nine major avocational categories: games; sports; nature activities; collection activities; craft activities; art and music activities; education, entertainment, and cultural activities; volunteer activities; and organizational activities. The plan that is developed must be considered tentative so that the patient and treatment team retain the flexibility to explore and revise activities as needed. Individuals may not be sure about an activity until they are thoroughly familiar with it.

Diagnostic Therapy

Skilled counseling may be necessary in helping the patient to accept an avocational goal (Overs et al., 1977) that is suggested by the diagnostic profile, and to try one of the activities. A.S. willingly accepted the two selected activities (swimming and tropical fish hobbyist activities) when he recognized that they would allow him to interact with his children and also use some of his pre-injury vocational skills. He even speculated that he might be able to use the tropical fish activity as a source of income.

In other cases, activities may be less readily accepted. Several activities within a general category may need to be tried before the patient selects an acceptable option. During this time, the patient and therapist must be free to explore the feasibility of a variety of activities; therefore, expenses should be kept to a minimum, particularly investment in materials.

Having tentatively set an avocational goal, the therapist must outline the types of treatment that are necessary to develop the individual's ability to engage in the activity comfortably and successfully. This may require the development of strategies to compensate for cognitive deficits (see Chapter 4) or adaptive equipment to compensate for motor impairments (see Chapter 2). The *International Directory of Recreation-Oriented Assistive Devices* (Nesbitt, 1986) is a valuable source of information on equipment and on the possibilities of adapting avocational activities to meet the needs of disabled individuals. Overs, O'Connor, and DeMarco (1974) have developed an index of avocational activities classified by environmental and social/psychological factors and impairment limitations (e.g., impaired memory, balance, hand movements). During this diagnostic therapy phase, the therapist also systematically explores the client's learning efficiency, need for prompts, cues, and physical assistance, and need for structuring of the task or of the environment. This phase is similar to the career exploration phase of vocational planning (Overs et al., 1977) since it allows the patient to become aware of the skill requirements of the selected avocational activities and their capacity to satisfy recreational needs. The patient and family are actively engaged in the process of setting goals and objectives. Family members may make specific requests so that their lifestyles are not compromised. For example, one family asked that activities be designed that could somehow integrate their severely impaired family member into their bowling league activities. This strong family interest became part of the patient's diagnostic profile and, because he also wanted to spend leisure time with his family, a goal and corresponding objectives were constructed to meet this family need.

THERAPEUTIC INTERVENTION

Establishing a Treatment Plan

Overall goals for avocational treatment are broad performance statements that specify the purpose of proposed activities and that are determined on the basis of the patient's diagnostic profile (Wehman & Schleien, 1981). Two important avocational goals for A.S. were

1. to develop family oriented activities in which A.S. can play an active role in directing and interacting with his children; and
2. to develop activities that can incorporate prior occupational knowledge into leisure tasks.

Treatment objectives identify the particular activities that are selected during the hypothesis-testing phase, the required skills and adaptations/compensations that are identified during diagnostic therapy, and the community conditions under which the activity will be performed. Objectives specify the skills and behaviors that must be acquired in order to achieve established goals (Edgington & Hayes, 1976; Mager, 1976; Wehman & Schleien, 1981). Treatment objectives for A.S. included the following:

1. A.S. will feed tropical fish accurately by following the steps specified in a specially designed "flip book" (5/5 consecutive trials).
2. In a role-play situation with the clinician assuming the role of one of A.S.'s children, A.S. will describe various aspects of fish anatomy and behavior.

3. In the home environment, A. S. will correctly feed fish at designated time periods (6/7 days, monitored by his wife).

The treatment plan must also incorporate relevant information about the community setting in which avocational activity will occur. Knowing the community constraints will allow the therapist-patient-family team to rule out activities or adaptations/compensations that are simply not feasible in the community, and will also allow the therapist to design simulations of community situations to enhance generalization of skills to those settings.

Treatment Considerations

Given the difficulty that most severely head injured individuals have learning new information and procedures and generalizing new skills to novel settings, training methods must be selected with great care. Training should proceed systematically through four phases: acquisition, proficiency, generalization, and maintenance (Wehman & Schleien, 1981). Selection of specific intervention procedures is based on information gathered during the evaluation, including diagnostic therapy and consultation with other rehabilitation professionals. For example, on the basis of the patient's cognitive profile, a choice is made between teaching new skills in an *involuntary* learning condition and teaching those skills by engaging the client's *deliberate* learning potential (see Chapter 4).

A great deal has been written in the past decade about instructional and training procedures for severely disabled individuals (Anderson, Hodson & Jones, 1974; Bender & Valletutti, 1976; Kazdin, 1975; Knapczyk, 1975; Wehman, 1979; Wehman et al., 1977; Wehman & Schleien, 1981) and, therefore, there is little need to repeat descriptions of these methods. Rather, the discussion in this section will be focused on two critical components of training: task analysis and generalization. The section that follows will discuss skills that we have found strongly related to the ultimate success of avocational programming: self-care and communication.

Task Analysis

Through precise identification of the component parts of a complex task, it is possible to isolate the behaviors that will be necessary for successful completion of an avocational activity (Wehman & Schleien, 1981) and thereby establish specific behavioral objectives and also a natural order of acquisition of those behaviors (Williams & Gotts, 1977). Selecting behavioral objectives on the basis of task analysis helps therapists avoid the random teaching of isolated leisure skills (Wehman & Scheien, 1981). Furthermore, for severely impaired individuals, careful sequencing and incremental integrating of cognitive and physical skills are important aspects of intervention. Thorough task analysis involves not only dividing a complex activity into the sequence of steps that comprise that activity, but also identifying the cognitive, perceptual, academic, psychosocial, and physical skills necessary to complete any of the steps.

Since the concept of a task component is relative — that is, for every component of a task there are subcomponents that could themselves be analyzed — there is no single "correct" analysis of a task. The size of the components appropriate for a given client depends on that client's processing and learning ability. If it is difficult for a client to comprehend or master a step in an activity, then the task analysis will need to be modified. Wuerch and Voeltz (1982) proposed the following general guidelines for revising a task analysis:

1. If the size of the step (component) is inappropriately large, then consideration should be give to:
   - branching the step into smaller responses
   - modifying the step so that an alternative behavior can be used
2. If an individual's handicapped condition precludes performance of the step, then consideration should be given to:
   - identifying another functional response to replace the step
   - eliminating the step or making it easier to accomplish
   - identifying a prosthetic device
   - designing the activity so that it is completed only in part by the patient

Because of his occupational history, A.S. wished to keep a tropical fish aquarium. His diagnostic profile suggested that the cognitive prerequisites for this activity would be problematic. To make a more precise determination of the feasibility of the activity and the training and compensations that would be required, the activity was first analyzed into component parts, and subsequently the cognitive aspects of each part were identified. Feeding the fish (itself a component of the activity of keeping an aquarium) involved the following steps:

1. Get the food (a jar of fish flakes):
2. Open the jar;

3. Measure the correct amount of food;
4. Place the food on a folded sheet of paper;
5. Close the jar;
6. Turn on the reflector light;
7. Raise the lid of the aquarium cover;
8. Place the food in the tank;
9. Close the lid of the aquarium cover;
10. Observe the fish to ensure that they are all eating;
11. Check to see that all the food is eaten within a specified time limit;
12. Remove any uneaten food; and
13. Return the food to its proper place.

Because of A.S.'s marked cognitive impairments, the second phase of the analysis process was to identify cognitive aspects of the task. While virtually all aspects of cognition are involved in the complex activities of daily life (see Chapter 4) we highlighted a small number of cognitive components of this task that would be particularly problematic for A.S.:

- ability to maintain attention to one task for at least 10 to 15 minutes
- adequate figure-ground perception
- ability to scan the fish tank visually
- ability to acquire, retrieve, and functionally use compensatory strategies for feeding the fish
- ability to identify and learn the feeding habits of various species of fish
- ability to solve problems independently (e.g., what to do when the fish do not eat) and to make sound judgments in the care of the fish

Identification of the thirteen components of the task allowed the team to teach small behaviors that could be learned quickly and without the frustration of repeated failure. Identification of the cognitive demands allowed the team to create strategies for A.S. that would permit him to complete the task despite cognitive deficits. To compensate for memory deficits, a 3"×5" flip book was developed to outline the steps in the task. A.S. used this book as he went through each step during the acquisition phase of treatment. Ultimately he learned the sequence of steps but only after a very large number of repetitions. A special timer was used to remind A.S. when to feed the fish.

To facilitate scanning, a series of paired colored tabs were attached to the tank (see Figure 8–1). A.S. was taught to start at the

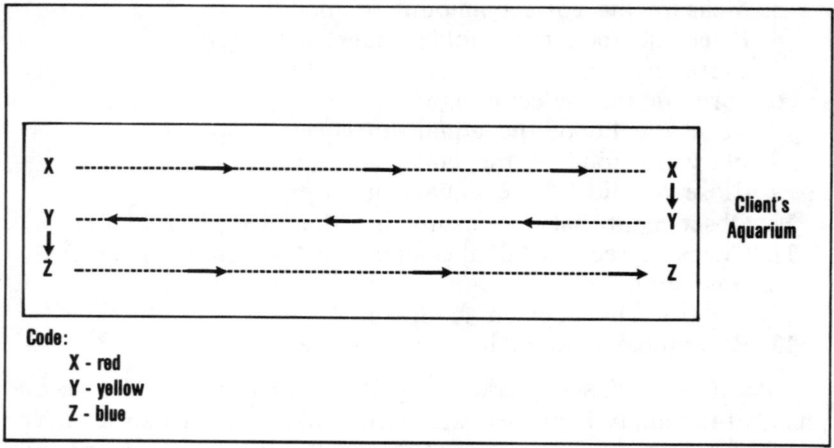

Figure 8–1. Cuing to facilitate screening.

top with the red dots proceeding left to right, then to follow the yellow dots from right to left, and to finish with the blue dots at the bottom from left to right. A resource book was developed for A.S. to enable him to make good decisions when faced with problems. Questions in his flip book (e.g., "Have the fish eaten all the food in 10 minutes?") were keyed to suggested solutions or courses of action in the resource book.

Generalization

Generalization involves transfer of stimulus control over a given behavior from specific instructions and prompts in a treatment setting to naturally occurring stimuli in the community setting. This process can be facilitated in a variety of ways, including systematic variation in the treatment environment, gradual fading of cues, and time delay techniques. Chapters 4 and 5 discuss generalization techniques in some detail.

Skills Related to Avocational Success

Self-Care Skills

As a rule, patients are less comfortable with avocational activities in a community setting to the extent that they are still dependent on others for basic activities of daily living — eating, toileting, dressing, and transferring. Since comfort is a fundamental factor in leisure activities, it is essential that self-care be addressed within an avocational program, and that training or adaptive devices be provided if the individual shows potential for improved functioning in these areas (Bigge with O'Donnel, 1976).

EATING: Oral motor and/or cognitive deficits may have long-term effects on the client's eating. Awareness of these problems and planned compensation can do much to facilitate successful reintegration into the community, while at the same time addressing safety considerations for the client. Possible problems in this area include:

- impaired chewing and/or swallowing
- limitations on the size or texture of foods because of impaired chewing and/or swallowing
- impaired sensation, resulting in an inability to detect food lodged in the mouth or on the lips or chin
- exceptionally fast or exceptionally slow eating
- "stuffing" the mouth with too much food at one time (related to impaired sensation/perception or impaired judgment)
- impaired hand and arm function, requiring the use of adaptive self-feeding equipment (e.g., scoop dish, built-up handle or strap on utensils, modified cup or straw)

It is not uncommon for cognitive-feeding problems to persist long after improvements in oral motor and upper extremity functioning have made self-feeding adequately efficient. Problems in the areas of initiation, attention, perception, and judgment may necessitate ongoing cuing to maintain effective and safe eating. The challenge for the community re-entry team is to recommend ways to ensure effective and safe eating without drawing undue attention to the individual or to the process of eating. Staff and family members involved in overseeing meals should be familiar with the patient's eating-related difficulties and with the least obtrusive compensations and cuing. Required physical or verbal cues should be given discretely and in a way that emphasizes similarities with conventional eating behavior. For example, individuals who cannot sense food on their chin can be given the respectful cue, "Here is a napkin for your chin" rather than the disrespectful cue, "You have food on your chin again; wipe it off." Offering a napkin to an adult is a common act of courtesy, whereas telling an adult, "Wipe your mouth," is unconventional and demeaning. Cutting up food for an adult is similarly attention getting and degrading since under normal circumstances only young children have their food cut up for them. Serving the food already cut into small pieces reduces attention to texture and size differences and to the individual's motor impairment. Family members can either prepare food in advance for use in community settings, or staff can be instructed in food preparation. Individuals who tend to "stuff" large quantities of food into their mouth can be paced with appropriately timed conversational questions rather than with constant verbal reminders to "slow down" or "swallow first" which can be attention getting and embarrassing. Again, conversation during a meal time is conventional, whereas telling an adult to "chew and swallow" is not. More obtrusive cuing and physical assistance may be necessary in cases of severe cognitive problems.

TOILETING: Efficient bowel and bladder management is an important aspect of being comfortable in the community. Specific management instructions should be given to the primary caretakers of individuals with impaired bowel or bladder control. Without this training, caretakers may be unwilling to take the patient on community outings.

Useful strategies for individuals with catheters include velcro or zipper openings in their pant legs to facilitate toileting. Disposable underpants may be a solution on those occasions when an adult who is incontinent ventures into the community. In both cases, the control and timing of intake may help with the management of bowel and bladder problems.

Procedures developed by staff to address toileting issues should be applicable to community settings and should be systematically taught to the patient and/or caretaker. Consultation among nursing staff, the physical therapist, and a community re-entry specialist is often required to develop a system that is most effective and functional in the community.

DRESSING: Dressing programs, traditionally implemented by occupational therapists, tend to focus on the physical aspects of dressing (e.g., pulling on slacks, buttoning buttons, tying shoes). With the goal of independence, these are important skills. In the context of community re-entry, it is equally important to focus on cognitive and aesthetic aspects of dressing. Inappropriate or unconventional attire calls attention to a disability as readily as a wheelchair or communication aid.

Following head injury, shallow thinking or impaired judgment can have a pronounced effect on dressing. This is illustrated by L.B., a head injured young man who planned to attend a baseball game as part of his avocational program. This was to be L.B.'s first independent community outing since the head injury. All details of transportation, tickets, and the like had been taken care of. However, L.B. had not discussed what to wear. Based on a weather forecast that he heard the night before the game, he decided to dress warmly. Later, he reported to his therapist that he had been miserable during the game because of the heat. It emerged that he had worn a heavy wool jacket despite temperatures in the 70s. He had inflexibly adhered to his one source of weather information and ignored the obviously more relevant information — the actual temperature. For future outings, the therapist prepared a decision guide for L.B. that included simple criteria for what to wear.

For individuals with physical limitations, specially designed outfits may provide an extra dimension of comfort and practicality. If an individual is limited to a wheelchair, clothing can be adjusted to the sitting position. Slacks should be a few inches longer to allow for the bend of the knees. Coats and jackets should have manageable front openings so that the individual needs a minimum of help when out in the community. Roomy front pockets that provide a secure and accessible place for needed articles are also useful.

TRANSFERS: For patients who are limited to their wheelchair, skill in transfers may "make or break" their community avocational program by allowing them to be independent in toileting and by opening a wider range of transportation. Three basic techiques are used for transfers: forward, sideways, and backward (Bigge with O'Donnel, 1976). Consultation with the patient's physical therapist would enable the avocational therapist to know which technique is preferable and to ensure that caretakers on community outings are similarly informed and trained.

Communication

Communication impairments following head injury may be severe and include an inability to speak intelligibly and a severely reduced ability to comprehend spoken or written language. Most often, however, head injured clients recover speech and the surface features of language (e.g., the ability to put sentences together grammatically), but continue to have difficulty (a) comprehending language if it is too complex or presented too rapidly, (b) finding words to express their thoughts, (c) expressing those thoughts in an organized way, and (d) conversing in a conventional manner. Conversational problems may take the form of rambling talk that moves unpredictably from topic to topic, lack of social initiation, or lack of inhibition which may result in language that is inappropriate or offensive. Since conversing is a primary means of establishing and maintaining social contact and since individuals whose conversational interaction is weak, bizarre, or offensive tend to become isolated socially, improved communication must be a focus of the avocational program Patients who cannot effectively initiate or terminate conversations, take turns, maintain topics of conversation, and inhibit socially inappropriate comments have considerable difficulty being accepted into a peer group even when avocational activities have been mastered. Improved verbal and conversational skills, then, increase the likelihood of success of the avocational program.

Knowledge of the peer group and avocational setting is useful in determining specific objectives for communication training. Furthermore, coached practice in communicative interaction in the identified setting is useful in promoting functional carry-over of learned skills. As was mentioned in the case of self-care skills, one of the goals of communication treatment is to highlight similarities between the patient and a selected peer group (Wolfensberger, 1972), and to reduce the isolation that accompanies unconventional communication.

Case illustration: E.S. was a 16 year old female, one year post-injury, who was scheduled for discharge from a rehabilitation hospital to a custodial care facility. She had severe motor impairment of both upper and lower extremities, but had functional use of her left hand. Cognitive problems included reduced arousal, attention, and initiation, and generally reduced intelluctual functioning. Although E.S. was capable of engaging successfully in and enjoying several leisure activities (e.g., board games), she did not initiate any of these activities. To compensate for this initiation problem, her therapist placed a list of well-rehearsed games on her lap tray along with her schedule. During free periods, a sequence of printed prompts was added to her lap tray. It began, "Do I feel like playing a game?" If the answer was yes, she was prompted to look next at the list of games. The next printed prompt was a conversation starter, "Would you like to play ________ with me? If the answer was no, then she was prompted to ask another person. If the answer was yes, then the next printed prompt was "Do you know the rules?" A general termination response was also included in the sequence of printed prompts, "Thanks, that was fun. Maybe we can do it again sometime." This sequence of utterances was practiced to habituation in role-playing situations and on the nursing unit with peers. Learning this sequence, even if it continued to require the printed prompts, had great practical significance for E.S., since it enabled her to initiate meaningful activities. At the custodial care facility, such initiation would be essential.

Without the social and cognitive stiumulation that these games provided for her, E.S. tended to either withdraw from social interaction or attempted to establish contact by endlessly repeating greetings ("Hi. How are you?") or by making comments like "I love you" repeatedly and indiscriminately. E.S. clearly desired social contact, but lacked conventional conversational strategies to establish and maintain contact.

Avocational therapy is a very useful context in which to provide communication intervention. We all tend to be more communicative when we have something meaningful and relevant to share. Communication is inevitably strained when two individuals have little in common and are not engaged in a mutually interesting activity. Enjoyable avocational activities often give the severely impaired individual something to talk about. Speech and language services may, therefore, be more effective for selected patients if the services are "disguised" within an avocational activity.

Communication aids must be considered for individuals with severe communication deficits. If communication partners are forced to "work" too hard in order to elicit or understand the patient's communication attempts, then they are likely to reduce their interaction with him or her. An important principle, therefore, in the selection of a communication system is that the system make it as easy as possible for caretakers and peers in the patient's natural setting to communicate effectively and quickly with the client. (Communication aids are discussed in Chaper 2).

Case illustration: S.M. was a 21 year old male with severe motor involvement. He was totally dependent for activities of daily living and mobility. Receptive language was adequate for conversational purposes, but S.M. had no functional speech. His spelling was adequate and he was taught to use a compact memowriter for interactive communication. This system afforded him flexibility (he could type whatever he wished) and accuracy (he could state exactly what was on his mind), but it was far from adequate for conversational purposes because it took S.M. several minutes to type a simple sentence. At times his communication partners did not have time to wait for him to generate his message. At other times, the process was simply too demanding of their patience. It was therefore decided that the communication system should have two components — a simple communication board that would allow quick communication of high frequency messages with one simple move, and the memowriter to be used for the expression of specific concerns or extended messages that could be typed out independently. It addition, since S.M. loved music, he was given a small tape recorder and a collection of tapes, and was taught to operate an adapted on/off switch. In addition to serving as a meaningful activity, the music became part of S.M.'s communication system; it served as a communication invitation to staff and visitors who walked by and at the same time established a topic of conversation that is meaningful for most people. The number of interactions initiated by staff and visitors increased significantly with the introduction of the tape recorder, and as a consequence, overall quality of life for S.M., who enjoyed social interaction, was enhanced.

Counseling

Despite its importance in the lives of severely head injured individuals, avocational programming often faces major obstacles that individually or collectively threaten its effectiveness. These include inadequate community resources for severely impaired people, hostile or indifferent community attitudes, and the refusal of funding sources to support avocational goals. Often, however, the chief obstacle is resistance from patients and families to focusing rehabilitative efforts on avocational goals. Head injured patients are typically young people who, before their accident, were completing their preparation for a vocational career or were beginning those careers. The aspirations and expectations of young people are high and preparation for failure and disability is nonexistent (Blazyk, 1983). This background, combined with the loss of coping ability that results directly from damage to the brain, creates complex adjustment problems that require the skills of a trained counselor. The three issues most commonly addressed are the individual's search for a new identity, role adjustment problems in the family (Shontz, 1975), and acceptance of avocational goals. Since these are issues for the patient and family members alike, the effectiveness of counseling services often depends on the willingness of both to participate in the process.

MARGINALITY. Marginality refers to the conflict between two identities: one that is desirable but not obtainable, and one that is available but unacceptable (Shontz, 1975). This state occurs when an individual values the identity associated with "normality" and devalues that associated with "disability." Individuals caught in this conflict may be resolute in refusing to admit that they have a functional limitation and are consequently handicapped (Wright, 1960). Denial and avoidance behaviors (e.g., refusing treatment) may be manifestations of marginality. Following head injury, the dynamics of denial interact in complex ways with an organically based inability to clearly perceive deficits and their functional implications.

Problems associated with marginality may be addressed by helping the patient to contain the loss (Gobble & Pfahl, 1985) and to channel maladaptive behavior into productive and effective action (Egan, 1982). In counseling sessions, the therapist encourages the patient to express feelings openly. The patient is assured that it is normal to mourn one's loss and experience depression. Cognitive re-structuring techniques (Burns, 1980) are used to help the individual focus on positive thinking and effective behavior change. An important step in this process is the development of positive coping behaviors which have their origin in the patient's ability to understand the futility of maintaining negative or irrational thinking patterns (Ellis, 1962). Furthermore, patients must develop a sense of personal worth and a recognition of the importance of self-fulfillment (Shontz, 1975; Wright, 1960). Goal-directed counseling is often effective in promoting behavior change by encouraging the individual to examine the results of maladaptive behaviors and formulate a plan for behavior change (Glasser, 1965).

Case illustration: D.M., a 30 year old female 3 years post-injury with cognitive and physical impairments including severe dysarthria, refused to consider avocational programming, which she viewed as associated exclusively with "mentally ill" and elderly people. By requiring D.M. to consider and discuss the consequences of her refusals to participate with friends in recreational activities, the counselor helped her to realize that the chief result of her refusal was extreme loneliness. When she recognized that her choice was between loneliness and establishing new social relationships, she agreed to explore avocational options.

Techniques of cognitive restructuring are also often useful in helping the patient to counter the effects of negative or irrational beliefs (Burns, 1980). The effectiveness of cognitive restructuring techniques depends in part on the individual's verbal and reasoning skills; patients with moderate to severe intellectual or receptive language deficits are inappropriate condidates for this type of counseling. These techniques are further discussed in Chapter 5. Counseling may be more effectively grounded in contractual arrangements in which the patient agrees to explore a specific activity for a certain amount of time and the counselor agrees to discontinue the avocational emphasis if the patient finds no value in the activity. This contractual process is illustrated by N.T., a head injured patient who initially wanted nothing to do with nonvocational goals. The first agreement specified that he would (a) attend therapeutic activities for a 2-week period and (b) record his positive and negative feelings about the activity. The counselor, in turn, agreed to discontinue avocational programming if N.T. were to find nothing positive in the selected activity. Using a series of contracts of this sort, N.T. continued in the program for 8 weeks, enabling the team to identify avocational activities that he considered meaningful and enjoyable.

Since families can be a powerful ally, it is often helpful to explain to them the issues related to marginality and solicit their support in working with the patient. Families may be experiencing their own conflict between the person they hope to have back and the person they now live with, which may result in their own denial of current deficits (Karpman et al., 1986). In this case, family counseling, described in Chapter 9, is recommended.

ROLE ADJUSTMENT. Problems resulting from revised or reversed family roles are a natural consequence of severe injury which results in long-term disability (Schlossberg, 1984). Referral to a family therapist is indicated when an inability to adjust to changed roles threatens the family system. An important goal of counseling is to help patients and their families understand the process of role adjustment and its implications for them. Deliberately taking and exploring the other's point of view may promote understanding of this process.

Case illustration: G.H. was a 36 year old male who had been the major provider for his family before his head injury. Since he was unable to return to work, his wife took a job. G.H. often complained that his wife had little time for him. She, on the other hand, felt that G.H. had become self-centered, had no appreciation for the work that she was doing, and devoted much of his energy to making people feel sorry for him. Through informational sessions and family counseling, the wife came to understand the pain that her husband experienced as a result of his inability to carry out what he felt was his primary family responsibility. They also explored ways in which he could help his wife with some household chores so that they would have more time to spend together. In addition, the avocational program for G.H. focused on activities (e.g., board games) that the family could do together.

ACCEPTANCE OF AVOCATIONAL GOALS. The issues of self-identity that we discussed under the heading of Marginality often result in resistance to avocational goals and activities. Overs et al. (1977) identified several counseling techniques that may be helpful in promoting client and family acceptance of avocational programming:

- Encourage discussion of pre-traumatic avocational activities and preferences;
- Explore feelings about avocational activities and about the value of avocational activity;
- In discussions with the family, actively promote avocational activity and its value for the patient;
- Give the patient and family specific information about avocational activities and community resources; and
- Use directive counseling techniques (Glasser, 1965) to engage the patient in an avocational activity.

Family members are asked to be a source of support for the patient at a time when their own coping resources may be seriously depleted. It is important to identify an individual in a family who is most capable of providing this support. At the same time, professionals must support family members by giving them information about community resources and services, by keeping them informed about head injury and its effects, by training them to implement effectively the management techniques of avocational program developing in therapy (see Chapter 4), and by allowing them to express their fears and frustrations in an atmosphere of acceptance and understanding. We routinely urge families to join the local chapter of the National Head Injury Foundation to broaden and deepen their own base of support. The search for meaningful avocational activity often causes families to experience frustration, irritability, depression, and social isolation which, combined with financial problems and transportation difficulties, necessitate active and ongoing support (Overs et al., 1977).

Community Re-entry

Avocational programming is incomplete if activities planned and rehearsed in therapy sessions are not satisfactorily implemented in the community. The avocational programming framework, discussed earlier, includes identification of community resources as an important aspect of the initial evaluation. Without this information, time in therapy can be wasted and the likelihood of transferring avocational activity from a rehabilitation setting to the community is substantially decreased (Wehman & Schleien, 1981). When community resources have been identified and avocational activities selected, the avocational therapist should gather detailed information about the setting in which the patient's leisure time will be spent so that effective treatment strategies can be developed to promote generalization to that setting. (Generalization is discussed at some length in Chapters 4 and 5). In addition, staff members of community facilities may need information about head injury and training in specific areas such as behavior management, self-care, and communication strategies.

The types of community services and resources needed depend on the avocational activities, the setting in which the activities will occur, and the nature and severity of the patient's impairment. Factors to be considered include the individual's safety, transportation needs, self-care skills, and communication skills. In their ideal form, support systems (e.g., family, friends, and support groups) provide the services and care needed by special populations (Bellack, 1984). In most cases, however, families and head injured patients are forced to cultivate resources so that individual needs of the patient are met while not imposing undue stress on the providers of such services. Follow-up services and direct consultation or intervention may be necessary following discharge from the rehabilitation facility.

Over the past decade, emphasis has been placed on the development of services and facilities to assist individuals with severe disabilities (Wehman & Schleien, 1981). Possible community resources for implementing avocational programs include church organizations, self-help groups (e.g., chapters of the National Head Injury Foundation), volunteer organizations, day activity program centers, community school programs, community associations (e.g., Young Men's Christian Association), rehabilitation organizations (e.g., United Cerebral Palsy Association), the Center for Independent Living, the National Handicapped Sports and Recreation Association, and concerned individuals. While many of the resources in this list are available in metropolitan areas, there may be few in rural areas. Experience working with head injured patients and their families points to an urgent need to develop more services in the community that have leisure or avocational activities as their focus.

SUMMARY

The goal of avocational programming for severely disabled head injured patients is to enhance viable career alternatives. Avocational programming is also recommended as a supplement for those individuals who have work potential. However, a very large percentage of severely head injured patients do not return to work (Gilchrist & Wilkinson, 1979; Oddy, 1984). Therefore, rehabilitation programs should enable them to engage in meaningful, productive, interesting — and fun — activities. The increase in patients' overall quality of life, including enriched social interaction, decreased stress and loneliness, improved interaction with family members, and increased fitness, may be incalculable.

REFERENCES

Adams, R., Daniel, A. & Rullman, L. (1975). *Games, sports and exercises for the physically handicapped.* Philadelphia: Lea & Febiger.

Amary, I. (1975). *Creative recreation for the mentally retarded.* Springfield, IL: Charles C. Thomas.

Anderson, R., Hodson, L. & Jones, R. (1974). *Instructional programming for handicapped students.* Springfield, IL: Charles C. Thomas.

Bellack, A. S. (1984). *Schizophrenia, treatment, management and rehabilitation.* Orlando: Grune & Stratton.

Bender, M., & Valletutti, P. (1976). *Teaching the moderately and severely handicapped* (Vol. II). Baltimore: University Park Press.

Bigge, J. L., with O'Donnel, P. A. (1976). *Teaching individuals with physical and multiple disabilities.* Columbus OH: Charles E. Merrill.

Blazyk, S. (1983). Developmental crisis in adolescents following severe head injury. *Social Work in Health Care, 8,* 55–67.

Bond, M. R. (1975). Assessment of the psychosocial outcome after severe head injury. In *Outcome of severe damage to the central nervous system: Ciba Foundation Symposium,* (Vol. 34, pp. 141–159). Amsterdam: Elsevier.

Brooks, N. (1984). Head injury and the family. In N. Brooks (Ed.), *Closed head injury: Psychological, social, and family consequences.* Oxford: Oxford University Press.

Bruckner, F. E. & Randle, A. P. H. (1972). Return to work after severe head injuries. *Rheumatology and Physical Medicine, 11,* 344–348.

Burns, D. D. (1980). *Feeling good: The new mood therapy.* New York: W. W. Morrow.

Edgington, C. & Hayes, G. (1976). Using performance objectives in the delivery of therapeutic recreation services. *Leisurability, 3,* 20–26.

Egan, G. (1982). *The skilled helper* (2nd ed.). Monterey, CA: Brooks/Cole.

Ellis, A. (1962). *Reason and emotion in psychotherapy.* New York: Lyle Stuart.

Gedde, D. (1978). *Physical activities for individuals with handicapping conditions.* St. Louis: C. V. Mosby.

Gilchrist, E. & Wilkinson, M. (1979). Some factors determining prognosis in young people with severe head injury. *Archives of Neurology, 36,* 355–359.

Glasser, W. (1965). *Reality therapy.* New York: Harper & Row.

Gloag, D. (1985). Rehabilitation after head injury — 1: Cognitive problems. *British Medical Journal, 290.* 834–836.

Gobble, E. M. & Pfah, J. C. (1985). Career development. In M. Ylvisaker (Ed.), *Head injury rehabilitation: Children and adolsecents.* San Diego: College–Hill Press.

Karpman, T., Wolfe, S. & Vargo, J. W. (1986). The psychological adjustment of adults and their parents following closed head injury. *Journal of Applied Rehabilitation Counseling, 17,* 28–33.

Kazdin, A. E. (1975). *Behavioral modification in applied settings.* Homewood, IL: Dorsey Press.

Knapczyk, D. (1975). Task analytic assessment of severe learning problems. *Education and Training of the Mentally Retarded, 16,* 24–27.

Kraus, R. (1973). *Therapuetic recreation service: Principle and practices.* Philadelphia: W. B. Saunders.

Lezak, M. D. (1978). Living with the characterologically altered brain injured patient. *Journal of Clinical Psychiatry, 39,* 592–598.

Mager, R. (1976). *Preparing instructional objectives.* Belmont, CA: Fearon.

Nesbitt, J. A. (Ed.). (1986). *The international directory recreation-oriented assistive device sources.* Marina Del Rey, CA: Lifeboat Press.

Oddy, M. (1984). Head injury and social adjustment. In N. Brooks (Ed.). *Closed head injury: Psychological, social and family consequences.* Oxford: Oxford University Press.

Oddy, M., Humphrey, M. & Uttley, D. (1978). Stresses upon the relatives of head injured patients. *British Journal of Psychiatry, 133,* 507–513.

Overs, R. P., O'Connor, E. & DeMarco, B. (1974). *Avocational activities for the handicapped.* Springfield: Charles C. Thomas.

Overs, R. P., Taylor, S. & Adkins, C. (1977). *Avocational counseling manual.* Washington, DC: Hawkins & Assoc.

Panting, A. & Merry, P. H. (1972). The long term rehabilitation of severe head injuries with particular reference to the need for social and medical support for the patient's family. *Rehabilitation, 38,* 33–37.

Romano, M. D. (1974). Family response to traumatic head injury. *Scandinavian Journal of Rehabilitation, 6,* 1–4.

Rosenbaum, M. & Najenson, T. (1976). Changes in life patterns and symptoms of low mood as reported by wives of severely brain injured soldiers. *Journal of Consulting and Clinical Psychology, 44,* 881–888.

Schlossberg, N. K. (1984). *Counseling adults in transition — Linking practice with theory.* New York: Springer Publishing Co.

Shontz, F. C. (1975). *The psychological aspects of physical illness and disability.* New York: Macmillan Publishing Co.

Super, D. E. (1976). *Career education and the meanings of work. Monographs on career education.* U.S. Department of Health, Education and Welfare, U.S. Office of Education.

Thomsen, I. V. (1984). Late outcome of very severe blunt head trauma: A 10–15 year second follow-up. *Journal of Neurology, Neurosurgery, and Psychiatry, 47,* 260–268.

Wehman, P. (Ed.). (1979). *Recreational programming for developmentally disabled persons.* Baltimore: University Park Press.

Wehman, P., Abramson, M. & Norman, C. (1977). Transfer of training in behavior modification programs: An evaluative review. *Journal of Special Education, 11,* 217–231.

Wehman, P. & Schleien, S. (1979). *Leisure skills curriculum for developmentally disabled persons.* Richmond, VA: School of Education, Virginia Commonwealth University.

Wehman, P. & Schleien, S. (1980). Relevant assessment in leisure skill training programs. *Therapeutic Recreation Journal,* 9–20.

Wehman, P. & Schleien, S. (1981). *Leisure programs for handicapped persons.* Baltimore: University Park Press.

Williams, W. & Gotts, E. (1977). Selected considerations on delivering curriculum for severely handicapped students. In E. Sontag, J. Smith & N. Certo (Eds.), *Educational programming for the severely and profoundly handicapped* (pp. 221–226). Reston, VA: Council for Exceptional Children.

Wolfensberger, W. (1972). *The principle of normalization in human services.* Toronto, Canada: National Institute on Mental Retardation.

Wright, B. A. (1960). Physical disability — A psychological approach. New York: Harper & Row.

Wuerch, B. B. & Voeltz, L. M. (1982). *Longitudinal leisure skills for severely handicapped learners.* Baltimore: Paul H. Brookes.

CHAPTER 9

Reactions of Family Members and Clinical Intervention after Traumatic Brain Injury

Pamela Klonoff
George P. Prigatano

Bond (1983) has recently summarized much of the empirical literature on the immediate and long-term effects of traumatic brain injury on the family of the patient. These studies have been helpful in providing a perspective on the varied consequences of traumatic brain injury for those who live with a brain injured person. However, there has yet to appear a description of the clinical intervention techniques used by out-patient rehabilitation staff working with families of brain injured patients. This can be elusive to empirical research because of the difficulties in quantifying such subjective information. Yet, a description of rehabilitation staff's techniques in working with families of brain injured patients is especially timely since there is a growing need for information to guide clinical activities as well as research in this area.

In this chapter, we will describe what some of the families we have worked with experience at intermediate and later phases of recovery (i.e., from 3 months to 10 years post-injury). We have found that family reactions to brain injury are heterogeneous, much like the patients'. They depend on a number of factors, including the coping styles of the family, the pre-injury role and personality of the injured patient, and the effects of the brain injury on behavior (e.g., personality and cognitive sequelae). The causes of stress on relatives produced by the patient's behavior will also be considered by reviewing both clinical experiences and relevant research data. Next, a model which conceptualizes coping styles of families will be presented. So called "functional" versus "dysfunctional" patterns will be described. Lastly, techniques of clinical intervention for effectively working with families will be suggested. From our work in the rehabilitation of brain injured patients, the authors have learned that for successful reintegration of patients into the home, community, and work, a strong working alliance with families is imperative. This can be achieved only with active family involvement in the rehabilitation process.

RESPONSES OF FAMILY MEMBERS TO BRAIN INJURY

Anecdotal reports are available which sensitively describe reactions families experience during the acute stages following brain injury. One such experience has recently been reported by a psychologist who is also the parent of a brain injured child (see Hock, 1984). Our experience has been primarily with families who have had the burden of care once the brain injured patient is discharged home. Typically, full-time supervision is required initially, and the entire family's routine is shifted to accommodate these demands. This results in feelings of anguish, confusion, and frustration. The end result is often marked disruption of family functioning. At the same time, family members are still likely to be in the grieving process, asking such questions as "How did this happen?" or "Why did this happen?" Throughout this early phase after discharge, however, hope generally continues that the patient will be restored close to his or her pre-injury state.

As the realization of the extent and permanency of the long-term cognitive, physical, and personality problems starts to emerge, there may be a sense of panic in the family about their ability to cope with or manage the situation. Often family members experience negative feelings towards their life circumstances and the patient, including hostility. Hostility often arises because patients are demanding and other family members' needs become subordinate to theirs (see Bond, 1983). The experience of hostility is especiallly common in the primary caretaker for whom the constant and extraordinary demands may become an overwhelming burden. Often hostility is combined with guilt for feeling or expressing these reactions. This further leads to depression or despair.

Research documenting these observations has been presented by Livingston, Brooks, and Bond (1985a, 1985b). They reported that relatives living with severely brain injured patients experience marked psychiatric problems, including anxiety, and marked dysfunction in the home 3 months and 12 months post-injury. In addition, Lezak (1978) has summarized many of the reactions that relatives experience when living with chronically disabled brain injured patients, including feeling trapped, socially isolated, abandoned by the extended family, and abused by the patient. These problems predictably result in family members becoming depressed, especially the primary caretaker.

Case illustration: An example of this is A.B., a 34 year old Navajo Indian who was a rodeo competitor and was injured when he was thrown from a horse on which he was riding bareback. Prior to the accident, he was employed as a sheet metal foreman. He sustained a severe brain injury, with an admission Glasgow Coma Scale score (Teasdale & Jennet, 1974) of 3. CT (Computerized Axial Tomography) scans indicated a right subdural hematoma over the fronto-parietal area. He had multiple neuropsychololgical sequelae, including significant memory problems and impaired abstract reasoning. As is often observed with traumatic brain injury, he was unaware of any cognitive changes. He also had a marked dysarthria and significant motor deficits (left sided clonus, ataxia and athetoid movements, and problems with equilibrium and posture), making him wheelchair bound. A.B. also showed dramatic personality changes, including irritability, disinhibition, impulsivity, and hypersexuality.

A.B. was discharged from the hospital to the care of his wife. They returned to their home in a small town in northern Arizona, and A.B. received out-patient speech and physical therapy. However, significant problems in managing A.B. in the home soon emerged. He was belligerent, had temper tantrums, and was at times both verbally and physically abusive toward his wife and children. He continued to be unaware of the extent of his difficulties and would try to insist on such activities as driving, which were beyond his capabilities. After approximately 6 weeks, his wife sought rehabilitation services more out of relief for herself and children .When interviewed she described herself as "exhausted" and "wrung out." She was obviously overwhelmed by his degree of deficits and her inability to understand and manage his behavior. She was understandably depressed over the sudden alteration in her life circumstances and the shift in her husband's role from a strong, equal partner in the relationship, to a very dependent, demanding, childlike person. It is often under circumstances such as these that families seek further rehabilitation for the patient.

CAUSES OF FAMILY STRESS AFTER BRAIN INJURY: RECENT RESEARCH FINDINGS

Research on the causes of stress on relatives of brain injured patients is starting to appear. This is important information for rehabilitation therapists to be aware of if they are to adequately help families cope with brain injured relatives.

A major cause of stress on the family following brain injury is personality change in the patient. Research studies have documented that relatives most frequently report emotional/motivational changes in their brain injured family member (Bond, 1983; Oddy, Humphrey & Uttley, 1978). McKinlay, Brooks, Bond, Martinage & Marshall (1981) have summarized ten frequently reported emotional problems at 3, 6, and 12 months post-injury according to relatives. Their findings are reproduced in Table 9–1. Note that a number of emotional difficulties were highly endorsed, including irritability, impatience, tension, anxiety, bad temper, depression, and "personality change." There was also a trend towards higher endorsement over time of irritability, impatience, and bad temper. Patients were described generally as more childish and inappropriate in their social behavior. A later study by Brooks and McKinlay (1983) further documents personality changes at 3, 6, and 12 months post-injury. A clear trend toward an increasingly wide variety of personality problems over a 12-month

Table 9–1. The Ten Problems Most Frequently Reported by Relatives as Being Present in the Patient (Percent Reporting)

Problem	3 months	6 months	12 months
Slowness	86	69	67
Tiredness	82	69	69
Irritability	63	69	71
Poor memory	73	59	69
Impatience	60	64	71
Tension and anxiety	57	66	58
Bad temper	48	56	67
Personality change	49	58	60
Depressed mood	57	52	57
Headaches	54	46	53

From McKinlay, W. W., Brooks, D. N., Bond, M. R., Martinage, D. P. & Marshall, M. M. (1981). The short-term outcome of severe blunt head injury as reported by relatives of the injured persons. *Journal of Neurology, Neurosurgery, and Psychiatry, 44,* p. 529.

period was reported. These results indicate not only that personality changes are significant stresses for the family, but that these problems may be exacerbated with time as patients are unable to understand and cope with residual cerebral deficits.

Klonoff, Snow, and Costa (1986) had relatives and close friends rate the behavioral and social role functioning of closed head injured patients 2 to 4 years post-injury. Ratings on the Katz Adjustment Scale — Relatives' Form (KAS-R) for 63 closed head injured subjects compared with age-appropriate normal control subjects and psychiatric patients are summarized in Table 9–2. Results indicate significant elevations in the R1 subscales of Belligerence, Verbal Expansiveness, Negativism, Suspiciousness, Withdrawal and Retardation, General Psychopathology, and Confusion. These results suggest that closed head injured patients, 2 to 4 years post-injury, were described by relatives and close friends as significantly more belligerent, slowed motorically, socially withdrawn, negative, socially obstreperous, suspicious, confused, and talkative when compared with age-appropriate norms (Hogarty & Katz, 1971). Similar findings have been reported by Prigatano, and others (1986).

The long-term nature of these personality problems is exemplified by the findings of Thomsen (1984). She reported that changes in behavior continued to be the most serious burden to relatives, 10 to 15 years post-injury. The emotional/motivational problems observed 2.5 and 10 to 15 years post-injury in forty severely head injured patients are summarized in Table 9–3. Changes in personality were rated by families as the most severe problems to cope with at follow-up. These results not only suggest that personality changes are highly enduring and disruptive, but that they can worsen with time, as noted above.

Several authors have attempted to identify which personality changes result in the greatest stress or "subjective burden" in relatives. Brooks and McKinlay (1983) reported that at 6 months post-injury, personality changes reflecting reduced control of temper, social withdrawal, and unreasonableness were significantly more frequent in the "higher burden group." By 12 months post-injury, in addition to the above characteristics, lack of energy, immaturity, insensitivity, and changeability were added to the list. They conclude that the increase in the number of characteristics by 12 months suggests the increasing extent to which relatives become aware of the pervasive nature of personality changes in the patients. Also, the relatives' ability to cope with these changes may decrease with time.

There is some evidence that spouses of brain injured patients experience considerable stress. Rosenbaum and Najenson (1976) compared reports of wives of open and closed head injured patients

Table 9-2. Mean Katz Adjustment Scale Scores (Relatives' Form) for the Total Sample, Normal Controls, and Psychiatric Patients

	Patient Population (n=63)		Normal Controls Age 20–29 (n=90)		Psychiatric Patients (n=133)	
Subscale	**Mean**	**S.D.**	**Mean**	**S.D.**	**Mean**	**S.D.**
R1:						
Belligerence	5.94*	2.31	4.86	1.03	5.44	1.88
Verbal Expansiveness	6.94*	2.03	5.99	1.48	6.98	2.46
Negativism	13.89*	3.82	11.84	2.61	15.30	4.47
Helplessness	5.21	1.30	4.78	1.16	8.44	2.91
Suspicious	5.05*	1.52	4.39	0.92	7.11	3.06
Anxiety	6.65	1.15	6.59	1.21	11.05	4.11
Withdrawal/Retardation	9.44*	3.09	8.09	1.84	12.29	4.10
General Psychopathology	37.79*	8.30	31.73	4.96	46.24	10.97
Nervousness	6.60	1.66	6.41	1.66	11.28	3.10
Confusion	3.54*	1.03	3.18	0.51	3.68	1.36
Bizarreness	5.54	1.13	5.41	1.05	7.25	2.51
Hyperactivity	4.84	1.62	4.37	1.21	6.82	2.33
Stability	31.08	4.00	30.99	4.75	26.03	5.82
R2	39.83	5.01	39.76	4.37	30.64	5.49
R3	38.94	4.82	39.68	4.13	38.91	5.77
R3–R2	2.54*	5.06	5.13	5.82	23.53	12.42
R4	45.54	7.20	45.52	4.99	51.70	6.11
R5	28.35	5.16	27.63	5.06	35.18	7.23

* $p<.01$, compared with age-appropriate norms.
From Klonoff, P. S., Snow, W. G. & Costa, L. D. (1986). Quality of life in patients with closed head injury, 2–4 years post-injury. *Neurosurgery, 19,* 735–743.

to wives of paraplegics and normal controls, one year post-injury. Head injured patients were described by their wives as more self-oriented, childish, demanding, and dependent. The patients took a smaller role in household responsibilities, especially in caring for their children. The wives also reported increased depression, significant loss in their social lives, and a reduction in sexual activity. Other authors have reported similar findings. Lezak (1978) reported that spouses live in "social limbo," experience significant role changes, often cannot divorce with dignity or good conscience, and have frustrated sexual and affection needs. Other research (Livingston et al., 1985a), however, has not supported the finding that wives undergo a greater degree of dysfunction than mothers of head injured patients, suggesting more research is necessary in this area.

Table 9-3. Problems at First and Second Follow-up

Problem	Percent after 2.5 years	Percent after 10–15 years
Poor memory	80	75
Changes in personality and emotion	80	65
Childishness	60	25
Emotional lability	40	35
Irritability	38	48
Restlessness	25	38
Disturbed behavior	23	20
Poor concentration	73	53
Slowness	65	53
Loss of social contact	60	68
Aspontaneity	43	53
Tiredness	28	50
Sensitivity distress	23	68
Lack of interests	20	55

From Thomsen, I. V. (1984). Late outcome of very severe blunt head trauma: A 10–15 year second follow-up. *Journal of Neurology, Neurosurgery, and Psychiatry, 47,* p. 264.

It should also be noted that some feelings and reactions of spouses may be elusive to empirical research because of their very personal nature. Walker (1972) reported that wives would report the personality changes in their brain injured husbands, but were hesitant to report changes in sexual functioning for fear of hurting their spouses' feelings. Post-interview letters from the wives confirmed their fear of embarrassing their husbands with information given in an interview.

An additional stress on the family is the long-term psychosocial differences of brain injured patients. One area of psychosocial difficulty is failure to return to work. Often the limiting factor in the ability to sustain a job following brain injury is not the severity of brain damage per se, but the concomitant personality problems. Emotional lability and post-psychotic states have been reported to be related to reduced work capacity (Bruckner & Randle, 1972; Gilchrist & Wilkinson, 1979; Weddell, Oddy, & Jenkins, 1980). In addition, Klonoff & Snow (in press) reported that employed severely brain injured patients reported significantly more difficulty with irritability with co-workers than less severely injured patients. Prigatano and others (1986) also have shown a close correlation between the ability to return to work and improvement in psychiatric status.

CONCEPTUALIZATION OF FAMILY REACTIONS

The above sections summarize reactions of family members to brain injured relatives and the primary causes of stress on relatives during the more chronic stages of recovery. Given this information, is there a way of conceptualizing family reactions that is useful in clinical practice? In our work and the work of others (Chaffee, unpublished; Power, 1985), coping styles have been conceptualized along two broad dimensions: (a) functional/expected versus (b) dysfunctional. In the former, despite the natural reactions of shock, sadness, and bitterness, the family eventually adapts to the existence of a brain injured relative. This is an extremely difficult process that involves the family eventually accepting the realities of the brain injury. They remain a responsive family while continuing with goals in their own lives. This also involves accurate self-appraisal of the limits of what family members can do and accurate appraisal of the strengths and weaknesses of the patient. Ultimately the family can recognize the real limits imposed by the patient's disabilities but maintain an appreciation of life's possibilities (Chaffee, unpublished).

Case illustration: The case of B.C. is an example of a functional family reaction. B.C. is a young man who sustained a severe brain injury as a result of a motor vehicle accident. Initial Glasgow Coma Scale score was 4. CT scan indicated hemorrhage in the left inferior frontal lobe and the midbrain. At one year post-injury, significant cognitive, personality, and motor problems persisted. Initially, B. C. was cooperative in therapy and at home. With time, however, as he became more aware of his residual deficits, he became more irritable, depressed, and demanding of the attention of others. Despite the family's difficulties at times coping with his cognitive and motor deficits and behavioral problems, there was increased awareness and acceptance by the family of the long-term effects of B. C.'s injury. At the same time, his mother eventually was able to return to her former job. His parents have also taken breaks from the responsibility of caring for B.C., in the form of short vacations. In their absence, other members of the immediate and extended family have helped with the care of B.C. Overall, by one year post-injury the family has been able to develop their own interests and goals, yet still continue to show a caring, supportive commitment to the recovery of B. C.

The second style of coping is considered more dysfunctional. Typically the patient becomes the focus of the family. Life centers around this patient. Associated with this is poor awareness and acceptance of the patient's residual disabilities. There may be "scapegoating," in which other family members, therapists, or associated circumstances are blamed as the cause of the patient's behavioral difficulties (Chaffee, unpublished). It should be noted that there is often a dynamic balance between elements of the functional and dysfunctional coping styles, which with time often resolve into predominantly one pattern or the other.

Power (1985) has described functional versus dysfunctional coping patterns in families with severely neurologically impaired members. He studied 49 families with a member with multiple sclerosis and described the positive coping strategies as including the ability to orient their lives to encompass new illness-related events with limited disruption of family functioning. The behavior of the patient, availability of financial resources, previous experience with family stress, individual resources, strength of religious convictions, and strong marital relations prior to the onset of the illness were also identified as factors which helped families cope.

Dysfunctional families on the other hand were described as neglecting customary family duties and responsibilities. There were tense communication patterns between family members, frequent misunderstandings of the important facts associated with the illness, and feelings of being overwhelmed and "trapped" associated with caring for the patient. Ongoing denial of illness was paramount, to the extent that treatment issues were often ignored.

Case illustration: An example of a dysfunctional family reaction was the case of the patient E.F. This middle-aged patient sustained a severe brain injury as a result of a fall from a horse. Initial CT scan indicated small hemorrhagic contusions with small ventricles. Follow-up CT scans indicated atrophy in the frontal lobes, right temporal lobe, and thalamic regions bilaterally. As a result of the accident she had significant motor, cognitive, and communication difficulties. She spent several months in an in-patient rehabilitation unit. During her hospitalization, her parents were with her almost continuously and she consequently became very dependent upon them. Her behavior became regressive and she would talk to them in a childlike way, e.g., refer to them as "mommy" and "daddy." Her parents encouraged this behavior and insisted upon attending and noisily interrupting many of her therapy sessions. They were very demanding and critical of nursing staff and therapists. Many rehabilitation team members tried to avoid them if possible. Her father's belligerent, aggressive style alienated the rehabilitation therapists and some physicians. Due to requests from therapists involved, weekly meetings were begun with the parents with a staff clinical neuropsychologist to help the parents begin to recognize that despite their concern for their daughter, they were having a negative impact upon the rehabilitation staff. As part of this, they were encouraged to be less controlling and to accord their daughter more independence.

When E.F. was transferred to an out-patient rehabilitation program, the parents continued to be demanding and controlling. Some therapists felt they could do nothing to please the patient or her family. Weekly meetings were instituted to confront this. The family dynamics that emerged revealed long-term problems between the husband and wife which were now being re-directed onto the patient and the therapists working with her. This contributed to their difficulty recognizing their daughter's need for independence and responsibility. Some progress was made, but at the time of discharge the family problems persisted. It was clearly a dysfunctional family style.

Another family reaction pattern which may be associated with a more dysfunctional family coping style is denial or unacceptance. Denial has been described as a defense mechanism employed to reduce psychic stress and the threat of reality (Beisser, 1979) and has been considered both functional and dysfunctional. Some authors feel that denial is at times helpful. Beisser (1979) stated that denial is functional if it promotes affirmative attitudes towards health. Often it is the means by which patients and families maintain hope (Luterman, 1985). In addition, Luterman stated that denial can be constructive if that is the only way the individual can cope with distressing news.

We agree that denial is a natural response to the initial shock of devastating news. However, it is our belief that the rehabilitation staff's responsibility is to slowly and gently help families face the long-term realities of brain injury. This is not done with a confrontive style, but by supportively pointing out misperceptions of reality at a pace the family can tolerate. Just as patients vary in their ability to face reality, so do family members. It is the responsibility of the rehabilitation therapists not to overwhelm patients and families, but not to lose sight of helping families cope with reality.

Several authors have described dysfunctional denial. Power (1985) stated that denial in some families precluded proper medical treatment and attention. Romano (1974) described the phenomenon of protracted denial of disability among head injured patients' families. Such denial was manifested in several ways:

1. *Common Fantasies:* There is the common fantasy that measurable improvement has occurred when there is no objective evidence to support this. Related to this is the common statement that if the patient tried hard enough, he or she would improve. This is illustrated by the patient E.F., described earlier. She had been a successful business woman previous to her injury. Her parents continued to insist that she would be able to return to her former career. They encouraged her to take up various aspects of her job responsibilities, despite her discouragement and *her* growing awareness that she had too many cognitive difficulties to successfully work as she used to. This fantasy persisted in the parents, despite attempts to show them results of neuropsychological testing and other examples of impaired intellectual functioning in her day-to-day functioning.
2. *Verbal Refusals:* These often take the form of insisting that the patients are no different than they had been prior to their injuries. Often families deny the presence of obvious physical, mental, and behavioral changes in the patients. This is well illustrated by a statement made by the wife of a successful professional who sustained a severe head injury and was in an obtunded state for several months. When an attempt was made to interview the patient and family, the patient was unable to respond in any way to the questions of the therapist. Instead, he lay on his side, drooling on the pillow. The wife turned to the therapist and said, "You know, ever since we've been married, my husband has always been a drooler when he sleeps." This comment in part reflects the spouse's difficulty in recognizing one major sign of the brain injury easily pointed out to her by rehabilitation staff. At times, relatives are willing to acknowledge one or two areas of deficit (often physical), but deny other limitations (often cognitive or behavioral changes).
3. *Inappropriate Responses:* When denial persists, families often are unable to respond appropriately to the patients' needs or behaviors. A common example of this occurs when relatives do not follow up on suggested compensatory strategies for behavioral or cognitive deficits, or express unrealistic plans or goals for the patient. An example of this was a plan by the family of a severely brain injured patient who had significant physical problems (including spasticity and clonus on the left side, and extremely slowed reaction time) to "adapt" a three-wheeler for him so he

could participate on family dirt-bike trips. A similarly unrealistic goal was expressed by another family member for her son to return to his pre-injury career as a professional golfer, when it was clear to the rehabilitation staff working with him, as well as the patient himself, that he had significant physical deficits which would make it impossible for him to accomplish this.

Romano (1974) suggested that the form and degree of denial over time have grave repercussions for the ultimate adjustment of the patient and family.

CLINICAL INTERVENTION WITH FAMILIES AFTER BRAIN INJURY

The preceding sections have summarized the reactions, stresses, and coping styles of relatives of brain injured patients during the chronic stages of recovery. Taken together, research and anecdotal information suggest that there are profound and enduring stresses on family functioning. This section will therefore focus on principles of clinical intervention with families of brain injured patients during these chronic stages of recovery. Topics and issues discussed with families are summarized in Table 9-4.

It has been our experience that a close working alliance with families is essential for successful neuro-rehabilitation. Successful neuro-rehabilitation is defined as having patients return to a state of independence in which they are productive (e.g., work) and contribute

Table 9-4. Clinical Intervention: Topics and Issues

1. A close working alliance with families is essential for the successful rehabilitation of patients.
2. The nature of frequent contact with relatives is both educational and supportive.
3. Families require clear definition of the goals of rehabilitation for the patient:
   (a) independence
   (b) productivity
   (c) satisfying love relationships
4. Families must learn to adjust to the effects of brain injury and begin to reconstitute their own lives, just as patients do.
5. To adequately address the needs of families, they must be worked with both in groups and individually.

to family or interpersonal life (e.g., mutually satisfying love realationship) (see Prigatano and others, 1986). Successful rehabilitation cannot take place only in the context of the rehabilitation facility; eventually it must generalize to the home, community, and when possible, the work place. In order to accomplish these goals, it is imperative to involve those individuals present in the home environment. For this reason, it is a requirement of our rehabilitation program that at least one relative (or individual who will be in close contact with the patient upon discharge) be involved in regular contact with our program.

In addition to the above general goal, there are several specific reasons for establishing a working alliance with family members. First, a good working relationship with the families provides important information for the rehabilitation team regarding the patient's functioning outside the rehabilitation setting. Second, good communication with and training of families encourages generalization of socially appropriate behavior and other skills acquired in rehabilitation to the extended environment. A third and very important reason is that families need a great deal of support and education regarding the acute and chronic effects of brain injury. This is necessary for them to learn to adjust to the effects of brain injury in a relative and begin to reconstitute their own lives. It takes guidance and support to find a balance between their needs and interests and those of the patient. This requires frequent interaction with families.

Our invitation to family members to be active members of the rehabilitation team begins with a listing of three goals of rehabilitation. The first goal is to reduce the confusion in the staff members' minds regarding the patient's strengths and weaknesses. The second goal is then to reduce the confusion in the family's mind. The third goal is to reduce the confusion in the patient's mind. Therefore the family is an important component of rehabilitation efforts. Once family members understand this, they typically are committed to working closely with rehabilitation staff members.

Work with family members is approached in several ways. It begins with the initial evaluation when patients are considered for participation in the rehabilitation program. Families' observations and concerns are incorporated in the evaluation, beginning with their participation in the intake interview. This is intended to set a tone of honest dialogue between the therapist, patient, and family members (see Prigatano, Pepping & Klonoff, 1986).

The process of family involvement continues by providing the patient and family with feedback regarding the neuropsychological test results, and even copies of the neuropsychological report if this is helpful. When patients are considered appropriate for participation in our rehabilitation program, one of the therapists gives family members a detailed description of the program, both in writing and verbally. This heightens the sense of inclusion of both the patient and family in the decision process.

When patients begin participation in our program, we provide a thorough orientation not only to the patient but also the family. It is often helpful to have family members attend the program for at least one full day in order to acquaint them with each therapy activity. Relatives are encouraged to revisit and attend individual family sessions for updatings regarding the patient's progress (or lack of it) in specific therapeutic activities. This is especially important for physical therapy, in which relatives may need regular input for managing physically disabled patients.

Family members are also required to participate in weekly relatives' groups. These meetings serve several purposes. Most importantly, they provide family members with an opportunity to share their experiences and frustrations with other family members who may have experienced similar situations. It also gives the less "seasoned" members an opportunity to learn about future issues that they may likely encounter. This may provide an important network of support beyond the therapists which is especially helpful when relatives experience some of the earlier described negative reactions towards the patient (e.g., hostility and frustration). Talking with other family members experiencing the same situation is often very therapeutic and provides an important source of support which helps relieve feelings of isolation and guilt experienced by individual family members.

Relatives' groups are typically conducted by a clinical neuropsychologist, with other therapists serving as co-therapists, including psychologists, social workers, and physical therapists. Often co-therapists are rotated, depending on the current needs of the families and/or patients. For example, for those patients with significant problems with mobility, physical therapists are involved in meetings, in order to answer families' questions and provide progress reports first hand to families.

A variety of topics is addressed within these sessions. These are summarized in Table 9–5. The overall goals of the program (i.e., to help the patient become independent and productive) are reviewed regularly. From an educational point of view, we provide information regarding the common neuropsychological, physical, and psychosocial effects of brain injury. This commonly includes discussion of personality changes and their etiology. To help families better understand the nature and etiology of personality disorders after brain

Table 9–5. Topics for Relatives' Group

1. Review of overall goals of the program
2. Education regarding common neuropsychological, physical, and psychosocial effects of brain injury.
3. Model of common personality changes:
   (a) reactionary
   (b) neuropsychological (e.g., frontal lobe damage, paranoia, and unawareness)
   (c) characterological
4. Report of patient's day-to-day functioning in the program and long-term prognosis
5. Acceptance by families of the patient's strengths and weaknesses
6. Inquiry regarding functioning of the patient at home
7. Education of and coping with (a) the "catastrophic reaction" and (b) unrealistic goals in patients
8. Changes in relationships with significant others
9. Importance of sharing the responsibility for the caretaking of the patient

injury, we use the classification scheme proposed by Prigatano and others (also see Chapter 1). This schema is presented in Table 9–6. Personality changes are classified as (a) reactionary problems, (b) neuropsychologically mediated problems, and (c) characterological styles. It is explained to families that personality characteristics are not limited exclusively to one category. Table 9–6 simply lists some typical examples of each category.

It has been our experience that family members frequently do not know that personality changes can be a direct result of the brain injury (neuropsychologically based changes). Often relatives must be educated to the fact that some personality changes have a relationship to the location and extent of brain damage, illustrated by those personality changes thought to be related to frontal lobe damage, including disinhibition, impaired judgment, rigid and concrete thinking, and childlike and inappropriate behavior (Luria, 1973; Stuss & Richard, 1982). Most of the severely brain injured patients we work with exhibit at least some of these personality characteristics, and they are often a major source of frustration for families. Helping relatives appreciate that these characteristics are at least in part organically based helps reduce their confusion as to why these behaviors occur.

A less common, but important example of organically based personality change, is paranoia. Research findings are presented to family members including the possibility that this change is related

Table 9–6. Schema for Typical Personality Disorders after Brain Injury

Reactionary Problems
Anxiety
Depression
Irritability
Mistrust of others
Hopelessness
Helplessness (i.e., more demanding attitude)
Anger
Social withdrawal
Phobias
Neuropsychologically Mediated Problems
Impulsiveness
Socially inappropriate comments or actions
Emotional lability (includes poor tolerance of frustration)
Agitation
Paranoia
Unawareness of deficit (or severity)
Childlike behavior (giddiness or insensitivity to others)
Misperception of the intentions or actions of others
Apparent lack of motivation
Hypoarousal
Characterological Styles
Obsessive or superorderly behavior
Hardworking attitude
Congeniality and friendliness
Social deceptiveness (psychopathic tendencies)
Desire to maintain satisfying interpersonal relations
Encouragement or discouragement of family support
Distrustfulness
Feeling not getting "enough" help from others and therapists
Avoidance of insight into self or discussion of personal topics
Enjoyment of upsetting others
Enjoyment of a dependent role
Defiant attitude (challenging therapist to go ahead and treat them if they can)

From Prigatano and others. (1986). *Neuropsychological rehabilitation after brain injury.* (pp. 45–46). Baltimore: Johns Hopkins University Press.

damage to the left temporal lobe and amygdala (Lishman, 1968). The possibility of organically based perceptual and cognitive disturbances which interfere with the interpretation of visual inputs from the environment (Pribram, 1971) is also discussed.

Another post-injury personality characteristic which may be a source of frustration or confusion to families is the patient's unawareness of residual cognitive and personality changes. The phenomenon of denial must be distinguished from unawareness. Denial is defined as an unwillingness to face something partially known and is considered a "psychological defense." Unawareness is defined as a lack of knowing secondary to brain dysfunction. We discuss with families the phenomenon of anosognosia, or "denial" of illness (Heilman, 1979) as an explicit example of organically based unawareness of deficit.

To help further explain the concept of unawareness, we present selected research findings to family members. For example, McLean, Dikmen, Temkin, Wyler, and Gayle (1984) reported a trend toward greater emotional distress in less severely head injured groups when compared with more severe groups. It was hypothesized that emotional distress was related to better awareness of deficit in the mildly injured groups.

The importance of improving patients' awareness of deficits for eventual psychosocial adjustment is also discussed. Research findings, such as those of Fordyce and Roueche (in press), can also be useful to present. These authors reported that patients who develop more realistic attitudes regarding the effects of their injuries show better psychosocial outcome with regard to work adjustment. To further clarify the neuroanatomical basis of many of the personality (as well as cognitive and physical problems), CT scans and Magnetic Resonance Imaging (MRI) scans are typically reviewed with families.

It has been our experience that the educative model, including presenting research findings and relevant patient data, provides explanations of why patients behave the way they do. The more the relatives understand the effects of brain injury, the more adequately they can cope with the patient's behavior. By reducing their confusion, ultimately, their degree of distress may be lessened.

In addition to educating families about brain injury during the relatives' group, we also bring families up to date regarding the patients' weekly progress in their rehabilitation. Often issues that the patients are struggling with are discussed, including depression and frustration over their lack of independence, their sense of loss, unawareness of deficits, and unacceptance of their current circumstances. Families are also apprised of the patient's progress in specific therapy activities. For example, the patient's progress in physical therapy may be discussed, or if the patient is involved in a volunteer work trial, an attempt is made to provide regular feedback regarding progress at the work site. Specific compensations utilized for problems (e.g., datebook for memory) are shared and reviewed with relatives in order to help with the generalization of use outside of the rehabilitation program.

During these discussions, families' difficulty with their own *acceptance* of the effects of brain injury often emerges. For example, it often takes family members several weeks or months to begin to accept the reality that their relative will have to be employed at a lower status job than pre-injury. This is especially evident during the early stages of discussion regarding the first volunteer work trial placement. A discrepancy between therapists and family members is often present, with family members having expectations that the patient perform a higher status position than the therapists consider appropriate.

Helping the family begin to accept the patient's deficits (and strengths) is a lengthy, complex process. It is an important challenge to the working relationship between the family and therapists; close contact and communication in group and individual settings are important in order to maintain the working alliance with family members.

In addition to providing feedback regarding our experiences working with the patient, another major focus of the relatives' group is to ascertain from the families how the week has gone and how the patient is functioning *outside* of the program. Questions asked include "How has the patient changed most since the accident?" and "How does the patient feel about the rehabilitation program?" Typical problem areas include interaction between patients and their families, patients' extrafamilial social relationships, their ability to do certain activities (e.g., driving, daily living activities), their judgment, and their safety awareness.

Often relatives raise specific concerns and inquire how best to manage a particular situation. One commonly raised concern is the frequent emotional outbursts that patients display in the home environment. Inquiry into the circumstances for this often reveals that the patient has become angry or frustrated about not being able to adequately perform a task. Relatives are introduced to the concept of the "catastrophic reaction" (Goldstein, 1952), in which patients become overwhelmed when they are confronted with tasks they are unable to perform as a result of the brain injury. Unable to cope with their confusion, patients become anxious and display a variety of responses, including angry outbursts (see Prigatano and others, 1986, for further discussion). Helping families (and patients) understand the nature of the patient's *own* catastrophic reactions often helps prevent their development. This involves structuring the environment in a way that does not inadvertently overwhelm the patient.

Another topic which frequently arises is how to respond to unrealistic statements that patients make about their deficits or abilities to perform functional activities. For example, patients may set deadlines to achieve various goals (e.g., returning to work, walking) and relatives may not be sure how to respond without upsetting the patient or causing a disagreement. In situations like this we encourage families to "stick to reality" with the patients, that is gently and supportively confront them with the truth. Sometimes if patients are determined to do something that is obviously beyond their current ability (e.g., drive or work), the situation may escalate into a confrontational situation in which the patient says "yes" and the family member insists on "no." Because of patients' difficulties with temper control, managing outbursts becomes a frequent problem for families in these instances. To help prevent this situation from developing, when patients make unrealistic demands, the relative is encouraged to acknowledge the frustration that the patient is experiencing, and gently explain that they are concerned and worried that the situation would become unsafe for the patient or the patient is getting "ahead of himself." This type of explanation communicates to the patient the caring feelings of the family member without chastisement.

Equally important communication skills that relatives are taught include how to compliment and support the patient when improvement in behavior is observed. This is especially important in situations in which patients are trying to modify socially inappropriate behavior (e.g., angry outbursts).

A benefit of discussing situations such as these in the relatives' group is that other families having experienced similar situations can provide their suggestions as well as support. It is at these times, when family members may feel worn down, that input from other families experiencing similar situations can be particularly encouraging.

We stress with families the importance of *sharing the responsibility* for the caretaking of the patient. In this context we discuss issues of burnout and present suggestions on how to overcome the sense of overwhelming burden the patient can at times place on the primary caretaker. Relatives are encouraged to take breaks and address their own needs. This may mean getting other family members involved in the caretaker role, or alternatively exploring resources in the community (e.g., nursing support). Often these suggestions are met with resistance, as relatives feel guilty at the idea of being away from the patient or pursuing some of their own interests and needs. However, it has been our experience that if only one person takes total responsibility for the care of a severely brain injury patient without relief, that relative eventually becomes exhausted, resentful, and frustrated. This may happen after one month, or after several years; the end result is that the family member may reach the point of wanting to abandon the care of the patient.

SUMMARY

Relatives of brain injured patients experience marked disruption in their lives following a severe brain injury in a family member. Reactions include shock, grief, anger, bewilderment, anguish, and guilt. Often many of these reactions persist as the family becomes aware of the patient's long-term deficits. In addition, research has demonstrated that the greatest sources of stress for relatives are the patient's personality changes. This is important information for rehabilitation therapists to be aware of and sensitive to if they are to adequately help families cope with brain injured relatives.

Our work with brain injured patients and their families has taught us that family reactions and coping styles are very heterogeneous. For successful reintegration of patients into the home, community, and if possible, work, a strong working alliance with family members is imperative.

It has been our experience that developing a therapeutic alliance with the patient's family can be a slow process. It can take several months, and the rehabilitation staff needs to persevere and obtain support from co-workers in terms of how best to work with the family. As stated earlier, if the staff has been unable to make adequate contact with the family, typically less is achieved in terms of educating and supporting both the patient and his or her family. With a true therapeutic alliance, relatives commonly report that they feel the rehabilitation staff has done as much or more to help them as they have done to help the patient.

REFERENCES

Beisser, A. R. (1979). Denial and affirmation in illness and health. *American Journal of Psychiatry, 136,* 1026–1030.

Bond, M. R. (1983). Effects on the family system. In M. Rosenthal, E. Griffith, M. Bond & J. D. Miller (Eds.), *Rehabilitation of the head injured adult* (pp. 209–217). Philadelphia: F. A. Davis Co.

Brooks, D. N. & McKinlay, W. (1983). Personality and behavioral change after severe blunt head injury — A relative's view. *Journal of Neurology, Neurosurgery, and Psychiatry, 46,* 336–344.

Bruckner, F. E. & Randle, A. P. H. (1972). Return to work after severe head injuries. *Rheumatology and Physical Medicine, 11,* 344–348.

Chaffee, P. (1986). *Family adjustment process.* Unpublished manuscript.

Fordyce, D. J. & Roueche, J. R. (in press). Different perspectives of disability among patients, staff and relatives during rehabilitation of brain injury. *Rehabilitation Psychology.*

Gilchrist, E. & Wilkinson, M. (1979). Some factors determining prognosis in young people with severe head injuries. *Archives of Neurology, 36,* 355–359.

Goldstein, K. (1952). The effect of brain damage on personality. *Psychiatry, 15,* 245–260.

Heilman, K. M. (1979). Neglect and related disorders. In K. M. Heilman & E. Valenstein (Eds.), *Clinical neuropsychology* (pp. 268–307). New York: Oxford University Press.

Hock, R. A. (Ed.). (1984). *The rehabilitation of a child with a traumatic brain injury.* Springfield: Charles C. Thomas.

Hogarty, G. E. & Katz, M. M. (1971). Norms of adjustment and social behavior. *Archives of General Psychiatry, 25,* 470–480.

Klonoff, P. S. & Snow, W. G. (in press). Employment outcome in a sample of Canadian closed head injury patients. NATCON.

Klonoff, P. S., Snow, W. G. & Costa, L. D. (1986). Quality of life in patients with closed head injury, 2–4 years post-injury. *Neurosurgery, 19*(5), 735–743.

Lezak, M. D. (1978). Living with the characterologically altered brain injured patient. *Journal of Clinical Psychiatry, 39,* 592–598.

Lishman, W. A. (1968). Brain damage in relation to psychiatric disability after head injury. *British Journal of Psychiatry, 114,* 373–410.

Livingston, M. G., Brooks, D. N. & Bond, M. R. (1985a). Patient outcome in the year following severe head injury and relatives' psychiatric and social functioning. *Journal of Neurology, Neurosurgery, and Psychiatry, 48,* 876–881.

Livingston, M. G., Brooks, D. N. & Bond, M. R. (1985b). Three months after severe head injury: Psychiatric and social impact on relatives. *Journal of Neurology, Neurosurgery, and Psychiatry, 48,* 870–875.

Luria, A. R. (1973). *The working brain.* New York: Penguin Books.

Luterman, D. (1985). The denial mechanism. *Ear and Hearing, 6,* 57–58.

McKinlay, W. W., Brooks, D. N., Bond, M. R., Martinage, D. P. & Marshall, M. M. (1981). The short-term outcome of severe blunt head injury as reported by relatives of the injured persons. *Journal of Neurology, Neurosurgery, and Psychiatry, 44,* 527–533.

McLean, A., Dikmen, S., Temkin, N., Wyler, A. R. & Gale, J. L. (1984). Psychosocial functioning at 1 month after head injury. *Neurosurgery, 14,* 393–399.

Oddy, M., Humphrey, M. & Uttley, D. (1978). Stresses upon the relatives of head-injured patients. *British Journal of Psychiatry, 133,* 507–513.

Power, P. W. (1985). Family coping behaviors in chronic illness: A rehabilitation perspective. *Rehabilitation Literature, 46,* 78–83.

Pribram, K. H. (1971). *Languages of the brain: Experimental paradoxes and principles in neuropsychology* (2nd ed.). Englewood Cliffs, NJ: Prentice-Hall.

Prigatano, G. P. and others. (1986). *Neuropsychological rehabilitation after brain linjury.* Baltimore: The Johns Hopkins University Press.

Prigatano, G. P., Pepping, M. & Klonoff, P. (1986). Cognitive, personality, and psychosocial factors in the neuropsychological assessment of brain-injured patients. In B. P. Uzzell & Y. Gross (Eds.), *Clinical neuropsychology of intervention* (pp. 135–166). Boston: Nijhoff.

Romano, M. D. (1974). Family response to traumatic head injury. *Scandinavian Journal of Rehabilitation Medicine, 6,* 1–4.

Rosenbaum, M. & Najenson, T. (1976). Changes in life patterns and symptoms of low mood as reported by wives of severely brain-injured soldiers. *Journal of Consulting and Clinical Psychology, 44,* 881–888.

Stuss, D. T. & Richard, M. T. (1982). Neuropsychological sequelae of coma after head injury. In L. P. Ivan & D. Bruce (Eds.), *Coma: Physiopathology, diagnosis, and management.* Springfield: Charles C. Thomas.

Teasdale, G. & Jennett, B. (1974). Assessment of coma and impaired consciousness. A practical scale. *Lancet, 2,* 81–84.

Thomsen, I. V. (1984). Late outcome of very severe blunt head trauma: A 10–15 year second follow-up. *Journal of Neurology, Neurosurgery, and Psychiatry, 47,* 260–268.

Walker, A. E. (1972). Long-term evaluation of the social and family adjustment to head injuries. *Scandinavian Journal of Rehabilitative Medicine, 4,* 5–8.

Weddell, R., Oddy, M. & Jenkins, D. (1980). Social adjustment after rehabilitation: A two year follow-up of patients with severe head injury. *Psychological Medicine, 10, 257–263.*

CHAPTER 10

Management and Advocacy

William R. Bauer
Jan Titonis *

Successful community re-entry for head injured individuals depends on a variety of factors. These include the severity of the residual deficits and the availability of services to address these deficits. Chapters 1 through 9 of this book discuss in detail the typical consequences of severe closed head injury on social, vocational, avocational, and academic functioning, and on the capactiy for independent living. This chapter includes a brief summary of resources most vital to successful community re-entry and explores how agencies and professionals can best meet the needs of head injured clients, from both clinical and management perspectives. Interagency networking is highlighted as an efficient way to consolidate existing services, capitalize on rehabilitative expertise that has developed to serve a variety of populations of disabled people, and provide continuity of care for individuals following a severe head injury. We recognize, however, that in most parts of the country existing services, even if successfully integrated, are insufficient, and where the services are available, it is too often the case that funding for individual clients is inadequate. Therefore, a summary of those issues that should be the focus of efforts in advocacy has been included. This book appropriately includes as its epilogue a personal account of one family's experiences with community re-entry, an account which we hope will remind us all that head injury rehabilitation is ultimately not about agencies, models of service delivery, professions, or laws, but rather real human beings whose lives have been shattered and whose efforts to put the pieces back together may be enhanced by our most creative efforts.

---

* Authorship listed alphabetically at authors' request.

COMMUNITY RE-ENTRY SERVICES

Head injured clients present with varying degrees of injury; varying rates of recovery, varying premorbid characteristics such as intelligence, levels of education, work history, and career goals; and varying support systems, including family. Compounding this variation is the notorious difficulty predicting eventual outcome early in the recovery process. Noting this, Ben-Yishay and Diller (1983) advocate a continuum of care for head injured clients, beginning with trauma care and extending through independent living services. For similar reasons, the Committee on Trauma Research (1985) proposed the development of tertiary rehabilitation systems connected to trauma centers for the management of brain injured patients. The head injured client may need services at any point in the recovery process, often well beyond initial hospitalization, for residual problems in cognitive, psychosocial, and physical function.

These residual deficits are well defined in the growing literature on outcome following head injury. Much of this literature is summarized in previous chapters. Forgetfulness, irritability, slowness, poor concentration, and fatigue are commonly reported by clients at follow-up. Several studies show that personality problems can persist indefinitely as the client and family struggle to adjust to residual disability and changed life style (Oddy, Coughlan, Tyerman & Jenkins, 1985; Weddell, Oddy & Jenkins, 1980). The degree of cognitive and psychosocial impairment is closely associated with changes in employment, leisure activity, social contact, and family life (Oddy, Humphrey & Uttley, 1978). These cognitive and psychosocial factors, more than physical deficits, prevent successful community re-entry: return to work, re-integration into the family, and resumption of social activity. Since the pattern of cognitive and psychosocial strengths and weaknesses, often in the absense of physical deficits, is not common to other disability groups of young adults, programs specifically designed to treat head injured clients may be critical to successful community re-entry.

Beginning with the initial hospitalization, a number of services may be necessary to support the extended process of community re-entry. After acute care, patients may go home or be transferred to a coma management program, other extended care program, inpatient rehabilitation program, or outpatient rehabilitation program. A common pattern of service delivery involves transfer from the acute care hospital to an inpatient rehabilitation center to outpatient services, including vocational rehabilitation, and finally to independent living. However, because of the extended duration of spontaneous recovery and the unpredictability of recovery and response to intervention, movement in any direction among programs and facilities is possible. It is, for example, not uncommon for the effectiveness of intensive rehabilitation programs to be increased if the client has struggled unsuccessfully with independent living or has faced the frustration of a period of time at home with no treatment and little activity prior to rehabilitation.

Comprehensive medical inpatient rehabilitation customarily includes medical and nursing services along with physical therapy, occupational therapy, speech-language therapy, cognitive rehabilitation therapy, neuropsychological services, psychosocial counseling, nutritional services, and work adjustment services. In large rehabilitation centers, it is essential to coordinate services to prevent duplication, assure a consistent approach to the person, ensure that information is shared with the family and with significant others, and facilitate discharge planning. These coordination activities can be the responsibility of a physician, program manager, or case manager.

Dramatic gains often occur during inpatient rehabilitation: ambulation is regained, speech returns, confusion and disorientation abate, independence in activities of daily living is established. However, problems in the cognitive areas addressed earlier may persist, even with intensive treatment. A person may, for example, be unable to independently or appropriately complete a work task, leisure activity, or social interaction because of reduced initiation, memory or organization problems, distractibility, or other form of cognitive weakness. Furthermore, emotional problems may actually intensify as the client becomes more aware of deficits and their implications. Finally, not all head injured individuals experience dramatic physical recovery during this period. Many are dependent on a wheelchair for mobility; many cannot speak or speak intelligibly; many are unable to care for their personal needs; many remain disoriented and confused.

When 24-hour care is no longer necessary and the client is discharged from inpatient rehabilitation, continued services are generally recommended. This may mean transfer to outpatient services at the same center; alternatively, discharge planners may look to other community services and resources. Eventually, the community will have to be explored for each individual and many potential problems may present themselves, including (a) the client's unwillingness to participate in what may appear to be inappropriate or unnecessary services; (b) programs designed for quite different populations and staffed by professionals with little experience or understanding of head injury; (c) admissions criteria that exclude otherwise appropriate clients; and (d) unavailability of transportation.

Community services for the head injured client may include:

- competitive employment
- vocational rehabilitation
- educational services
- sheltered workshop
- therapeutic activity center
- volunteer work
- independent living programs
- adjustment counseling

Neurologic injury is more costly than other types of injury and produces a greater need for organized systems of acute, subacute, restorative, and rehabilitative care. However, the cost of these services is estimated at one-tenth of the cost of custodial care with repeated hospitalization (Committee on Trauma Reesarch, 1985).

Competitive Employment: Most head injured clients who are beyond the stage of recovery characterized by significant confusion and processing problems want desperately to return to their previous level of employment. Often clients whose deficits are not obvious cannot or will not identify or accept these deficits and hence return to work despite professional recommendations to the contrary. Although painful, failure on the job may be the only way to convince the client that further services are necessary.

Vocational Rehabilitation: Vocational services, necessary for most severely injured clients, may include work adjustment, vocational evaluation, vocational training or retraining, and specialized placement services with long-term job support (see Chapters 5 and 6). Vocational rehabilitation centers designed primarily to serve mental health/mental retardation clients may be unable to program successfully for head injured clients who often require a very flexible approach to vocational evaluation and training due to uneven ability profiles, and a long-term program to accommodate their need for psychosocial counseling and the development of strategies to compensate for specific cognitive deficits. Furthermore, vocational specialists inexperienced in head injury rehabilitation easily misinterpret impaired initiation, slowness, fatigue, uninhibited behavior, and disorganization as behavioral problems rather than as direct consequences of the brain injury. Finally, if the program treats a number of mentally retarded clients, the head injured individual may feel out of place socially and actively resist the program. These considerations indicate the need for specialized vocational services of the sort outlined in Chapters 5 and 6.

Higher Education: We have worked with head injured young adults who have returned to college and successfully completed their course of studies. However, given the pace and volume of work required in most college settings and the resulting stress, most head injured students, including those whose performance on neuropsychological assessment is not significantly depressed, either fail, drop out, or require special services (e.g., tutorial services) and strategies (e.g., tape recording lectures) to succeed. We also urge students to consider a reduced schedule for a least the first term. Community colleges often offer special programs for students with learning problems, including support services and less challenging course work. For some head injured students, it is essential to choose an entry-level training program, such as food service, child care, or nurses aide training. (Special education for head injured adolescents is discussed in Chapter 3.)

Sheltered Work: For clients who lack the skills necessary for competitive employment, higher education, or vocational training, sheltered work can be considered. Often, however, fine motor incoordination or slowness precludes the client's involvement if the workshop operates on a contractual basis with production quotas. Furthermore, head injured clients may react negatively to the social environment of the workshop (see Chapter 6).

Therapeutic Activity Center: Therapeutic activity centers can be explored for those clients who do not meet sheltered workshop criteria. However, many of these centers were developed for clients who are unable to work because of serious mental illness. Few head injured individuals carry a primary psychiatric diagnosis and therefore fail to meet the admission criteria. Also, like sheltered workshops, activity centers may not be socially appropriate for head injured clients. Chapter 8 explores other avocational options for those who are severely injured.

Volunteer Work: Volunteer work offers the head injured client an opportunity to be active and perform a useful service without having to meet production standards. It also makes possible increased social interaction outside the home. Churches, hospitals, and libraries have been good settings for volunteer placement and are often able to match a task to an individual's abilities.

Independent Living: Independent living programs are as vital to successful community re-entry as vocational and avocational programs. Many head injured clients lived alone before the injury and will need to do so again. In other cases, marital separations occur after the accident and different living arrangements must be found. It is often not possible or, indeed, desirable for head injured adults to live with older parents. Independent living programs can teach clients safety and social judgment skills, money management skills, attendant care management, and other skills discussed in Chapter 7. In addition, independent living counselors can help secure adequate housing and transportation.

Adjustment Counseling: Ongoing adjustment counseling is often necessary for both the head injured client and the family as they struggle to forge a new life style. Serious depression is not uncommon during the re-entry process. Chapter 9 identifies a number of unique characteristics of the counseling process for head injured individuals.

The primary need, then, is not necessarily for the development of new types of programs, but rather (a) for the replication of excellent programs in underserved parts of the country and (b) for existing programs to have the skill and flexibility to meet the community re-entry needs of head injured individuals by combining, modifying, and customizing those existing programs. This point is underscored in a survey reported by The Committee on Trauma Research. In Houston, with a population of 3.5 million, there are 875 newly brain injured persons annually (five times the number of spinal cord injuries). However, there are only 45 beds in two institutions which are specialized to serve these people and in a given year there are fewer than 100 persons admitted (Committee on Trauma Research, 1985).

Education and training of professionals and flexibility in program development, implementation, and timing are the keys to successful programming, both for new and established programs. Adequate education and training of staff makes possible an understanding of the dynamics of recovery, prevents misinterpretations of the behavior of head injured individuals, and leads to the implementation of appropriate intervention strategies, particularly in the area of cognitive dysfunction (see Chapter 3 and 4). Given such training, programs that previously could not meet the needs of head injured clients can do so. Furthermore, agencies that have developed programs appropriate for head injured individuals frequently find that the new intervention techniques and strategies are often quite applicable to other populations of clients as well. Individualizing programs for a small number of head injured individuals within a larger program need not be overwhelming — and relatively small efforts of this sort (e.g., providing a job coach during the first few weeks or months of competitive employment) can mean the difference between a successful and an unsuccessful return to community life.

Flexibility in admission criteria and program structure is also an important consideration if programs are to meet the needs of head injured people. A number of factors must be considered in determining a head injured client's appropriateness for a particular program. These include length of time following the injury, neuropsychological data (including a general intelligence measure), and behavioral and physical limitations, if any. An intelligence quotient alone should never be used as an admission criterion. Some head injured persons test well but function poorly in a stressful academic or work setting. Others do not perform well on psychometric evaluation, but because of the recovery of skills learned pre-traumatically, they are able to function at a higher level than the test results would predict. The need for flexibility in admission criteria and programming is illustrated by substance abuse treatment programs. Most programs rely heavily on verbal skills, which may be weak following head injury. However, treatment for substance abuse may also be essential for individuals with weak verbal skills, and therefore, creative modification of the standard treatment regimen may yield very important results.

Time is both friend and foe of head injured clients. Because recovery following head injury can proceed for years, some clients may, with adequate support and intervention, reach a level of employment or independent living that was considered out of the question as late as one year post-injury. However, time becomes an enemy when progress is slow and rehabilitation professionals or third party payers expect a certain amount of progress in a limited amount of time. Recovery following head injury is often characterized by periods of apparent plateau followed by unexpected progress. Premature discharge from a program can, therefore, deny the individual needed services.

NETWORKING

Realizing the rehabilitative needs of head injured individuals and the variety of available services is, in most cases, only the beginning of the client's and family's search. Often obstacle after obstacle is presented in the form of rigid systems that fail to incorporate the needed services in an effective delivery system. Each agency or institution seems to specialize in one area or another, and very few can offer a continuous treatment plan that spans the needs of the client from acute care through physical and cognitive rehabilitation and on to a successful return to the family, job, and community. Furthermore, most systems are committed to "what they do" rather than to what the client needs, and very few agencies have joined together to fill in the gaps between what they are able to do well and what others can offer to the client. Considering the entrenched patterns of service delivery in combination with the special needs of many head injured clients, it may seem to the family that a full-service delivery system is an impossible dream. But this need not be the case. Individual and group efforts can overcome many of the problems encountered in the search for total rehabilitation, and overcoming the rigidity of existing systems may be a primary goal in this search.

Since the needs of the head injured client are such that a battery of specialized treatment procedures is necessary for an effective continuum of services, it may be unrealistic to expect all or even a majority of agencies to offer so complete a program. That does not, however, mean that they cannot join with other agencies to respond to the variety of needs presented by their clients. In fact, to do otherwise is to ignore the responsibility of any service provider to render services that take into account both previous services delivered and the ongoing needs of clients following discharge from that agency. It also makes good business sense to develop arrangements that provide a reliable referral system among those agencies that typically see head injured clients at different stages of the rehabilitation process or for different categories of rehabilitative services. This integration of agency resources to contribute to the individual needs of clients is typically called "networking."

In some areas, scarcity of specialized manpower can limit the program potential of a single agency, whereas in others there may be a need to reduce duplication of services. Many agencies find themselves in need of some specialized service which they are not currently able to provide. The most obvious advantage of interagency agreements is the resulting ability of each agency involved to provide a broader continuum of care and spectrum of diversified services. Many freestanding rehabilitation facilities, for example, consider it unnecessary or undesirable to enter areas of treatment in which they lack experience or ability but nevertheless find that those services would benefit their clients if they were part of a broader service offering. By teaming with another agency that provides such service, they are able to accept their traditional clients while adding the "next step" in treatment through networking.

In addition to increasing client service, such agreements may also open new markets. A small freestanding facility that offers traditional medical rehabilitation, for example, might benefit from an agreement with an agency specializing in cognitive rehabilitation, thus opening their facility as a first step for treating head injured clients and assuring those clients a continued service stream through referral to their networking partner. The partner, in the same case, need not change its structure to provide medical rehabilitation and benefits from referrals provided by the collaborative agreement. The effective utilization of each agency's services is thus maximized, and the added economies of scale benefit both.

Successful networking arrangements begin, of course, with planning, and effective planning depends on several important concepts. In addition to recognizing the need for expanding systems of service delivery, each agency involved must be convinced that its needs and character will be respected and retained. Generally, the key administrators in the decision to enter into networking arrangements are the chief executive officers of the agencies involved. Often CEOs travel in the same circles, belong to the same professional organizations, and, since they share similar concerns in their day-to-day activities, understand each other's problems and needs. If they happen to socialize outside their professional roles, so much the better! Someone must initiate the proposal, and the greater the degree of comfort between the CEOs involved, the greater the chance that a networking arrangement will succeed.

Having decided to explore the possible benefits of interagency collaboration, the CEOs typically appoint a group of key staff members to further define needs and expectations. Objectives must be agreed upon by each agency, and resources, be they fiscal, physical, or human, must be identified. Before any program begins, it is also necessary to establish procedures for continued planning, monitoring, and evaluating.

Since no single planning model can accommodate the diverse needs of various agencies, a flexible orientation to planning may prove to be the most appropriate approach. Different levels of interagency coordination should be considered, recognizing that the integration of services to eliminate gaps in a client's program is different from the integration of administrative structures to facilitate operational coordination between two or more agencies. In addition, planning on the systems level must focus on broader systems of services beyond the administrative constraints of the agencies involved (Martinson, 1982).

Having decided that a networking arrangement may present opportunities to expand or improve programs, it is useful to explore the possible problems or restraining forces before entering into the agreement. In some cases, a history of competitiveness may make networking difficult, or there may be a lack of organizational structure to bring agencies together around mutual interests. On a more clinical level, lack of experience with interdisciplinary communication or a lack of staff time to devote to the joint effort can hinder progress. If the staff members lack agreement on the objectives, target population, roles, responsibilities, or lines of communication or authority, inconsistent treatment is likely to result. Key positions must be filled by people familiar with and committed to the joint program, and staff turnover problems must be managed to prevent confusion about the function of the collaboration.

In some cases, a successful beginning may lead to one agency or the other adopting an "I don't need you anymore" attitude or the feeling that they can now compete alone. Such attitudes lead to sporadic relationships which are generally destructive to an ongoing networking arrangement. If all parties do not continue to cooperate at all levels, divisions can easily lead to the eventual failure of the program. Attempts to achieve specific individual or subgroup advantages may compromise general program objectives. External agencies or purchasers of service may be the first to spot weaknesses in this area.

Experience indicates that the primary barrier to successful planning and implementation of collaborative effort is lack of communication. Effective communication among individuals associated with the delivery system may be the most important single factor in the success of such collaboration. In this area, too, the commitment demonstrated by CEOs and key staff members will set the tone for the rest of the professional staff. It is important for all parties that their agency leaders demonstrate that they want the networking arrangement to work and that they are willing to offer ongoing guidance, support, and resources. If necessary, agencies considering networking may use facilitators trained in group dynamics to support the effort by motivating participants toward a collaborative philosophy. Johnson, McLaughlin, and Christensen (1982), Magrab and Elder (1979), and LaCour (1982) offer comprehensive discussions of important considerations in interagency collaboration.

One example of an effective collaborative agreement exists in Pittsburgh, Pennsylvania, involving The Rehabilitation Institute of Pittsburgh, the Vocational Rehabilitation Center of Allegheny County (VRC), and United Cerebral Palsy Association of Pittsburgh (UCP). As a freestanding rehabilitation center and specialty hospital, the Institute recognized the need to expand its services to head injured clients needing vocational training and placement as well as training in independent living. As a freestanding vocational rehabilitation agency, VRC recognized the need to offer its head injured clients the cognitive rehabilitation and other therapies necessary to succeed in work training and placement. For their part, UCP recognized the possibility of expanding their services to include head injured clients in their independent living program. By developing a collaborative agreement, these agencies, together, provide a continuum of services to their clients. Through interagency referrals, joint treatment, and shared staffings, clients may participate in any or all of the programs, as either inpatients or outpatients, depending on their needs. Early in their rehabilitation, head injured clients begin to develop cognitive strategies at the Institute that prepare them for the types of training and placement services offered by the Vocational Rehabilitation Center and for return to their communities. The Institute also provides counseling, physical therapy, occupational therapy, speech-language therapy, and work adjustment services necessary for success in the vocational setting and for successful independent living. Clients referred to VRC may spend part of their time at the Institute to continue treatment for those cognitive or motoric deficits that interfere with progress in the vocational areas. As patients progress to the point at which they are ready to benefit from a community living arrangement, staff members from UCP and the Institute communicate goals and also techniques that may assist in achieving the goals.

There are, of course, other examples of networking agreements that work in the best interests of the head injured clients they serve, and although networking may be more common in acute care hospitals, more and more rehabilitation agencies are using the networking concept to develop and refine service delivery systems. As illustrated in Figure 10–1, The Rehabilitation Institute of Pittsburgh's Head Injury Program has moved from a single agency offering highly specialized but somewhat limited services to the focal point in a network that enables clients to receive comprehensive, coordinated services along a much broader continuum. In many domains of rehabilitative treatment and in many areas of the country, however, head injured clients and their families continue to be underserved and, consequently, need to apply what they have learned through their experience to make the needs of head injured individuals known and to assist existing systems in their efforts to meet those needs. As in so many other areas of health and human services, the consumer advocates may well be the driving force behind improved comprehensive services for individuals who have suffered severe head injury.

ADVOCACY

Having identified the needs of clients and families and examined traditional resources and possible adaptations to existing programs, it

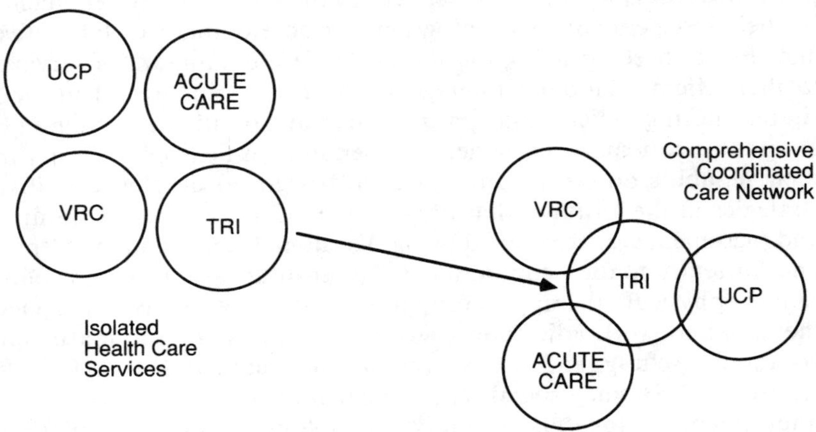

Figure 10–1. An illustration of how isolated agencies can create a network of agencies to deliver care in an integrated manner. TRI — The Rehabilitation Institute of Pittsburgh; VRC — Vocational Rehabilitation Center of Allegheny County; UCP — United Cerebral Palsy.

is necessary to determine an appropriate agenda for efforts in advocacy. Unlike cancer or heart disease, head injury is not yet a household word. Although in the United States, 500,000 to 700,000 people are hospitalized each year as a result of head injury and 70,000 of these injuries are severe (Committee on Trauma Research, 1985), their consequences are little understood by the general public. In fact, head injured patients often fail to attract the attention they deserve (Jennett & Teasdale, 1981). The task of education and advocacy will, at least initially, fall largely upon those individuals and families immediately affected and those health care professionals who serve them. Although it may seem an insurmountable task, it helps to remember that other significant milestones for handicapped individuals, such as P.L. 94-142, the Education for the Handicapped Act, did not always exist either. This important legislation, like many other major political changes, was initiated by a small group of families and professionals. The education of individuals is followed by the education of local communities, and ultimately the political system can be made to respond. One excellent source of information on advocacy, "Self-Advocacy: How to be a Winner," is available from the National Information Center for Handicapped Children and Youth.

Individual efforts begin with head injured clients and their families testing and changing the delivery systems encountered in their own communities. Different areas of the country are at quite different stages of sophistication in the services offered to head injured clients. Acute care hospitals, rehabilitation centers, vocational agencies, and schools vary widely in their ability to meet the unique needs of the individual affected by head injury. Each opportunity, each success, provides learning that can be transferred to other situations and to the advocacy activities that are needed.

One of the most useful resources is the National Head Injury Foundation (NHIF), which maintains information on available services in various areas. Involvement of family members and head injured individuals in NHIF serves many purposes, not least of which is collective advocacy. "Through their involvement in such an organization, family members can be involved in decision making and plans for the future regarding head trauma treatment" (Sachs, 1985, p. 23).

The establishment and maintenance of a head injury registry should also be a national priority, as should integration of services offered by public agencies. One such effort by the Office of Special Education and Rehabilitation Services would establish responsibility for a continuum of services among many publicly funded agencies on behalf of head injured individuals. In their 1985 report on traumatic brain injury, the Rehabilitation Services Administration (RSA) outlined a number of problems and concerns across the United States and suggested a directon for integrated efforts on the part of the numerous public agencies. Among their chief concerns was the need for each state to have a plan for comprehensive service delivery to individuals affected by severe head injury and the development of advocacy groups to bring the special needs of this group to the attention of state legislatures (Department of Education, 1985).

Research needs to be expanded and focused on the needs of the head injured population, both pediatric and adult. Neurosurgical advances may decrease the amount of secondary brain damage, pharmacologic advances may provide us with better answers to stubborn treatment questions in basic areas of cognitive and behavioral functioning, and efficacy research may determine what techniques are most effective in teaching cognitive and psychosocial skills. Figure 10–2 dramatically illustrates the neglect of research at the level of the federal government in the area of injury. Agencies such as the National Institute for Handicapped Research and the Veteran's Administration have been influential in sponsoring significant research projects, and various other public and private agencies have

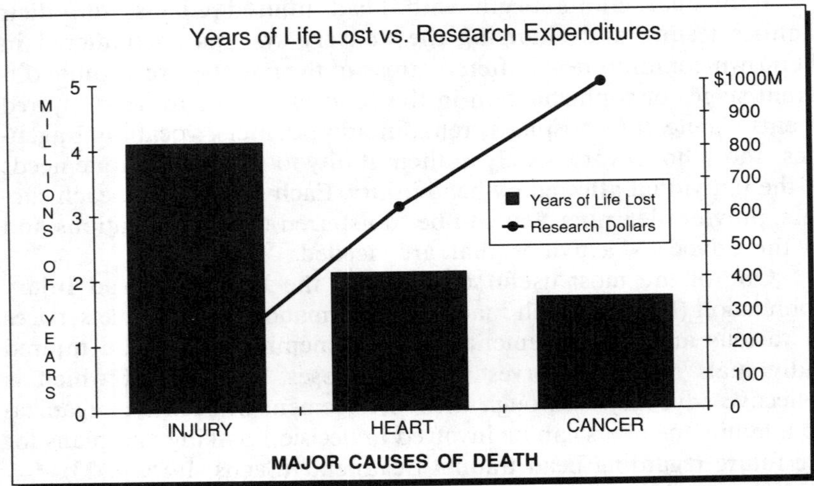

Figure 10–2. Research expenditures compared to impact in terms of mortality: injury, heart disease, and cancer. Information taken from *Injury in America* (1985).

begun to recognize the need for answers to the many questions in the largely uncharted territory of traumatic brain injury. As suggested in the Department of Education (1985) report, significant priorities include the areas of prevention, rehabilitation in the acute phase and early post-coma period, and in the period one year post-trauma. Of these priorities, perhaps the most important is prevention.

Many states have strengthened their drunk driving laws, the national speed limit remains at 55 mph despite efforts in some areas to increase it, and some states now have laws requiring the use of seat belts. These measures undoubtedly help prevent some head injuries. As a nation, however, we have not been successful in mandating passive restraint systems, such as air bags in motor vehicles, and despite the many public service campaigns and other efforts aimed at encouraging the use of seat belts, effective methods have not yet been found to ensure that this simple preventive measure will be taken by both drivers and passengers.

Substance abuse on the highway continues to be an area in which education aimed at the prevention of head injuries is needed. About 50 percent of brain injuries are caused by motor vehicle accidents, and a quick scan of almost any daily newspaper shows that there are far too many vehicular accidents involving drivers under the influence of alcohol or other drugs. This sad fact indicates that an effective method to discourage such abuse has not yet been found.

Safety during sports activities has also shown itself to be an area in need of improvement. In addition to recognizing the need for more effective helmets and other protective equipment, we must concentrate on educating the public to the dangers of young people participating in strenuous contact sports such as football prior to adequate physical maturation, muscle development, and training. Safety, rather than winning, must become the priority in the arenas of competitive sports for young people.

Emphasis must also be placed on the improvement of safety standards in work places. Occupational safety, along with improved equipment, can contribute to the prevention of head injuries resulting from industrial accidents.

In addition to those areas noted, advocacy groups need to lobby for research in the growing field of cognitive rehabilitation therapy. Such questions as "What is cognitive rehabilitation therapy?" "Does it do any good?" "Which treatment techniques are most effective?" and "Should it be defined as a separate field of rehabilitation?" are not yet satisfactorily answered. Answers to these questions may then logically initiate inquiry about how to provide training in this area.

Although at the present time there is no clearly identified preservice or inservice preparation for individuals practicing or wishing to practice in this growing field, experience suggests that an interdisciplinary approach may yield the greatest gains for those who have suffered a severe head injury. The uniqueness of each individual both prior to and after such an assault requires the services of many specialists in medicine and rehabilitation, and the treatment issues involved cut across many professions. Without an interdisciplinary approach, fragmentation of service delivery seems unavoidable. While it is not perfect, this team concept seems to hold the most promise for delivering integrated services to the head injured client.

Since many individuals affected by severe head injury are young adults (between 16 and 21 years of age), we must also strive to make the special education systems in our states aware of the educational needs of the head injured population in this age group. Too often, individuals who have suffered a severe head injury are treated as exaggerated learning disabled or socially and emotionally disturbed young adults rather than given the cognitive training they need for success in the educational and vocational environments. Whether services are delivered in separate classrooms or within existing regular or special education settings, such services must be aimed at the particular needs of the head injured individual. (These issues are further discussed in Chapter 3.)

Along with advocating better programs, those interested in the welfare of head injured individuals must lobby for comprehensive medicare, medicaid, insurance, and SSI benefits. The funding stream for acute care, rehabilitation services, and skilled nursing care needs to be uninterrupted and flow directly with the client. Only when comprehensive funding is available can we hope for comprehensive service agreements that will provide all the services necessary to treat head injured individuals and also undertake research to improve the success rate in their treatment.

One of the important objectives of research and improved funding must be the development of assistive devices and other high technology aides to enable the head injured individual to function effectively despite significant physical deficits and return to the most productive lifestyle possible. The success of new technology, however, may indeed rest upon the creation of funding streams that allow devices to follow the client to the home and work place rather than remaining a luxury to be explored exclusively in the rehabilitation setting. Manufacturers in rehabilitation-related fields of technology must be urged to make and market at reasonable prices the types of adaptive equipment that research and practice show to be useful. An interesting discussion of these subjects and their relationship to rehabilitation in general appears in Bowe (1980).

The management of and advocacy for programs for head injured individuals have become important issues in treatment. Along with education aimed at preventing head injury and improving clinical skills in treatment, we must work toward providing the appropriate environment for cooperative agreements and networking. Much of this can be done through a strong advocacy system that takes advantage of existing resources and encourages their use in creative and efficient ways. These goals will be most effectively achieved by a coalition of individuals who have suffered head injury, their families, and the professional community interested in comprehensive rehabilitation.

REFERENCES

Ben-Yishay, Y. & Diller, L. (1983). Notes toward a systems approach to the rehabilitation of the traumatically brain injured. In *Working approaches to remediation of cognitive deficits in brain damaged persons* (Rehabilitation Monograph No. 66). New York: New York University Medical Center, Institute of Rehabilitation Medicine.

Bowe, F. (1980). *Rehabilitating America.* New York: Harper & Row.

Committee on Trauma Research. (1985). *Injury in America: A continuing public health problem.* Washington, DC: National Academy Press.

Department of Education. (1985). *Report on issues relating to traumatic brain injury.* Washington, DC.

Jennett, B. & Teasdale, G. (1981). *Management of head injuries.* Philadelphia: F. A. Davis & Co.

Johnson, H. W., McLaughlin, J. A. & Christensen, M. (1982). Interagency collaboration: Driving and restraining forces. *Exceptional Children, 48,* 395–399.

LaCour, J. A. (1982). Interagency agreement: A rational response to an irrational system. *Exceptional Children, 49,* 265–267.

Magrab, P. & Elder, J. (Eds.), (1979). *Planning for services to handicapped persons: Community, education, health.* Baltimore: Paul Brooks.

Martinson, M. C. (1982). Interagency services: A new era for an old idea. *Exceptional Children, 48,* 389–394.

Oddy, M., Coughlan, T., Tyerman, A. & Jenkins, D. (1985). Social adjustment after closed head injury: A further follow-up seven years after injury. *Journal of Neurology, Neurosurgery, and Psychiatry, 48,* 564–568.

Oddy, M., Humphrey, M. & Uttley, D. (1978). Stress upon the relatives of head injured persons. *British Journal of Psychiatry, 133,* 507–513.

Sachs, P. R. (1985). Beyond support: Traumatic head injury as a growth experience for families. *Rehabilitation Nursing, 10,* 21–23.

Weddell, R., Oddy, M. & Jenkins, D. (1980). Social adjustment after rehabilitation: A two year follow-up of patients with severe head injury. *Psychological Medicine, 10,* 257–263.

Epilogue

A Letter to Professionals Who Work with Head Injured People

Beth B. O'Brien

Head injuries happen to people — most often young people whose limitless dreams and aspirations are shattered and whose families are called on to assume a role the dimensions of which are often beyond comprehension and for which they are not prepared. This is the fundamental reality underlying rehabilitation. This epilogue, a letter written by the mother of a head injured young man, is added to place in proper perspective all of the professional considerations presented in this book. Ultimately, models, theories, and techniques of rehabilitation, as well as agencies, policies, and organizations all have their point only because of real people struggling to recreate meaning and fulfillment in their lives.

John, my 20-year-old son, has moved away from the protective world of hospitals, home, and family, and into the world of relative independence and autonomy. He is now living 600 miles from home at the Center for Comprehensive Services in Illinois. He is willingly learning how to be independent, he is maturing emotionally, and he is finally beginning to adjust to his disability! Considering the extent of his injuries, I often wonder how we managed to get this far. "Life after head injury may never be the same." That is what they say at the National Head Injury Foundation, and it's the truth! John is a different person and so is his mother. The event that threw our lives into chaos 6 years ago has changed us in ways that are hard to calculate. I still get that awful feeling in my stomach every time I think about his accident. John was simply crossing the street, something he had done a thousand times before, when the car hit him. He was barely a teenager. He was a really good soccer player, captain of his wrestling team, a happy, social boy with a rich life ahead of him. As for me, I had just applied for admission to a master's program in social work. I wanted to work with cancer patients; John's father, my husband, had died of cancer just 3 years earlier.

I have learned a great deal in these past 6 years. I've made mistakes and have been angry and frustrated; I've struggled with people who didn't seem to care and with agencies that had nothing to offer. But I've also had success and have met the most caring people in the world and have found agencies that would move heaven and earth to help people in need. I want to share some of our experiences with you and let you know how we survived during these 6 years and how we sometimes even flourished. Perhaps these experiences will help you in your work with head injured people and their families. What I think and write now is, of course, filtered through time and change. I can't say for sure what I needed at each stage of our recovery, and I surely can't say what every other family or every other head injured persons needs.

John was in a "coma" for 6 months. It was 2 more months before we moved him from the acute care hospital to the rehabilitation center in August 1981. The tears that never seemed to stop tell me something now about how confused I was and how frustrated I felt with a system that seemed unable to recognize our needs or that was simply ill-equipped to help survivors of severe head injury.

It seems silly now that I asked the neurosurgeon only a week after the accident when John would be able to come home. I had no idea of the magnitude of the problem. And the neurosurgeon made no attempt to begin my education. Six months later, another hospital physican told us, "What you see is what you get. When are you taking John home?" Since we had had him home for one- and two-day visits, I knew I could not handle him at home. How could they possibly ask me to do that? And with no preparation? They made no suggestions about where John could go for more rehabilitation, or even about how to find home care services. No brochures, no lists of agencies in the area, no names to call.

Perhaps they didn't consider John a candidate for rehabilitation: he could not walk, talk, dress, or eat with any semblance of independence. But we had hope. Thank God we had hope! Suppose we had given up?

Some of that hope came from good folks at the acute care hospital. The Sisters of Mercy pulled me through many bad days and even more bad nights. Their quiet presence, their invitations to prayer and to lunch gave us hope, strength, and a little perspective. They visited John daily, and although some say that he was taking in no information at the time, I believe that this was very important for him. John wrote a poem just before the accident that expressed his great, child-like faith:

Who's up there?
Why is He up there?
How did He get there?
Maybe he flew up there.
I'm just glad He's up there.

I heard about a local rehabilitation institute quite by accident, from a friend whose classmate knew something about the agency. I called to see what I could possibly do with John. What followed were 4 years of mainly positive experiences, with John first as an inpatient and later as an outpatient and student in the agency's special education center.

I knew nothing about rehabilitation or home care or, for that matter, about head injury. Like most people, I had some ideas about heart attacks and strokes, but I had absolutely no frame of reference for head injury. My anxiety did not go away when John was admitted to the rehabilitation center: the intake unit seemed disorganized, crowed, and casual, a sharp contrast to the formal and efficient hospital we had just left. Perhaps the staff assumed that I knew what was going on; head injury had been part of our lives for 6 months, and I had initiated John's admission without professional help.

My usual strategy for dealing with big problems is to fill my head with information. Other people have different needs: some need a hug and a reassuring voice above all; others need guidance and direction. But I wanted information. The first hospital had taught me nothing about brain damage; and the books that I found in the local library were of little help. During those long months of acute care, when I wondered if John would ever wake up, I wanted to learn about head injury: What happened to my son's brain? What would he be like? What happens to families in this situation? How do they cope?

Perhaps I'm kidding myself, but I feel strongly that if I had had some simple printed material that disucssed these issues I would have been much less anxious and would have had more confidence in attacking a force that seemed at the time to be both indomitable and incomprehensible. My introduction to rehabilitation would also have been much more comfortable if I had had a better understanding of the roles of the professionals treating John and how I was going to fit into the big picture. Although visiting was unlimited and I was invited to observe and even participate in therapy sessions, my lack of understanding almost gave me the feeling that I was not supposed to fit in.

Since it's important for me to appear to be in control, it was very hard for me to admit that I did not understand what I was being told. The first formal meeting with the staff of the center was a nightmare. It was brutally demoralizing to face a set of professionals who had very important information and not be able even to understand their titles, much less their jargon. "Physical therapy" and "speech therapy" made some sense to me, but what did "occupational therapy" mean? Wasn't it a bit early to be thinking about occupations? And what was "cognitive rehabilitation therapy"? And Aphasia? Apraxia? Agnosia? When they first mentioned John's "premorbid" characteristics, I thought maybe they were predicting his death! These strange and bewildering words made me feel uneducated and uncomfortable and initially formed a barrier between me and the staff.

Under the extraordinary stress caused by traumatic brain injury to a member of family, people do not hear well, and they remember less. Furthermore, what they are emotionally capable of comprehending changes over time. Printed materials — a layman's glossary of terms, simple descriptions of head injury and of the treatment program, guidelines for what family members can do to help — are very useful. They can be studied, digested piecemeal, shared with friends, and returned to when a new stage of acceptance makes possible a deeper processing of the information.

Meeting other people who had already experienced what I was going through was enormously helpful to me. Meeting Jean Bush, for instance, was a major breakthrough. Jean and her husband Gerry also have a head injured son. In their search for answers they had met people in the Boston area who were forming a group, the National Head Injury Foundation. The information that I started to receive became a lifeline. I knew I wasn't alone. But what we all discovered was that there simply was not much information available. The highly sophisticated medical system that had saved our sons' lived had little to tell us about how to rehabilitate them.

That was how I began my association with NHIF, my route to sanity through all the stress. We all have different needs, but I believe that the Foundation can be a vital support for head injured persons, their families, and professionals. Head injury causes isolation, and a support group is good medicine; helping others cope with and solve their problems is also therapeutic. NHIF meetings may be the only place where our problems are understood. Local chapters provide support to people at all stages of recovery and make information available about all aspects of head injury. Meetings are an opportunity to share experiences and first-hand knowledge about local resources; they also create the supportive context families need to confront their denial of the injury. Most families are like me; they know nothing about head injury and have never before met a family struggling with its consequences. Sharing with other families helps them to ease their fears of the unknown and strengthen their conviction that they can handle the crisis. Working with the NHIF chapter to locate resources, to educate the community about the problems of head injury and the needs created by it, and to advocate the development of resources can create a focus for fragmented lives and a safety valve for frustration. The meetings have helped me and many other families I have known over the past 5 years grow and become more stable.

They have also helped John. In order to foster free expression of thoughts, feelings, and frustrations, we generally split into two groups — one for family members and one for head injured individuals. During the drive home after one of these meetings, John said, "What a great meeting we had — too bad I can't remember what it was about." And John had useful ideas to contribute. I'll never forget an NHIF meeting we attended several years ago. A professional spoke to the group and closed by asking if there was anything that her organization could do for the support group. In his characteristically uninhibited way, John said with no hesitation, "Start a dating service!" Just recently I read an article in *Disabled USA* about Handicapped Introductions, a dating service for disabled people. John was ahead of his time.

The most difficult part of John's injury for both of us has been his terrible loneliness. He yearns for the companionship of other young people, for the activities that are important for anyone his age. If you have any doubts that your work to promote active community re-entry for head injured young people is of value, put them to rest. You help to give meaning to their lives.

I knew instinctively that John's reintegration into his community would be the key to his rehabilitation. It was not easy. It was not easy for either of us to expose his new self to a sometimes unkind and sometimes thoughtless world. It was not easy to confront a community that did not understand the anger of a traumatized teenager. It was not easy for the people John knew before his accident to understand and accept occasionally angry, offensive, and inappropriate behavior from their old friend.

But John absoutely needed to be part of the normal world of teenage activities. I swear we tried everything: the city parks recreation program, Easter Seals camp, young peoples' group at church, bowling, music lessons, YMCA day camp, sled skiing, horseback riding, cooking, amateur photography, and cactus gardening. The cactus garden was a catastrophe. It's hard to believe that we hadn't anticipated the result of combining a cactus with significiant tremors! The amateur photography wasn't a howling success either for the same reason, despite countless hours of work by the creative staff at the rehabilitation agency to mount the camera on John's wheelchair so he could use it.

Helping John become a part of the teenage world had its notable moments, especially during outings and vacations. John's favorite activity has always been fishing. Despite the tremors, he has been able to relearn fishing, except for baiting the hook. Handling nightcrawlers is not exactly my line of work. On one fishing expedition there were no other fishermen available to bait the hook, and I wasn't having an easy time of it. Finally, in frustration I dumped all those worms on the dock and chased them with the hook until I got one. After that it was only shrimp and minnows for bait, but I did learn from a friendly fisherman how to bait a hook. John was very proud of me.

Camping vacations through the local Easter Seals organization were also a successful adventure. The first year, John was gone for 10 days while I took a needed vacation. My first 3 days were ruined by a stomachache. When I picked John up at camp, I learned that he had spent the first 3 days in the infirmary with a stomachache! It was the first time we had been separated in the 3 years since his accident. When John's second year at the camp ended — and with no stomachaches for either of us — the camp director told me that he had not been looking forward to John's return to camp because his attitude and behavior had been so difficult the first year. But John had changed so much that the camp staff had actually enjoyed his presence.

A vacation to Florida also stands out in my mind. The beaches at Daytona appealed to John because the surface is hard enough for a wheelchair, and the boardwalk allowed great access to young people and activities. John, whose desire to drive has been about as intense as his desire for a girl friend, had his heart set on trying one of the three-wheeled all-terrain vehicles that are used on the beach. He nagged until I relented. In his excitement, he went much too fast, hit a sand gully, and went head over heels. After the paramedics declared no one hurt, John sheepishly admitted that maybe he wasn't quite ready for driving yet. All this time I, of course, had been wondering if my judgment was as impaired as his, but at least the "Why can't I drive?" issue was diffused for another week.

Without these activities, John's life would have been empty, and despair would have consumed him. How did we find useful activities? The staff of the rehabilitation center were very helpful. They knew that walking, talking, and relearning how to read and do math do not exhaust the interests of a teenage young man. They adapted equipment and taught John to compensate for his disability when necessary, and they constantly explored new areas of possible interest. They also made a great suggestion early in his rehabilitation, a personal computer at home. The time he spent was therapeutically useful, but, more importantly, he liked it, it was a fun way to spend his leisure time, and it was an activity that he could do with friends.

When it came to finding community activities, on the other hand, I had to rely largely on my own instincts and resources. I investigated everything that seemed even remotely possible. I searched the newspapers, the telephone book, and the public library. And I mainly asked friends for help. I would never have survived without my friends.

Friends! I've known from the time of my husband's death how essential a support system is for me. I am an independent person, but I knew that at the time of John's accident I had to ask friends for help and accept their help. I am sure there are times when your greatest contribution to a family will be your encouragement to seek support and accept help from friends. Teach them how to build a support network.

I think I needed my friends most when I saw John suffering and there was little I could do. Including John in community activities was a frightening challenge. He hurt deep inside when he saw other teens going off to school, playing sports, attending dances, hanging out uptown. His hurt nearly broke my heart. I was angry. I guess I still have some very real anger. John and I can't face the world alone. This is when friends are needed and tested. The best friends are those who are open, honest, practical, and caring. They will invite you and your son to a holiday party when they know that you would otherwise be alone. So what if John propositions one of the guests? My friends handle it with love and understanding.

New friendships developed as a result of my taking John to sports events at his former high school, but there were some problems friendships couldn't resolve. In trying to integrate John back into his community, I began with activities that had been most important for him. He was always a good athlete and still knew many of the players on the teams. The high school officials were very cooperative. They gave us a special parking place and allowed John to watch the games from the field. For John, this was great fun and great therapy. He was with people who knew him, who were patient with him, and who accepted him most of the time. The crunch came after the games were over: John had to go home with his mother while the others partied or hung out downtown. It was not that I insisted that John go home with me; rather, it was just too much for the young people to include John in the after-game activities. John thought that if he could drive, everything would be O.K. His frustration led to horrendous outbursts; his fury was uncontrollable. Driving remains the one issue that makes his frustration violent. I wonder if he will ever accept the verdict that he can never drive.

I'm sure I don't need to tell you that the care-giver's life is filled with stress. Professionals have told me from the beginning that I need to "take care of myself." This is very true and their advice is sound. I have experienced myself and have seen in others the terrible toll that this stress takes on family relationhships. I have regret and guilt concerning the amount of time I devoted to John to the exclusion of my other children. Care-givers need information about the dynamics of stress on families — spouses and siblings — as well as specific advice on how to acquire respite and attendant care. There have been many times when I needed and wanted time away from John, and there have been an equal number of times when John needed companionship other than mine. He resented attendant care as "babysitting" unless the person was around his own age. I tried nursing services and answered personal ads in the newspapers; we even ran ads for help through university employment offices. Many of the recruits were people my age (heaven forbid, another mother!); John rejected others as misfits. And it was exhausting explaining to every new person the little I knew about head injury and behavior management.

The best answer to my need for relief was always calling on a friend of John's. Yes, John developed his own small support system. There are a few, very special young people with an understanding and compassion beyond their years. They are still an integral part of our lives and our support system. The great thing about young people as care-givers is that they do things: they play cards, go out for pizza, take in a movie, attend special events. John enjoyed this. But it was never a complete answer for him because he was still not in control. John will not feel that he has a solution until he is in control of what he does.

John's cognitive and social problems have always been the most troubling for both of us. Weak memory, difficulty in taking in new information, poor judgment, social inappropriateness, uninhibited behavior: the impact of these problems seems to outweigh by far John's considerable physical deficits. John couldn't understand why his old friends deserted him, why he couldn't drive like everyone else, why he couldn't have a beer, why he couldn't have a girl friend, why he couldn't go to school at his old high school.

John wanted so much to return to his school. He thought he could handle it. I regularly listed the many reasons why it wouldn't work; I carefully explained the importance of the special school at the rehabilitation center; I pointed out that we were very lucky to have such an excellent resource close to home. My explanations fell on the deaf ears of a teenager who has little respect for his mother's wisdom. When John was at the rehabilitation center, he was happy. It was only when he was back home, thinking about his life and feeling his loneliness, that he missed his old school.

What have I learned about being an advocate for my son and successfully acquiring the best community services? For me, it has been important to become knowledgeable about head injury and to become actively involved with organizations that can help. I am active at the local, state, and national levels of NHIF. I have read many of the recently published books on head injury. I have attended as many conferences as possible. This has been a labor of love — love for John and for all of the other head injured people I have come to know. In a way John is one of the lucky ones: he has good funding, and he is one of the 5 percent of head injured people who are receiving services. But what about the rest? Professionals and families must continue to fight for services and funding for the remaining 95 percent.

I am 48 years old. Who will take care of John when I cannot? He will always need supervision. He will always need help to be part of the community. I need to think about his long-term needs and how he can grow. He was 14 when he had the accident. After 4 years at home, it was clear that my 18 year old was in many ways still 14. He was not maturing. As hard as I had tried to bring his life into a normal pattern, he was not maturing. He needed the independence that is normal for 18 year olds. I had raised my other children to be independent and to be ready to go away to college at 18. It was hard for me to accept that cutting the apron strings was equally necessary for John. College was out of the question. But what then? The thought of his leaving gave me my old stomachache. Who would kiss him goodnight? But then how many 18 year olds are kissed goodnight by their mothers?

John needed an independent living program that focused on his self-responsibility and his social and emotional maturity. The program would need to address issues like sexuality, peer group relationships, and independence. I knew it would be best for John to struggle with these issues away from home. It was painful at the beginning to drag him around to several facilities that couldn't meet his needs. Fortunately, we found one that could. We chose the Center for Comprehensive Services on the basis of its reputation, its long association with NHIF, and conversations I had had with others who had made similiar decisions. I was also guided by the NHIF guidelines for choosing a rehabilitation facility.

John has been in Carbondale now for 7 months and has recently moved to the Center's Transitional Living House. I would say his adjustment to leaving home took at least 5 months. The staff told me that homesickness would be a major hurdle, and it was. But I promised them I would not take him out of the program no matter how many tears of anguish either of us shed. To some degree, I was prepared for this transition by our experience during the last few weeks of John's inpatient rehabilitation. He would cry, rage, complain, and demand to move home, but I knew I had to be strong.

I began this letter by saying that John is now maturing emotionally, learning to be independent, and beginning to adjust to his disability. It has been a long row to hoe, and the work is far from done. John and I have both changed; we have both grown. I am now in the master's program that I first applied to 6 years ago. My goal when I am done is to continue to be an advocate for head injured people, and their families. We have come far, we have far to go. We need your help.

Author Index

A

Abelson, R., 159, 214
Abraham, J., 286, 299
Abramson, M., 351, 352, 363, 379
Adamovitch, B., 180, 182, 210
Adams, J. H., 4, 21
Adams, R., 351, 377
Adkins, C., 351, 352, 353, 354, 358, 361, 362, 374, 375, 378
Amary, I., 351, 377
American College of Sports Medicine, 69, 71, 74
American National Standards Institute, 67, 74
Anderson, J., 89, 95, 101, 130
Anderson, R., 363, 377
Anderson, T., 270, 296
Antrobus, J. S., 136
Arnold, S., 279, 298
Arthur, G., 222, 257
Astrand, P. O., 69, 74
Arthelstan, G., 266, 297
Auerbach, S., 180, 182, 210
Ausubel, D. P., 245, 253
Aves, D. K., 287, 292, 295, 296
Avezaat, C., 27, 75
Ayres, A. J., 36, 74

B

Baddeley, A., 95, 130, 142, 210
Baer, D. M., 233, 241, 257
Baker, E., 158, 210
Baker, L., 36, 74
Balicki, M., 128, 134
Bandura, A., 119, 130
Barbera, M., 153, 211
Barrett, J. E., 67, 76
Barth, J. T., 2, 22, 221, 230, 256, 277, 298
Bartlett, F. C., 94, 130, 158, 210
Basmajian, J. V., 36, 74
Batellan, J., 44, 76
Baxter, R., 107, 130
Bean, J., 27, 76
Behrman, M., 192, 210
Beisser, A. R., 390, 400
Bell, J., 116, 134
Bellack, A. S., 376, 377
Bellamy, G. T., 238, 239, 254, 257, 299
Bender, M., 363, 377
Benson, D. F., 158, 214
Benton, A. L., 1, 4, 21, 87, 95, 97, 134, 153, 212, 221, 255, 260, 296
Ben-Yishay, Y., 3, 20, 88, 108, 119, 130, 137, 140, 189, 210, 227, 243, 244, 245, 250, 254, 257, 261, 263, 278, 290, 296, 297, 324, 345, 404, 418
Bergen, A., 53, 74
Berroll, S., 242, 254
Bigge, J. L., 367, 369, 377
Biggs, S. J., 196, 211, 212, 214
Bisanz, J., 116, 132, 133
Black, J., 112, 130, 242, 256
Blazyk, S., 372, 377
Blyth, B., 26, 74
Bobath, B., 36, 74
Boll, T. J., 221, 230, 256, 277, 298
Bolton, B., 257
Bolton, S. D., 57, 74
Bond, M. R., 1, 7, 20, 26, 75, 105, 130, 133, 174, 210, 211, 213, 221, 254, 298, 305, 345, 346, 349, 350, 377, 381, 382, 384, 386, 400, 401
Boone, L., 294, 297
Booth, B. J., 36
Botterbusch, K. F., 229, 254, 271, 272, 280, 297, 298
Bowe, F., 418
Bower, G., 95, 130
Bowers, D., 16, 21
Bowers, S., 27, 74
Braakman, R., 27, 75
Bracy, O. L., 192, 210

Brainerd, C., 135, 213
Brigance, A., 311, 345
Brooks, D. N., 1, 8, 9, 20, 87, 95, 96, 97, 101, 130, 131, 383, 384, 385, 386, 401
Brooks, N., 105, 133, 156, 210, 221, 254, 345, 350, 377, 378
Brouwer, W., 88, 131
Brown, A. L., 94, 95, 96, 97, 116, 131, 158, 159, 210
Brown, D., 213
Brown, J., 136
Bruce, D., 402
Bruckner, F. E., 221, 254, 277, 297, 349, 377, 387, 401
Bruyn, A. W., 22, 23
Buenning, W., 153, 211
Burns, D., 185, 210
Burns, D. D., 246, 254, 373, 377
Burns, M. S., 182, 210
Butters, N., 95, 131

C

Calliet, R., 30, 74
Campione, J. C., 116, 131
Cantor, 112, 131
Carlston, D., 112, 133
Carper, M., 128, 134
Caton, W., 26, 27, 75
Ceci, S., 94, 116, 131
Cermak, L., 95, 130, 131, 133, 135, 136, 158, 210, 212, 214, 215
Certo, N., 379
Chadwick, O., 2, 22
Chaffee, P., 388, 389, 401
Chapman, L. R., 5, 6, 7, 21
Chi, M. T. H., 100, 116, 131, 159, 210
Chiulli, S., 158, 214
Chomsky, N., 89, 131
Christensen, M., 412, 419
Clark, E., 174, 210
Clark, H., 174, 210
Clovers, M., 296, 297
Cofer, C. N., 95, 131
Cohen, J., 227, 254
Cohen, S., 107, 124, 125, 126, 130, 131
Colangelo, C., 53, 74
Cole, J. C., 29, 75, 261, 274, 298, 302, 303, 304, 325, 345, 346
Cole, M., 135
Cole, P., 211
Collins, A., 213
Committee on Trauma Research, 404, 406, 408, 414, 416, 419
Condeluci, A., 295, 297, 312, 320, 322, 336, 345
Connis, R., 290, 299
Cook, D. W., 257
Corthell, D. W., 294, 297
Costa, L. D., 385, 386, 401
Coughlan, T., 9, 10, 22, 305, 346, 404, 419
Cowood, L. T., 223, 254
Craik, F. I. M., 94, 95, 131, 132, 158, 210, 212
Craine, J. F., 96, 132, 137, 211
Crewe, N., 266, 297
Crosson, B., 153, 211
Crovitz, H. F., 153, 211
Crowder, R., 90, 93, 132
Csongradi, J. J., 49, 76
Cull, J. G., 222, 254, 255
Cuvo, A. J., 227, 231, 241, 257

D

Daniel, A., 351, 377
Dashiell, S. E., 57, 74
DeJong, G., 302, 309, 322, 345
DeKosky, S. T., 16, 21
DeLoach, C., 310, 320, 345
Delwaide, P. J., 36, 76
DeMarco, B., 361, 378
Department of Education, 415, 416, 419
Deutsch, D., 100, 132, 133
Deutsch, J. A., 100, 132, 133
Diehl, L. N., 205, 208, 211
Dikman, S., 221, 254
Dikmen, S., 397, 401
Diller, L., 88, 108, 119, 130, 132, 137, 140, 153, 189, 210, 211, 227, 243, 244, 245, 250, 254, 257, 261, 263, 278, 290, 297, 404, 418
Dodd, D., 90, 132
Dollard, J., 119, 134
Donaldson, W., 136
Dowrick, P. W., 196, 211, 212, 214
Doyle, D., 4, 21
Doyle, M., 36, 74
Ducker, C., 301, 345
Dustman, R., 88, 92, 108, 132, 140, 211
Duyvis, J. D., 43, 76

E

Ebbesen, B., 133
Ebert, V., 96, 136, 157, 215
Edgington, C., 362, 377
Egan, G., 373, 377
Eichler, J. J., 43, 74
Elder, J., 412, 419
Elliot-Faust, D., 116, 135, 153, 213
Ellis, A., 185, 211, 244, 247, 254, 373, 377

Emery, G., 185, 211
Enders, A., 44, 49, 75
Estes, W. K., 135
Ewing-Cobbs, L., 2, 21
Ezrachi, O., 3, 20, 88, 108, 130, 137, 140, 189, 210, 227, 243, 257, 261, 263, 278, 290, 297

F

Farber, S. D., 36, 75
Fawber, H. L., 295, 297, 320, 322, 336, 345
Fensterman, K., 72, 75
Ferguson, S. M., 15, 21
Feuerstein, R., 119, 132, 158, 164, 169, 182, 183, 211, 232, 234, 255
Field, J. E., 223, 255
Field, T. F., 223, 255
Flamm, L., 15, 21
Flavell, J. H., 93, 111, 115, 116, 132
Fletcher, J. M., 2, 21
Fordyce, D. J., 8, 21, 128, 135, 193, 213, 221, 227, 243, 246, 250, 256, 261, 262, 263, 271, 278, 290, 297, 298, 303, 304, 345, 346, 397, 401
Forrest-Pressley, D., 116, 135, 153, 213
Foster, R., 311, 345
Fowler, R., 278, 297
Fox, S. M., 69, 70, 75
Fry, R., 256, 257, 271, 299

G

Gajar, A., 231, 255
Galambos, J., 112, 130
Galbraith, S., 27, 75
Gale, J. L., 397, 401
Gans, J. S., 2, 21
Gardner, D. C., 249, 255
Gardner, H., 15, 21
Gazzaniga, M., 249, 255
Gedde, D., 351, 377
Geller, R., 242, 256
Gerrein, J., 131
Gerring, J. P., 124, 135
Ghatala, E., 116, 134
Gianutsos, R., 128, 132, 153, 158, 211
Gibson, E. J., 92, 93, 132
Gilchrist, E., 2, 3, 21, 221, 255, 277, 297, 349, 377, 387, 401
Ginzberg, E., 246, 255
Giordani, B., 2, 22, 277
Giordani, M. A., 221, 230, 256
Gitomer, D., 116, 132
Glang, A. E., 192, 212
Glasgow, R. E., 153, 211
Glasser, W., 244, 245, 249, 250, 255, 373, 375, 378
Glenn, M. B., 221, 222, 242, 255
Gloag, D., 349, 378
Glover, A. T., 178, 212
Gobble, E. M., 373, 378
Goethe, K., 260, 297
Gogstad, A., 261, 263, 298
Goldstein, A. P., 244, 245, 255
Goldstein, G., 230, 255
Goldstein, K., 5, 21, 398, 401
Gordon, F., 116, 132
Gordon, P., 112, 133
Gordon, S., 112, 136
Gordon, W., 88, 132, 153, 211, 261, 263, 297
Gotts, E., 364, 379
Gouvier, W. D., 29, 75, 261, 274, 298, 303, 304, 325, 346
Graham, D. I., 4, 21
Grant, H., 27, 75
Gretz-Lasky, S., 295, 297, 320, 322, 336, 345
Grice, H., 174, 177, 211
Griffith, E. R., 26, 29, 75, 130, 210, 211, 213, 254, 298, 345, 346, 400
Gronwall, D., 97, 132, 242, 255
Gross, Y., 22, 402
Grossman, R. G., 1, 4, 7, 21, 87, 95, 97, 134, 153, 212, 221, 255
Gudeman, H. E., 96, 132, 137, 211
A guide to job analysis, 223, 255
Gummow, L., 88, 92, 108, 132, 140, 211

H

Haack, D., 27, 76
Haarbauer-Krupa, J., 109, 132, 143, 151, 163, 193, 211, 220
Hackler, E., 287, 298
Hagen, C., 104, 132, 159, 211, 332, 333, 345
Hagen, D., 192, 212
Hagen, J., 133, 134, 213
Hahn, H., 320, 342, 345
Haigh, B., 215
Halper, A. S., 182, 210
Hamilton, D., 133
Harden, R., 311, 347
Hardy, R. E., 222, 254, 255
Harris, J. E., 108, 132, 140, 157, 212
Harter, S., 119, 132
Harvey, M. T., 153, 170, 211
Hastie, R., 112, 133
Hastorf, A., 112, 133
Hayes, G., 362, 377
Heiden, J., 26, 27, 75
Heider, F., 120, 133
Heilman, K. M., 15, 16, 21, 23, 397, 401

Helffenstein, D., 193, 195, 212, 248, 255
Heller, K., 244, 245, 255
Henderson, J., 180, 182, 210
Henry, K., 109, 132, 143, 151, 193, 211, 220
Higgins, E., 174, 212
Hintzman, D. L., 90, 93, 94, 133
Hock, R. A., 382, 401
Hodson, L., 363, 377
Hogarty, G. E., 385, 401
Holland, A. L., 89, 135, 159, 186, 214, 215, 328, 346
Holland, J. L., 245, 246, 255
Holyoak, K., 112, 133
Horn, R. W., 153, 170, 211
Horner, R. H., 238, 254
Hosford, R. E., 195, 197, 212
Howe, M., 94, 116, 131
Humphrey, M., 221, 243, 255, 350, 378, 384, 401, 404, 419
Huppert, F., 95, 133

I

Imes, C., 192, 212
Ingram, A., 159, 213
Inhelder, B., 95, 134
Inman, D. P., 238, 254
Isen, A., 112, 133
Istominia, G. N., 116, 133
Ivan, L. P., 402

J

Jacobs, H., 302, 318, 336, 345
Jacoby, L., 158, 212
Jaffe, M., 28, 75
Jane, J. A., 2, 22, 221, 230, 256, 277, 298
Jefferson, G., 174, 214
Jenkins, D., 7, 9, 10, 22, 23, 305, 346, 387, 402, 404, 419
Jennett, B., 26, 27, 75, 105, 107, 133, 304, 345, 383, 402, 414, 419
Jennett, G., 303, 345
Johns, D., 215
Johnson, H. W., 412, 419
Johnson-Laird, P. N., 214
Jones, E. E., 120, 133
Jones, R., 363, 377
Joyce, C., 124, 125, 131

K

Kagan, N., 195, 212, 248, 255
Kail, R., 116, 133, 134, 213
Kanouse, D. E., 133
Kaplan, E. F., 158, 214
Kapur, N., 156, 212
Karan, O. C., 299
Karpman, T., 350, 374, 378
Katch, F. I., 70, 75
Katch, V. L., 70, 75
Katz, M. M., 11, 21, 385, 401
Kausler, D. H., 90, 133
Kavale, K., 88, 133, 189, 212
Kazdin, A. E., 212, 363, 378
Kelley, H. H., 133
Kelly, G. A., 245, 255
Kendall, P. C., 152, 212
Keogh, B. K., 178, 212
Kessen, W., 135, 213
Kiely, B., 194, 214
Kinsbourne, M., 94, 96, 101, 133, 136, 157, 158, 214, 215
Kintsch, W., 95, 133
Kjellman, A., 261, 263, 298
Klonoff, H., 2, 23
Klonoff, P. S., 1, 12, 22, 277, 298, 385, 386, 387, 393, 401, 402
Knapczyk, D., 355, 363, 378
Knott, M., 36, 75
Kozol, H. L., 17, 21
Kraat, A., 43, 75
Kraus, M., 290, 298
Kraus, R., 352, 378
Kraut, R., 174, 212
Kregel, J., 291, 299
Kruesi, E., 94, 134, 158, 213
Kurlycheck, R. T., 192, 212
Kurze, T., 26, 27, 75

L

LaCour, J. A., 412, 419
Lahey, B., 212
Lakin, P., 3, 20, 88, 108, 130, 137, 140, 189, 210, 227, 243, 245, 250, 254, 257, 261, 263, 278, 290, 297
Laurie, G., 312, 316, 346
LeBlanc, M. A., 49, 76
Leftoff, S., 8, 21
LePoole, J. B., 43, 76
Levin, D., 11, 12, 22
Levin, H. S., 1, 2, 4, 7, 21, 22, 87, 95, 97, 134, 153, 212, 221, 255, 260, 297
Levin, J. R., 116, 134, 213
Lewin, W., 28, 75
Lewinsohn, P. M., 153, 211
Lesak, M. D., 96, 134, 221, 243, 255, 256, 261, 263, 286, 298, 349, 350, 378, 383, 386, 401
Lincoln, N., 96, 131
Ling, P. K., 15, 21
Lipsitz, N., 286, 299
Lishman, W. A., 7, 8, 21, 221, 256, 397, 401

Livingston, M. G., 383, 386, 401
Lockhart, R., 95, 132
Lodico, M., 116, 134
Long, C. H., 29, 75, 261, 274, 298, 303, 304, 325, 346
Luria, A. R., 395, 401
Luterman, D., 390, 401
Lyerty, S. B., 11, 21
Lynch, R. T., 244, 256, 259, 298
Lynch, W. J., 189, 212, 242, 256
Lytel, R. B., 280, 298

M

Maas, A., 27, 75
MacEacheron, A., 290, 298
Mager, R., 362, 378
Magrab, P., 412, 419
Malec, J., 153, 158, 213
Maltzman, I., 135
Mandler, G., 160, 213
Mann, J., 222, 257
Markman, E. M., 116, 134
Marshall, L., 27, 74
Marshall, M. M., 384, 401
Marshall, T., 28, 75
Martinage, D. P., 384, 401
Martinson, M. C., 411, 419
Mastrilli, J., 28, 75
Matheson, J. M., 277, 298
Mattis, S., 156, 214, 259, 299
Mattson, P., 88, 133, 189, 212
Mauss, W. K., 242, 256
May, V. R., 242, 256
Mayer, R., 90, 93, 135
McArdle, W. D., 70, 75
McDonald, E. T., 43, 75
McDonald, J. R., 242, 256
McFarlane, B., 242, 257
McGonagle, E., 128, 134
McGowan, J., 222, 256
McGuinness, D., 15, 22
McKinlay, W. W., 8, 9, 384, 385, 401
McLaughlin, J. A., 412, 419
McLaughlin, P., 238, 257
McLean, A., 397, 401
Meers, G. D., 226, 256
Meichenbaum, D., 119, 134, 155, 175, 179, 213, 241, 244, 256
Mercer, C. D., 232, 241, 256
Merrett, J. D., 242, 256
Merry, P. H., 350, 378
Mesulam, M. M., 4, 21
Miller, E., 326, 346
Miller, G., 116, 135, 153, 213
Miller, G. A., 100, 134
Miller, J. D., 75, 130, 210, 211, 213, 254, 298, 345, 346, 400
Miller, N. E., 119, 134
Miller, P., 88, 92, 108, 132, 140, 211
Mills, M. E., 195, 197, 212
Mills, V., 28, 75
Minderhoud, J., 27, 75
Minters, F. C., 304, 346
Mischel, W., 112, 131
Mithaug, D. E., 238, 256
Moely, B. E., 94, 134, 158, 213
Moffat, N., 109, 131, 132, 136, 147, 156, 157, 158, 212, 213, 214, 215
Mogil, S. I., 182, 210
Molitor, C., 28, 75
Montgomery, J., 36, 59, 74, 75
Moreines, J., 95, 130
Morgan, J., 211
Moser, L., 163, 211
Muir, C., 205, 213
Murphy, P., 311, 347
Musante, S., 265, 271, 296, 298
Mussen, P. H., 134

N

Najenson, T., 286, 299, 350, 378, 385, 402
National Association of Rehabilitation Facilities, 293, 298
National Head Injury Foundation, 310, 314, 336, 346
National Task Force on Special Education, 124, 134
Neale, H. C., 43, 74
Nelson, A. W., 134
Nesbitt, J. A., 361, 378
Newmark, S. R., 242, 256
Nisbett, R. E., 120, 133
Norman, C., 351, 352, 363, 379
Norman, D. A., 94, 95, 134
Norton, J. A., 27, 76

O

O'Connor, E., 361, 378
O'Connor, G., 299
Oddy, M., 7, 9, 10, 22, 23, 221, 243, 255, 305, 346, 350, 356, 378, 384, 387, 401, 402, 404, 419
Odom, G., 296
O'Donnel, P. A., 367, 369, 377
Office of Technology Assessment, 58, 75
Okun, B. F., 244, 245, 256
Orr, W. C., 15, 22
O'Shea, B. J., 44, 76
Osipow, S. H., 246, 256
Ostrom, T., 133
Overs, R. P., 351, 352, 353, 354, 358, 361, 362, 374, 375, 378

P

Palmer, C. D., 128, 134
Pang, D., 122, 134
Panikoff, L., 324, 346
Panting, A., 350, 378
Papert, S., 192, 213
Parker, K., 36, 74
Parkin, A., 96, 134
Patterson, C. H., 250, 256
Pearson, D., 156, 212
Pellegrino, J., 116, 132, 159, 213
Pepping, M., 1, 12, 22, 221, 227, 243, 246, 250, 256, 261, 263, 271, 278, 290, 298, 304, 346, 385, 393, 402
Perry, J., 30, 75
Peterson, P. L., 148, 153, 213
Pfah, J. C., 373, 378
Pfluger, S., 302, 346
Pharm, D., 27, 76
Phil, M., 156, 214
Piaget, J., 89, 94, 95, 119, 134, 158, 213
Piasetsky, E. B., 3, 20, 227, 243, 245, 250, 254, 257, 261, 278, 297
Pickard, J., 27, 75
Piercy, M., 95, 133
Poeck, K., 15, 22
Pollock, M. L., 69, 70, 75
Porter, T., 222, 256
Postman, L., 94, 95, 96, 134, 158, 213
Power, P. W., 388, 389, 390, 402
Pressley, M., 116, 134, 135, 153, 213
Pribram, K. H., 15, 16, 22, 397, 402
Prigatano, G. P., 1, 2, 3, 4, 5, 8, 11, 12, 13, 14, 15, 16, 21, 22, 87, 88, 89, 106, 107, 108, 109, 128, 135, 137, 141, 180, 193, 203, 205, 213, 221, 227, 243, 246, 250, 256, 261, 262, 263, 271, 278, 290, 297, 298, 303, 304, 345, 346, 385, 387, 393, 395, 396, 398, 402
Pyke, H. F., 196, 214

Q

Questad, K., 153, 158, 213

R

Randle, A. P. H., 221, 254, 277, 297, 349, 377, 387, 401
Rapp, R., 27, 76
Rattok, J., 3, 20, 88, 108, 130, 137, 140, 189, 210, 227, 243, 245, 250, 254, 257, 261, 263, 278, 290, 297
Rayport, M., 15, 21
Read, S., 112, 130
Reale, L., 158, 210
Reese, H. W., 131, 133, 210, 213
Reitan, R. M., 113, 135, 221, 254
Resnikoff, D., 195, 212
Revel, G., 279, 298
Rhoades, K., 124, 125, 131
Richard, M. T., 395, 402
Rimel, R. W., 2, 22, 221, 230, 256, 277, 298
Roberts, A., 28, 75
Rodahl, K., 69, 74
Rohwer, W. D., 158, 213
Romano, M. D., 350, 378, 390, 392, 402
Rood, M., 36, 76
Rosen, C. D., 124, 135
Rosenbaum, M., 286, 299, 350, 378 385, 402
Rosenthal, M., 75, 130, 205, 210, 211, 213, 221, 222, 242, 254, 255, 298, 345, 346, 400
Ross, B., 3, 20, 88, 108, 130, 137, 140, 189, 210, 227, 243, 245, 250, 254, 257, 261, 263, 278, 290, 297
Ross, E. D., 16, 22
Roueche, J. R., 8, 21, 221, 227, 243, 246, 250, 256, 261, 262, 263, 271, 278, 290, 297, 298, 303, 304, 345, 346, 397, 401
Rullman, L., 351, 377
Rummelhart, D., 101, 135, 167, 213
Rusch, F. R., 238, 256
Russell, W. R., 1, 22
Rutherford, W. H., 242, 256
Ruthven, L., 230, 255
Rutter, M., 2, 22

S

Sachs, P. R., 415, 419
Sacks, H., 174, 214
Salamone, P., 233, 257
Sanborn, C. J., 196, 214
Sanborn, D. E., 196, 214
Sanderson, D., 36, 74
Sands, H., 304, 346
Sankovsky, R., 222, 257
Sapir, E., 89, 135
Sarazin, F. F., 158, 214
Sattely, C., 76
Sax, A., 226, 257
Schacter, D., 95, 135, 157, 158, 213
Schank, R., 159, 214
Schauble, P., 195, 212
Schegloff, E., 174, 214
Schinsky, L., 42, 76
Schleien, S., 351, 352, 357, 358, 362, 363, 364, 375, 376, 379
Schlosberg, H., 245, 257
Schloss, C. N., 231, 255
Schloss, P. J., 231, 255

Schlossberg, N. K., 374, 378
Schultz, A., 43, 75
Schwab, L., 312, 346
Schwartz, A. H., 192, 214
Schwartz, M. D., 112, 131, 210, 217
Schwartz, M. L., 15, 21
Sechrest, L. B., 244, 245, 255
Shaffer, D., 2, 22
Shoben, E., 112, 135
Shontz, F. C., 243, 257, 350, 372, 373, 378
Siegel, A., 116, 133
Siegler, R. S., 90, 135
Siegler, S., 131
Silver, S., 3, 20, 88, 108, 130, 137, 140, 189, 210, 227, 243, 257, 261, 263, 278, 290, 297
Silverman, F., 34, 76
Silverman, J., 15, 21
Sitver-Kogut, M., 43, 75
Skelly, M., 42, 76
Skillbeck, C., 192, 214
Skinner, B. F., 119, 135
Small, R., 26, 27, 75
Smirnov, A., 94, 96, 135, 158, 162, 214
Smith, C., 256, 257, 271, 299
Smith, E. E., 94, 101, 135
Smith, J., 379
Smith, P. C., 242, 257
Smith, R. K., 289, 299
Snell, M. E., 232, 241, 256
Snoek, J., 105, 133
Snow, W. G., 277, 298, 385, 386, 387, 401
Sontag, E., 379
Sowers, J., 290, 299
Spence, J. T., 213
Spence, K. W., 213
Srull, T., 130, 133, 135, 136, 212
Staff, 307, 346
Stahl, M. L., 15, 22
Stokes, T. F., 233, 241, 257
Stolov, W., 296, 297
Stuss, D. T., 158, 214, 395, 402
Sublett, D., 242, 256
Sullivan, D., 163, 211
Sunderland, A., 140, 157, 212
Super, D. E., 244, 246, 257, 349, 378
Swing, S. R., 148, 153, 213
Symington, D. C., 44, 76
Szekeres, S., 89, 109, 132, 135, 143, 151, 159, 163, 193, 211, 214, 220, 328, 346

T

Tabaddor, K., 156, 214, 259, 299
Tarpy, R., 90, 93, 135
Taylor, S., 351, 352, 353, 354, 358, 361, 362, 374, 375, 378
Teasdale, G., 27, 75, 107, 133, 383, 402, 414, 419
Temkin, N., 397, 401
ten Kate, J. H., 43, 76
Tenney, Y. I., 116, 136
Thedore Poister Associates, 344, 346
Thomas, S., 308, 347
Thompson, C. K., 231, 255
Thompson, D. M., 94, 136, 158, 214
Thompson, G. B., 2, 23
Thompson, L., 290, 299
Thompson, M. M., 315, 346
Thomsen, I. V., 10, 11, 23, 28, 76, 221, 257, 287, 299, 349, 378, 385, 387, 402
Thuedt, J., 311, 346
Tibbs, P., 27, 76
Titonis, J., 126, 131
Tobis, J. S., 287, 298
Tomkins, S., 94, 136
Traumatic Coma Data Bank Project, 2, 23
Trower, P., 194, 214
Tulving, E., 94, 95, 132, 135, 136, 157, 158, 210, 214
Tyerman, A., 9, 10, 22, 305, 346, 404, 419

U

Umphred, D., 36, 76
Underwood, B. J., 95, 134
U. S. Department of Labor, 273, 299
Uttley, D., 350, 378, 384, 401, 404, 419
Uzgiris, I. C., 131
Uzzell, B., 22, 402

V

Valenstein, E., 15, 16, 21, 23, 401
Valins, S., 133
Valko, A., 28, 75
Valletutti, P., 363, 377
van den Burg, W., 29, 76, 156, 214
Vanderheiden, G. C., 74
van Wolffelaar, P. C., 88, 131
Van Zomeren, A., 29, 76, 156, 214
Vargo, J. W., 350, 374, 378
Vecht, C. J., 27, 75
Vicker, B., 43, 76
Vinken, P. J., 22, 23
Vocational Rehabilitation Center, 287, 293, 299
Voeltz, L. M., 364, 379
Vogelsburg, T., 290, 299
Voss, D., 36, 75
Vygotsky, L. S., 89, 136

W

Wahlstrom, P. E., 305, 346
Walker, A. E., 387, 402
Walker, G., 310, 320, 345
Walls, R., 311, 346
Warren, S. A., 249, 255
Wason, P. C., 214
Wechsler, F., 193, 195, 212, 248, 255
Weddell, R., 7, 23, 387, 402, 404, 419
Wehman, P., 233, 238, 257, 279, 290, 291, 298, 299, 351, 352, 357, 358, 362, 363, 364, 375, 376, 379
Weiner, B., 120, 133, 136
Weir, W. S., 158, 214
Weisberg, R. W., 90, 136
Weiss, L., 289, 299
Weisst, M., 26, 27, 75
Weizmann, F., 131
Welks, D., 124, 125, 131
Wenker, T., 322, 345
White, D. A., 44, 76
White, R. M., Jr., 90, 132
Wilcox, B., 239, 257
Wilkins, R., 310, 320, 345
Wilkinson, M., 2, 3, 21, 221, 255, 277, 297, 349, 377, 387, 401
Williams, J. R., 49, 76
Williams, W., 290, 299, 364, 379
Wilmore, J. H., 69, 70, 75
Wilson, B., 109, 131, 132, 147, 157, 212, 213, 214, 215
Wincour, G., 158, 214
Wittmeyer, M., 67, 76
Wolfe, S., 350, 374, 378
Wolfensberger, W., 238, 257, 308, 313, 321, 346, 347, 352, 370, 379
Wolff, H. G., 5, 6, 7, 21
Wood, B. C., 221, 227, 243, 246, 250, 256, 261, 263, 271, 278, 290, 298, 304, 346
Wood, F., 94, 95, 96, 101, 133, 136, 157, 215
Wood, R. L., 88, 92, 136, 158, 215
Woodworth, R. S., 245, 257
Woosley, T., 311, 347
Wortis, J., 215
Wright, B. A., 372, 373, 379
Wright, E. C., 11, 12, 22
Wrightson, P., 97, 132, 242, 255
Wuerch, B. B., 364, 379
Wyer, R., 112, 130, 133, 135, 136, 212
Wyler, A. R., 397, 401

Y

Ylvisaker, M., 21, 75, 89, 107, 109, 130, 131, 132, 134, 135, 143, 151, 159, 186, 193, 211, 214, 215, 220, 328, 346, 378
Young, B., 27, 76
Young, R. R., 36, 76

Z

Zahara, D. J., 227, 231, 241, 257
Zane, T., 311, 346
Zangwill, O. L., 141, 215
Zazula, T., 156, 214, 256, 299
Zeigarnik, B. V., 159, 215
Zeiner, H. K., 12, 15, 22, 227, 243, 246, 250, 256, 261, 263, 271, 278, 290, 298, 304, 346
Zeiss, R. A., 153, 211
Zide, E., 3, 20, 278, 297
Zinchenko, P., 96, 135
Zivanovic, C., 288, 299
Zorn, G., 275, 299

Subject Index

A

Academic assessment. *See* Educational assessment
Academic deficits, 17
Academic placement. *See* Educational programming
Activities of daily living, 36. *See also* Self-care skills
Adapted equipment. *See* Compensatory device
Advocacy, 323, 403–418
Affective disorders. *See* Personality disorders
Aggressive behavior, 187
Agitation, 14
Alcohol abuse and head injury, 416–417
Amnesia. *See* Memory deficits; Post-traumatic amnesia
Amygdala, 4, 15
Anxiety, 7, 16, 29–30, 194, 383–384
Aphasia, 15–16. *See also* Cognitive rehabilitation
Apraxia of speech, 31
Aprosodia, 15
Applied behavioral analysis. *See* Behavioral disturbances, treatment of
Arousal deficits, 14–15, 91–92
Architectural barriers, 315, 337–340
Articulation, deficits of. *See* Motor deficits, treatment of
Assessment, avocational. *See* Avocational evaluation
  cognitive. *See* Cognitive assessment
  educational. *See* Educational assessment
  vocational. *See* Vocational evaluation
Ataxia, 28
Attendant services, 321–322
Attention, 91–92
Attentional deficits, 14–15, 31, 87–88, 92, 142
  treatment of, 137, 158, 216, 228, 329, 340–341, 365
Attribution, 112, 120, 173
Augmentative communication, 32–34, 38, 42–46, 49, 52, 54–57, 62, 64, 371–372
  psychosocial factors and, 32–34
Automobile accidents, as cause of head injury, 416–417
Avocational evaluation, 352–358
  cognitive functioning and, 355–356
  community resources and, 354
  interest/motivation and, 357–358
  leisure history and, 353–354
  physical functioning and, 356
  psychosocial functioning and, 356–357
Avocational programming, 349–377
  avocational hypothesis and, 358–361
  communication skills and, 369–372
  community re-entry and, 375–377
  counseling and, 372–375
  diagnostic profile and, 358, 359–360
  generalization and, 366
  principles of, 351–352
  self-care and, 366–369
  therapeutic intervention and, 361–375
  treatment plan and, 361–363

B

Basal ganglia, 4
Behavioral assessment, 230, 231
Behavioral management. *See* Behavioral disturbances, treatment of
Behavioral modification. *See* Behavioral disturbances, treatment of
Behavioral disturbances, 5, 175, 260, 304
  treatment of, 19, 175, 178, 231
Behavioral skills, 230

Biofeedback, 30, 36
Bossiness, 36
Bowel and bladder care. *See* Self-care skills
Braces, 36
Brain damage, diffuse, 141

C

Cardiovascular conditioning, 30, 68–73, 223, 241–242
Career development theory, 246
Casts, 34, 36
Catastrophic reaction, 5, 395, 398–399
Characterological styles, 8-9, 396
Chronic pain syndrome, 29–30, 72
Cognition, aspects of, 89–104
Cognitive assessment, 106–107, 113–114, 355–356
Cognitive behavior modification, 119, 176, 178
Cognitive deficits, 87, 91–104, 138, 175, 259, 261–262
  motor recovery and, 26–28, 30–31
  personality disorders and, 5–8, 17–20
Cognitive recovery, stages of, 104–106
Cognitive rehabilitation, clinical direction of, 126–130
  cognitive development and, 114–117
  compensatory strategies and, 108–109, 140–156, 216–220, 267–268
  computer training and, 172, 189–193
  content of, 111–113
  counseling and, 187–188
  forms of, 107–111, 156–158
  goals of, 89, 113–118, 120–122
  individualization and, 120–122
  principles of, 122–124
  program summary, 127
  training procedures and, 118–122, 132–220
  video therapy and, 193–196, 246–247, 252
  vocational programming and, 264
Communication aids/devices. *See* Augmentative communication
Communication disorders, 31, 369–372. *See also* Cognitive deficits; Cognitive rehabilitation; Motor deficits
  motor deficits and, 31
  treatment of, 172–180, 195
Community re-entry services, 404–409
Community resources, 287–293, 312–324, 376, 406–409, 421–430
Compensation, environmental, 108
Compensatory device, 25, 32–34, 38–68
  available aids and, 38–49
  community settings and, 65–66
  compatability of, 49
  evaluation for, 51-59
  funding and, 58-59
  pacing and, 63-65
  seating and positioning and, 53-54
  training and, 59-68
Compensatory strategy. *See* Strategy, compensatory
Competitive employment, 292–293, 406
Comprehension deficits, treatment of, 217–218
Computer assisted cognitive retraining, 172, 189–193
Concussion. *See* Postconcussion syndrome
Confusion, 104–105, 161, 203
Consistency, 123, 204
Conversational disorders, treatment of, 92, 109, 174–180
Cooperativeness, 13, 32, 174
Counseling, 223, 243–250, 276, 321, 372–375, 408–409. *See also* Psychosocial intervention
  acceptance and, 374–375
  marginality and, 372–374
  role adjustment and, 374

D

Daily living, activities of. *See* Self-care skills
Decision making, 184–189, 252
Denial, 7, 389–392, 397. *See also* Unawareness of deficits
Depression, 7, 11, 16, 194, 382–383
Devaluation, 308
Diffuse brain damage. *See* Brain damage, diffuse
Dysarthria, 31
Dyskinesia, 28
Dictionary of Occupational Titles, 273

E

Educational assessment, 126
Educational programming
  cognitive deficits and, 124–126
  community schools and, 124
  compensatory strategies and, 126
  diagnostic teaching and, 124
E. I. du Pont de Nemours & Co., 294
Electric wheelchair. *See* Power mobility
Electrical stimulation, 30
Electronic communication devices. *See* Augmentative communication
Electromygraphy (EMG) biofeedback. *See* Biofeedback
Emotion, 4
Emotional problems. *See* Personality disorders; Psychosocial intervention

Employer incentives. *See* Vocational placement
Encoding. *See* memory
Environmental control, 44, 47–49, 57
Environmental therapy, 203-205
Equipment. *See* Compensatory device
Executive functions, 102–104, 143, 187–189, 349
  deficits of, 87, 97, 138
    treatment of, 176–178, 182–189
Exercise programs, 68–73

F

Facial recognition, 16
Family education and training, 106, 205–207, 329–400
Family reaction to head injury, 8–11, 381ff., 421–430
  denial and, 390–392
  dysfunctional response and, 389–390
  functional response and, 388–389
  unacceptance and, 390–392
Family stress, 381–388
  causes of, 384–388
Family therapy, 207, 392–400
Feature analysis. *See* Semantic feature analysis
Federal targeted job tax credit. *See* Vocational placement
Fine motor treatment. *See* Motor deficits, treatment of
Flaccidity, 28
Frontal lobe damage, 3-5, 14–17, 32, 102, 158, 383, 388, 395
Functional electrical stimulation, 30, 36
Functional-integrative performance, 90, 103–104
Functional-integrative treatment, 110–111

G

Generalization, 103, 107–108, 110, 123, 125, 141, 150–153, 164, 178–180, 182, 206, 240–241, 269, 393
Genesis Manufacturing Co., 288
Glasgow Coma Scale, 1, 383, 388
Glasgow Outcome Scale, 26, 105
Goal setting, 102, 109, 139–140, 144, 249–250
Gross motor treatment. *See* Motor deficits, treatment of
Guilt, 382

H

Headache, 29, 384
Head injury
  incidence of, 414
  long-term needs and, 302
  mild, 29, 277
  New York University Head Trauma Program and, 278, 290
  Neuropsychological Rehabilitation Program at Presbyterian Hospital and, 278, 290
Heteromodal association cortex, 4–5
Higher education, 407
Hippocampus, 4
Homemaker support. *See* Independent living supports
Hostility, 7, 382
Hypertonicity. *See* Spasticity
Hypokinesis, 15

I

Independent living, 301–344
  counseling and, 321
  definition of, 302
  future directions and, 336–344
  history of, 307–310
  supports and, 319–324
Independent living settings, 312–319
  continuum of placements and, 313
  cost and, 344
  domicillary homes and, 314
  family homes and, 318–319
  group homes and, 315–316
  guidelines for determining, 328, 335–336, 337–341
  independence and, 318
  institutions and, 312–314
  supervised apartments and, 316–317
  transitional apartments and, 317–318
  transitional aggregate settings and, 314
Independent living supports, 319–324
  advocacy and, 323
  attendant services and, 342
  counseling and, 321
  homemaker/chore supports and, 322
  medical care and, 322
  respite services and, 323
  training and, 320–321
  transportation and, 323
Information processing. *See* Cognitive deficits; Cognitive rehabilitation
Inhibition, 102
Inhibition, deficits of, 5, 14–15, 32, 102, 383
Initiation, 102, 151–152
  deficits of, 6, 14, 16, 32, 102
Input control, treatment of, 217
Insight therapies, 261
Insomnia, 29
Intellectual deficits. *See* Cognitive deficits

Interdisciplinary programming, 32, 49, 88, 123, 128–129, 141, 152, 173, 187–188, 226
Interface. *See* Switch
Interpersonal process recall, 195, 248–249
Irrational thinking patterns, 247–248
Irritability, 4, 7–11, 13, 15–16, 29, 383–384
Ischemia, 4

J

Job analysis, 272, 280
  cognitive factors and, 280, 282–284
Job placement. *See* Vocational placement
Job training, 222

K

Katz Adjustment Scale, 11–13, 385–386
Knowledge base. *See* Memory

L

Language deficits. *See* Cognitive deficits; Communication disorders
Language organization, deficits of, 87
Language therapy. *See* Cognitive rehabilitation
Learning deficits. *See* Cognitive deficits; Memory deficits
Learning theory, 119
Leisure activity. *See* Avocational programming
Limbic system, 4–5, 14–17
Long-term memory. *See* Memory

M

Management, head injury programs. *See* Program management
Mediated learning, 119, 234–237
Memory assessment, 96
Memory, aspects of, 93–97, 156
  deficits of, 7, 10, 29, 87, 93–97, 138, 142, 384
    treatment of, 105–106, 137, 156–172
  Metacognition, 96, 109, 116, 126–127, 143–144, 148, 161–162, 164, 185, 234–237
Metaphor, 154, 250
Minor brain injury, 29
Mobility aid. *See* Power mobility
Motivational problems, 14–16, 32, 384
Motor deficits, 26–28, 102, 259, 303–304. *See also* Physical deficits
  treatment of, 35*ff,* 356
Motor speech treatment. *See* Motor deficits, treatment of

N

National Head Injury Foundation, 415
Networking, 409–413
Neurobehavioral deficits. *See* Cognitive deficits, Motor deficits; Behavioral disturbances
Neuromuscular deficits. *See* Motor deficits; Physical deficits
Neuropathology, 3–5, 14–16
Neuropsychological assessment. *See* Assessment
Neuropsychologically mediated personality problems, 8–9, 14–17, 395–396
Nonspeech communication. *See* Augmentative communication
Normalization, 308
  principal of, 308

O

Occupational therapy. *See* Cognitive rehabilitation; Motor deficits, treatment of
Organization, 97–98, 101, 159–160
  deficits of, 87, 98, 159
    treatment of, 156–172, 219
Orientation, deficits of, treatment of, 216
Outcome following head injury, 2–3, 277–279

P

Paranoia, 8, 15, 395
Pathophysiology, 3–5, 14–16
Perception, 92–93
  deficits of, 93
Persistent vegetative state, 26–27
Personality, cognitive deficits and, 5–8
  effects of head injury on, 1–3, 8–11
  pretrauma, 1–2, 16–17, 17–20
Personality disorders, 1–3
  characterological, 8–9, 395–397
  cognitive deficits and, 5–8, 175
  family reaction and, 384–388
  neuropsychologically mediated, 8–9, 14–17, 395–397
  pretrauma factors and, 17–20
  reactionary, 8–9, 14, 16–17, 395–397
  treatment outcome and, 11–13
Pharmacologic intervention, 30, 35–36
Physical conditioning, 25, 30, 68–73. *See also* Work conditioning
Physical deficits, 26–30. *See also* Motor deficits

cognitive deficits and, 26, 30–32
psychosocial deficits and, 32–34
rehabilitation of, 35*ff*
Physical therapy. *See* Motor deficits, treatment of; Physical deficits, rehabilitation of.
Postconcussion syndrome, 29
Posttraumatic amnesia, 1, 7, 97
Power mobility, 34, 38–42, 49, 54–55, 63
Prevocational programming. *See* Vocational programming
Problem solving, 98–100, 146, 151–152, 328–331
deficits of, 100, 138
treatment of, 180–189, 219
Processing deficits. *See* cognitive deficits
Program management, 128–130, 403–418
Proprioceptive neuromuscular facilitation, 36
Project with Industry, 293
Psychiatric disorders, 16–17
Psychosocial adjustment, 8–11. *See also* Personality disorders
personality disorders and, 8–11
physical recovery and, 32–34
Psychosocial dysfunction. *See* Personality disorders
Psychosocial intervention, 13–14, 104, 112, 139, 154, 172–180, 265–271, 372–375
Psychosocial issues, 261–262, 356–357
Psychotherapy, 13–14, 154

R

Rancho Los Amigos levels of cognitive recovery, 104
Reactionary problems, 8–9, 14, 16–17, 395–397
Reality of orientation. *See* Orientation
Reasoning, 98–99, 180–182
deficits of, 98–99
treatment of, 180–189, 219
Rehabilitation Institute of Pittsburgh, 216, 412–413
Respite services, 323
Response system, 102–103
Reticular activating system, 14–16
Retrieval. *See* Memory
Retrograde amnesia, 101
Rigidity, 28
Role adjustment. *See* Counseling

S

Scapegoating, 389
Seating and positioning, 53–54
School. *See* Educational programming
Seizures, posttraumatic, 15
Self-awareness. *See* Self-evaluation; Unawareness of deficits
Self-care skills, 222, 236, 366–369
Self-evaluation, 265–267
Self-monitoring deficits, treatment of, 140–156, 175–178
Semantic feature analysis, 163–164
Sensory integration, 36
Serial casting. *See* Casts
Sexual disturbance, 15, 387
Sheltered employment, 287–289, 407
Short-term memory. *See* Memory
Sign language, 42
Sister Kenny Institute, 292
Sleep disturbance, 15
Social cognition, 111–113, 252
deficits of, 172–173
treatment of, 172–180
Social isolation, 11, 13–14, 221, 383
Spasticity, 28, 36, 72
Special education. *See* Educational programming; Cognitive rehabilitation
Speech-language pathology. *See* Augmentative communication; Cognitive rehabilitation: Motor deficits, treatment of
Splints, 36
Storage. *See* Memory
Strategy, compensatory, 108–109, 119, 140–157, 164, 169–172, 194, 216–220, 328, 329, 330, 331
Structured activities, as cognitive rehabilitation, 196–203
cognitive factors of, 198–202
content/academic factors of, 198–202
psychosocial factors of, 198–202
Supported work, 290–291
Switch, 40–41, 45–50, 63–64

T

Task analysis, 117–118, 197–202, 326, 363–366
Temporal lobe damage, 3–5, 8, 14–16, 397
Therapeutic activity center, 407
Therapeutic milieu, 14
Thought organization. *See* Organization
Transitional employment, 291–292
Tremors, 28
Transportation, 323, 354, 369, 375–376

U

Unawareness of deficits, 10, 14, 33, 65, 102, 109, 123, 129, 142–143, 147,

Unawareness of deficits *(continued)*
193–194, 383, 397. *See also* Self-evaluation
Unemployment, 221
United Cerebral Palsy, Inc., 412–413

V

Valorization, 308
Verbal expression deficits. *See* Augmentative communication; Cognitive rehabilitation
Verbal fluency deficits. *See* Cognitive rehabilitation
Verbal thought organization. *See* Organization
Video games, 189
Video therapy, 193–196, 246–247, 252
Visual-perceptual deficits, 16, 28, 93
Visuomotor deficits, 16
Visuospatial deficits, 16, 93
Vocational evaluation, 222, 271–274, 276
assessment techniques of, 223, 227–232
commercial evaluation systems and, 271
Vocational Evaluation and Work Adjustment Association, 226
Vocational goals/objectives, 269–270, 274–276
Vocational outcome, 2–3
Vocational placement, 222, 270, 277–294
competitive employment and, 292–293
employer incentives and, 294
family suppport and, 284
federal targeted job tax credit and, 294
follow-up services and, 295
future directions for, 295
issues of, 279–285
job analysis and, 280
job site and, 281, 284
modifications and, 289
Project with Industry and, 293
sheltered employment and, 287–289
staff support and, 284
supported work and, 290–291
transitional employment and, 291–292
Vocational rehabilitation, 3, 223, 259, 406–407
counseling and, 223
service delivery model, 263–271
stages of programming, 264–271
vocational behaviors and, 222, 224–226
Vocational rehabilitation agencies, 294
Vocational Rehabilitation Center of Allegheny County, 226, 252, 261, 287, 290, 293, 412–413
Vocational skills, 222
Vocational therapy, 223, 232–241
acquisition phase of, 234–238
diagnostic assessment and, 233
generalization phase of, 239–240
proficiency phase of, 240–241
Volunteer work placement, 289, 407

W

Wechler Intelligence Scale for Children — Revised, 19
Word retrieval deficits, treatment of, 218
Working memory. *See* Memory
Work Abilities, 224–225
Work adjustment, 222, 226, 276
counseling and, 222–250
diagnostic assessment and, 223, 227–232
goals of, 222
methods of, 223
Work conditioning, 223, 241–242
Work endurance, 230, 242–243
Work proficiency factors, 227, 229–232
work quality and, 229
work rate and, 229
work tolerance and, 230
Worker's compensation, 228